Helping Your Hyperactive/ Attention Deficit Child

HELPING YOUR HYPERACTIVE/ADD CHILD

REVISED, 2ND EDITION

John Taylor

Prima Publishing

Library of Congress Cataloging-in-Publication Data

Taylor, John F.
Helping your hyperactive/add child /
John F. Taylor.
—Rev. 2nd ed.
p. cm.
Previous edition published under title: Helping your hyperactive child.
Includes bibliographical references and index.
ISBN 1-55958-423-8
ISBN 0-7615-0868-6 (pbk.)
1. Attention-deficit hyperactivity disorder—Treatment.
2. Self-control in children. 3. Self-esteem in children.
4. Adjustment (Psychology) in children. 5. Child rearing.
I. Taylor, John F., Helping your hyperactive child. II. Title.
RJ506.H9T36 1994
618.92'8589—dc20 93-23554
CIP

99 00 01 02 AA 10 9 8 7 6 5 4
Printed in the United States of America

How to Order

Single copies may be ordered from Prima Publishing, P.O. Box 1260BK, Rocklin, CA 95677; telephone (916) 632-4400. Quantity discounts are also available. On your letterhead, include information concerning the intended use of the books and the number of books you wish to purchase.

Visit us online at http://www.primapublishing.com

To Tammi, Brian, Dana, Beth, Sharon, John,
Amy, Michael, and especially to Linda

FOREWORD

Chronic hyperactivity and distractibility can be a nightmare for everyone affected by the behavior. The "victims" include the children themselves, their despairing parents, and their perplexed and frustrated teachers.

Children who have difficulty filtering out distractions, staying on task, focusing their attention, inhibiting their impulses, and controlling their bodies invariably function in school at a level significantly below their potential. Because of their negative school experiences, many of these children erroneously conclude they are hopelessly inept and incompetent.

For many years, physicians, psychologists, and educators described chronically distractible children whose behavior is characterized by poor impulse control and often purposeless movement as hyperactive. Extensive clinical and classroom observations ultimately led professionals to make an important differentiation: *although most hyperactive children are inattentive, not all inattentive children are hyperactive*. The relatively new terminology, *Attention Deficit Disorder with Hyperactivity* and *Attention Deficit Disorder without Hyperactivity*, underscores this important distinction and permits a more precise diagnosis.

In a class of thirty students, each child should theoretically require approximately 3% of the teacher's time and energy. The child with ADD who demands 10% of the teacher's energy destroys this important equation. Teachers who must continually monitor, supervise, and control the child with ADD are reluctantly thrust into the role of drill sergeants. They realize they are depriving their other students of their fair share of instructional time. Many of these teachers become frustrated, demoralized, weary, and resentful.

Parents can also become frustrated, demoralized, weary, and resentful. Being forced to deal every day with counterproductive and self-sabotaging behavior can wear down the patience and fortitude of even the most well-intentioned parent.

As an educational therapist who has evaluated and treated over 8,000 underachieving and learning disabled children during the last twenty years, I have seen my fair share of children with ADD. In fact, our organization built its reputation on working with ADD children using a wide range of intensive behavior modification and academic remediation strategies.

From an educator's perspective, the presenting profile of children with ADD is classic. The children struggle to remember and follow written and verbal instructions, to write legibly, to spell accurately, to decode language, to read with comprehension, to sit still, to stay on task, and to control their bodies. The net effect for the vast majority of these children is almost invariably marginal academic performance, poor self-confidence, and, in extreme cases, frustration, despair, and feelings of inadequacy and hopelessness. It should be no surprise that many ADD children learn to hate school. Seven hours a day of poor performance and reprimands can break the will and spirit of any child.

The parents of ADD children are also on the receiving end of a continual stream of negative feedback. Everyone seems to blame them for their child's nonadaptive, stress-producing behaviors. The clear implication is that the child is misbehaving because they are doing an inadequate job of parenting. These parents are often confused about the issues, overwhelmed by the choices they are expected to make, unsure of their prerogatives, pained by their children's actions, and fearful about the future.

If you are one of these despairing parents or teachers, take heart. Meaningful, substantive help is now available thanks to Dr. John Taylor. This highly skilled and insightful family psychologist has written what is undoubtedly the definitive parent-oriented book about this enigmatic and often debilitating condition called ADD.

He has not only compressed a vast quantity of information into *Helping Your Hyperactive/Attention Deficit Child*, he has also succeeded in making the book highly readable and has managed to include a wealth of practical, workable strategies for dealing with the problem. It is impossible for parents to read this book without acquiring a comprehensive understanding of the issues, causes, and solutions to the problem of ADD. Dr. Taylor has covered all the bases.

The more parents understand about ADD, the more actively and intelligently they can participate in the process of helping their child. Their intervention is vital if destructive, and often permanent, psychological and ego damage are to be avoided. In my opinion, no responsible parent of a child with Attention Deficit Disorder can afford not to read this invaluable book.

Lawrence J. Greene, Ph.D.
Executive Director, The Developmental
Learning Center, San Jose, CA

CONTENTS

Introduction

When interviewed about what it was like growing up, adults who were hyperactive as children view their hyperactivity as an aspect of life that affected their social and family relationships, their school performance, and their self-esteem. The attention deficit hyperactivity syndrome colors an individual's experiences in every arena of life. It has had many names, the most current reflecting the key symptoms of hyperactivity and attention disorder—attention deficit hyperactivity disorder, abbreviated in this book as ADHD.

ADHD is the most common child psychiatric disorder and accounts for at least half of all referrals to child guidance clinics. From 5 to 10% of the children in the United States are afflicted with this syndrome. With such other conditions as diabetes, heart disease, and high blood pressure, it shares incompletely understood causes and outcomes and a range from very mild to very severe. Early indications are often not recognizable, and controversy surrounds almost every aspect of the topic.

As its apparent incidence increased over the past few decades, research findings have confused professionals, and, with advancing research, many of those findings have been found to be false. Although this syndrome represents the most written about child behavioral psychological disorder, there is a giant gap between current academic research knowledge and what has been conveyed to parents for direct application to ADHD family settings. Inconsistent and inaccurate professional training continues to spawn disagreement and controversy about almost every aspect of this disorder, from initial diagnosis to the difficulties that an adult with ADHD can expect. ADHD is still grossly underrecognized, misdiagnosed, and incorrectly managed.

Anyone who has a family member with a chronic medical problem quickly realizes the importance of readable, accurate, and nontechnical sources of information. Many texts aimed at the general public are superficial, incomplete regarding treatment practices and controversies, and silent on key issues of family life such as the marital relationship, parents' feelings, and sibling rivalry.

I have attempted to present the latest information while avoiding scientific jargon so that this book can serve as a reservoir of current knowledge. If you share the relevant sections with the professionals working with your family, your child's progress will be much enhanced. When all who are involved have trust and confidence in their knowledge base and share common points of reference, it will facilitate the coordination of efforts.

In my nearly two decades of work with hyperactive children, adults, and adolescents, I have learned to respect the potency of the biochemistry of the nervous system. In general, I find it best to use biochemical treatment combined with psychological and academic efforts. A simplistic treatment approach will not bring the benefits you and your child need and deserve.

During the 1950s, 1960s, and early 1970s, only one biochemical treatment was used with any degree of success—prescribed stimulant and antidepressant medication. Not until the early seventies was the startling discovery made that limiting exposure to certain chemicals capable of interfering with normal brain chemistry processes can greatly reduce hyperactivity symptoms. Some professionals and researchers in this field prefer to cling to a narrow viewpoint that admits prescribed medication as the only effective form of biochemical treatment. Experience and familiarity with controlling chemical exposure, however, has provided me with a broader view of how to facilitate normal biochemical processes in the nervous system to alleviate hyperactivity symptoms. Throughout this book I refer to "biochemical treatment program," which means either using prescribed medication or controlling exposure to irritant chemicals that often cause ADHD symptoms to flare up.

Because medication is the more common method, I have included guidelines for using medication. During this discussion I assume that you prefer medication as the treatment method. I do not append each sentence with "or, if that doesn't work, consider using the chemical exposure control method." Please feel free, however, to consider that option if it seems to fit your child's situation.

There is very little agreement among physicians on a host of factors surrounding medication treatment of ADHD, and the resource guides they use are not always accurate. To create a more realistic picture of the best practices, I have included instructions for adjusting dosage level and controlling for side effects.

The frank discussion of adverse reactions to medication is not intended to scare you away from obtaining needed help. Bear in mind that almost all forms of therapy are associated with some risks. These risks, however, may be less serious than the consequences of ignoring true therapeutic needs. Information about side effects helps prepare you for their possible occurrence while alleviating fears or anxiety stemming from any inaccurate information you may have received about these medications.

Although the backbone of the ADHD syndrome comprises abnormalities in the nervous system, the flesh of the disorder consists of psychological factors. Hyperactive children have good days and bad days, just as everyone else does. They grow angry and rebellious if mistreated, they become criminal if neglected and/or abused, they are excited and pleased when they receive sincere appreciation and acknowledgment of their efforts, and they become discouraged and want to quit if faced with continued frustration and failure. I urge you to remain open-minded about the possibility that several factors may combine to influence behavior and mental efficiency.

I have included guidelines for preventing and overcoming the most common and troublesome disciplinary situations that occur with hyperactive children, including away-from-home times. The emphasis must be on orderly routines, clear communication of feelings and needs, and close family relationships based on mutual respect. After-the-fact parenting just doesn't work with ADHD children and adolescents. Throughout this book I provide information to help you deal with current problems as well as prevent future difficulties.

Research clearly shows that orderly family processes and firmness help an ADHD child adjust successfully. The relationship between you and your child is far more critical and powerful than any relationship your child could ever establish with a teacher, physician, psychologist, counselor, or other helping professional. Therefore, I have included elaborate discussion of how to relieve marital stresses, sibling rivalry, and the emotional roller coaster that parents experience in coping with a hyperactive child. In addition, I have provided an entire chapter on how to join or organize a support group, and Appendix C lists several support organizations and sources of additional information about attention deficits and hyperactivity.

Hyperactivity poses severe stresses on a marriage; I have witnessed divorces stemming from arguments about how to deal with a hyperactive child. The misbehavior, chaos, and stress can be relentless and overwhelming. Intense sibling rivalry is the norm for families with a hyperactive child. Your family will become more united or more divided in response to hyperactivity; its effect will not be neutral. The focus throughout this book is on strengthening the self-esteem of parents and children along with rebuilding harmony among family members. Everyone can share a sense of mission and purpose, a common goal of working to counter a shared stress.

Most public school teachers face hyperactive children every school year, and a significant proportion of those children are taking prescribed medication or attempting to control chemical exposure. Teachers, however, are probably the most overlooked and underused professionals with the potential to help the hyperactive child. I have included three chapters on school adjustment along with numerous suggestions for how teachers can fulfill their central role. I have also provided forms by which they can assist in diagnosis, monitor the progress of biochemical treatment, and communicate to you about your child's emotional, social, and academic adjustment at school.

Lack of a consistent, agreed-upon knowledge base among professionals and parents can cause uncertainties and misconceptions. Sensational articles in popular periodicals and newspapers only make things worse. Highly biased articles, both for and against both types of biochemical treatment, have fueled bitter controversy and clouded issues. Because there are few comprehensive references for parents, teachers, and health care providers about medication and controlling for chemical exposure, this book devotes considerable attention to answer these questions about hyperactive children, adolescents, and adults.

Making diagnostic and treatment information available in this format does not mean that nonmedical caregivers should preempt a medical role. School personnel should not make medical diagnoses or recommend to parents that the child should definitely be placed on a certain type and dosage of medication. Teachers can be helpful to physicians by providing much needed feedback about response to treatment and diagnostic information about ADHD with the aid of the forms provided in this book. The school is only one part of a team effort that also involves you, health professionals, mental health care services, and perhaps social welfare agencies. Management of your child, with or without the use of prescribed medication, should involve an individualized, comprehensive, and cooperative effort among helping professionals and your family.

You have a choice of several levels of awareness and intervention toward the difficulties your child is experiencing. After reading Chapter 1, for example, you might decide your child displays several traits cataloged there, yet still not conclude the ADHD disorder is an accurate label. You might also agree those traits are causing many difficulties for your child and other family members, yet conclude those difficulties can and should be overcome without biochemical intervention. If you choose to forgo any direct biochemical alteration and put all your effort into training your child to adapt, you can still use this book as your guide. It shows you how to help your child develop better self-control, temptation resistance, social skills, study habits, decision making, friendship building, relaxation techniques, anger control, assertiveness, problem solving, and various other skills for day-to-day functioning that are most at risk among hyperactive children.

This book provides a panoramic catalog of the stresses faced by the family and many suggestions for relieving those stresses. Although addressed primarily to parents, it is also intended to be useful to members and students in all of the helping professions, as well as to friends, relatives, caregivers, child care providers, church group leaders, and others who assist hyperactive children or members of their families. It can also become source material for a discussion group or college course on hyperactivity and attention deficits. A group of parents meeting weekly, for example, can share their experiences and approaches, discussing two chapters each week with the aid of the study and discussion questions in Appendix A. Such a discussion group does not require a professional leader.

My goal is that this book will provide practical assistance for parents and others who want to understand and help the hyperactive individual.

1

Understanding Hyperactivity and Attention Deficits

Attention Deficit Hyperactivity Disorder **(ADHD)** is the most common psychiatric disorder among children. Yet, it is mishandled in every conceivable way, with thousands of children, adolescents, and adults incorrectly diagnosed and thus denied the benefits of correct treatment. Its symptoms are not necessarily obvious and start at various times. Some give indication of the disorder before they are born; others are not suspected of having it until their preteen years. The disorder overlaps with several other conditions, further confusing physicians and mental health professionals who attempt to provide a diagnosis. The traits discussed in this chapter are the most common symptoms of hyperactivity and attention deficits. Although they are applicable to people of all ages, I will emphasize their manifestation in children's behavior.

Often misdiagnosed as "emotionally disturbed," hyperactive children create havoc in the home and at school. Parents must fend off numerous criticisms as well as "suggestions" from relatives, neighbors, teachers, medical professionals, mental health professionals, and school personnel. There are few solid answers—only more questions as the child's behavior continues to create severe problems for the entire family.

The number, severity, and types of symptoms differ from one child to the next, each of whom shows a unique pattern of behavior and personality. There are, however, certain similarities among ADHD children.

A COMMON SYNDROME WITH MANY NAMES

ADHD was described as early as 1845 by the German physician Heinrich Hoffmann in his classic *Der Struwelpeter* (Slovenly Peter), a collection of humorous moral tales for children. The heroes were drawn from his observations of children, including "Fidgety Philip."

In 1902, one researcher, Dr. G. F. Still, described the behavior of a group of apparently hyperactive children. He knew of no medical reasons for their behavior and made no mention of their educational needs or social skills. He expressed one of the classic lines of unfair criticism most consistently leveled against parents of ADHD children: that part of the problem was "deficient training in the home."

In 1923, subsequent to an acute encephalitis outbreak at the end of World War I, a researcher, F. G. Ebaugh, chastised physicians for confining their concern to medical management and for not showing enough interest in providing the parents of this large group of brain-damaged children and adolescents with genuine assistance for their disruptive behavior. Ebaugh was perhaps the first to publish a professional paper recognizing ADHD as a long-term problem requiring cooperation and intervention by several professional disciplines.

Over the past four decades, dozens of labels have been used for a collection of traits that has come to be known as attention deficit hyperactivity disorder. Most children who have most of these traits show them most of the time; the types, number, and level vary within each child from moment to moment and from situation to situation.

Recent popular names for the syndrome include attention deficit disorder (ADD), ADD with hyperactivity (ADD-H), ADD without hyperactivity (ADD-noH), brain damage syndrome, dyslexia, functional behavioral problem, hyperactive child syndrome, hyperkinesis, hyperkinetic impulsive disorder, learning disabilities, minimal brain damage syndrome, minimal brain dysfunction syndrome, minimal cerebral dysfunction syndrome, minor cerebral dysfunction syndrome, postencephalitic disorder, and specific learning disabilities.

I have observed four overlapping conditions that deserve special attention. All involve the simultaneous occurrence of another condition along with ADHD: (1) ADHD-sa, the simultaneous occurrence of ADHD and numerous allergies and sensitivities, is discussed in Chapter 5; (2) ADHD-ld, the simultaneous occurrence of ADHD and learning disabilities, is discussed in Chapter 10; (3) ADHD-cd, the simultaneous occurrence of ADHD and a conduct disorder; and (4) Tourette's syndrome are discussed later in this chapter. An individual can have any combination of overlapping conditions.

Research studies consistently point to a 5 to 10% proportion of children who have the syndrome. Some experts believe the true number is closer to 20% of the general population. In a recent study of over 9000 children in the Midwest, the prevalence of children who have been medically diagnosed as hyperactive was about 3%. The prevalence of undiagnosed sufferers, based on data from teachers and parents, was estimated at about 4%. In a comparable study in Canada, the overall prevalence of ADHD was 5%. Of the children referred to mental health clinics in the United States, 3 to 5% are diagnosed as having ADHD.

Differing prevalence rates from nation to nation have resulted from differing methods of defining and cataloging ADHD symptoms. When these differences are taken into account, the prevalence rates for most European countries, China, and Australia coincide reasonably with those in North America.

Surveys employing teachers' and parents' ratings generally find a 10 to 30% prevalence of ADD (with and without hyperactivity) in school-age populations.

CHARACTERISTICS OF ADHD CHILDREN

Many characteristics of ADHD children are socially appropriate and desirable. Their spontaneity, zest, tirelessness, enthusiasm, intensity, curiosity, stimulating brashness, and life-of-the-party energy have their useful moments and serve as social catalysts.

There is probably a link between ADHD and giftedness. These children have rich imaginations and can quickly generate new and different ideas. They seem always to have their psychological antennae out and are aware of nuances and sensations others miss. They can combine unrelated ideas in novel ways so their art productions and written compositions show a special measure of creativity. When they are successfully treated biochemically, these personal expressions display even greater variety, depth, and attention to detail. Some of the most creative persons in history, including Thomas Edison, apparently had this disorder.

Remember that no hyperactive child will have all of the traits discussed in this chapter. The following are general trends that are more consistently shown by ADHD than by non-ADHD children. The majority of hyperactive individuals lead successful, well-adjusted lives.

ADHD is difficult to diagnose because, like all behavior disorders, it tends to appear gradually. Neurological and physiological studies indicate that ADHD sufferers have a wide range of biochemical imbalance and uniqueness. Symptoms phase in and out in various settings and change somewhat from moment to moment. Often there has been no previously normal behavior pattern for parents or professionals to use as a basis of comparison in deciding which of the actions are symptoms of ADHD. The child often seems mentally alert, smiling, energetic, and interested in contact with others. One of the most difficult aspects of this disorder is deciding how much of the unusual behavior is "normal."

The apparatus and procedures for measuring such key ADHD traits as attention span and reaction time are elaborate and expensive and are currently confined to experimental use. There is no simple test for ADHD. Physicians cannot measure blood or urine to assess biochemical imbalances in the nervous system of these children. The most accurate diagnostic method is a review of the child's history and behavior at home and at school.

Imagine giant decks of 200 cards each for all children. On each card is a trait of the ADHD syndrome and its overlapping conditions: difficulty following teacher's instructions, bedwetting, entering sister's bedroom without permission, flitting from one activity to another. Each child receives some cards from the deck that represents particular behaviors. Some children receive only a few cards. Others might receive over 100 cards. Those who receive many cards have enough traits to become noticeably different from most other children. Even though two ADHD-identified children might have the same number of cards—say, 103—the collection of traits that one child has is different from the array occurring in the next child.

Compared with ADHD girls, ADHD boys are generally more likely to be overactive, too aggressive, too disruptive, and referred for child guidance services. Both ADHD girls and ADHD boys are physically active and rowdy, with the girls being tomboyish. Among ADHD children 60 to 80% are boys.

The following sections discuss the clusters of mental, physical, and emotional traits that comprise the ADHD syndrome. Not all ADHD individuals have all of these symptoms, but most have a majority of them. Although many of these traits appear in most children from time to time, they indicate the ADHD syndrome when they appear consistently, the child is unable to change them, and they don't stem from psychological causes or from the ADHD-imitator conditions discussed in Chapter 2.

Mental Difficulties

DISTRACTIBILITY. As you read this paragraph, you are blocking out millions of messages. Your brain is preventing you from being aware of the majority of information it is receiving. You can ignore this flood of messages from every sense organ and every location in your body because you have a "gatekeeper" that allows only relevant, useful, and important information into your conscious awareness.

ADHD children have a faulty gatekeeper. They have little ability to block out noises in order to concentrate. A noise outside the window, a cough, or a dropped pencil are equally as important as what the teacher is saying. One mother describing her 9-year-old said, "He can't tune out sounds. The sound of a fly drives him crazy."

Stimulation from experiencing the feel of cloth rubbing against skin, created by wiggling in the chair, is as important as eating; tiny marks and scratches on books and desks command attention as much as assigned reading passages; the pattern of colors on the wall is just as important as remembering the chores to be done.

ADHD sufferers are poor at focusing concentration, channeling effort, and saving energy for useful purposes. It is as if they are drawn magnetically to any stray flash of light, any noise, or any internal body signal. The result is a short attention span and a tendency to be distracted by whatever is unimportant and irrelevant and to flit from activity to activity, discontinuing efforts before each task comes to a proper completion. They seem overly aware and alert, but about the wrong things.

Motivation plays a large role in determining attention to a task. Parents and teachers consistently have trouble differentiating between the circumstances in which ADHD children *can't* focus and those in which they *aren't interested* in focusing. The result is that the focusing of attention is variable from one situation to another. These children are especially distracted when mental discipline or self-restraint is needed, as when functioning in a group or performing a difficult or uninteresting task. Participant sports, television shows, videotapes, and computer games and instructional programs all feature enough novelty, movement, and fascination to command the sustained interest and attention of most hyperactive children.

Confusion. ADHD children have trouble recognizing an object that stands out from the background, perceiving both as a blurred unity. This trait applies to handling ideas. They are poor at prioritizing, recognizing what is important, and making decisions based on the relevant factors. They don't assign priorities or values consistent with reality, but instead base decisions on distorted perceptions of self, others, and circumstances. These children have trouble organizing and arranging schoolwork; for example, they may be tempted to go skateboarding on the night before an important exam. They might appear scatterbrained, absentminded, and forgetful. Performance varies, so that they seem to learn something one day but completely forget it the next.

These children have trouble understanding ordinary conversations or lectures, especially sorting out details, listening for key information, and sifting through what the other person is saying for points of agreement. They are confused by instructions, especially those involving three or four steps in a row.

They have difficulty computing logically. They can become sidetracked and enamored with one unimportant detail. Faulty reasoning ability leads to poor impulse control, decreased ability to plan and predict consequences of their own actions, weak social judgment, and impaired academic skills. They might make sweeping claims and confident statements without backing them up with reasonable observations or details.

Their perception is selective. They tend to notice and remember only the specific parts of personal experiences that fulfill hopes, wishes, or prior beliefs. They might make contradictory statements without being aware of the inconsistencies. When asked how well school is going, they might recall high grades on one or two homework assignments while forgetting the many failed tests and homework assignments not turned in or graded low. Their impression is that all is well, and the report card, reflecting the true overall performance level in class, shocks and confuses them as well as their parents.

Faulty Abstract Thinking. Concept formation, or abstract thinking ability, is poorly developed in ADHD children. Since they have difficulty restating a sentence or paragraph in different words, their note taking is often inept. They have difficulty understanding what they read. Abstract subjects like mathematics are especially difficult for them to grasp.

These children have trouble thinking hypothetically in "what if" fashion or understanding cause and effect in "if . . ., then . . ." reasoning. Rather than using an example as a general guideline, they personalize or misinterpret it. After hearing the method used by two children to settle an argument, the ADHD children might not understand how those methods could possibly apply to them, because they themselves were not involved in the argument.

Because these children are especially weak in social situations involving abstract concepts, they interpret the teacher's reminder to sit still and stop bothering nearby students as a personal insult that has no basis other than "the teacher is picking on me."

Fragmenting an experience is another symptom of the syndrome. They have trouble learning and applying information from previous experiences to current ones, and often appear lost and confused when asked to apply a previously learned tactic to a new situation. They might claim not to know a geography fact because they haven't been there. They might not be able to do something they have watched other children do, simply because they themselves have never done it before.

They have trouble handling nonroutine situations that require putting together pieces of information from a past experience or current circumstance in order to handle a new situation. In emergencies or crises, ADHD children sometimes do not know how to behave and what steps to take. These children need to have a routine and close and direct supervision to cope with new or ambiguous situations.

Inflexibility. Hyperactive children lack flexibility in their approach to situations. They have trouble switching from one activity to another and tend to adjust poorly to changes in their surroundings. Rearranged furniture or a new day-care environment can bring on tantrums.

These children persist in their approach and point of view despite new information, and they reject better solutions even after several unsuccessful attempts with their current approach.

Poor Verbal Skills. Finding the words with which to express their thoughts and feelings is difficult. Stuttering and stammering sometimes result from their inability to deal with emotion through language. Though they might understand some concept, they still do poorly on tests because of difficulty remembering the correct words and piecing them together in a proper sequence to express the complete idea. Despite the belief that so-called normal girls do better than boys in thinking and language skills, ADHD girls often have more problems with those skills than ADHD boys.

Aimlessness. Hyperactive children appear inconsistent and unpredictable, always keeping parents, teachers, and siblings off balance. One of the most common reports from parents is never knowing what to expect. These children lead disjointed, chaotic lives. They seem unable to accommodate to change or to the needs of others. They seem to profit little from past errors, so they continue to make academic and social blunders. Acting without stopping to consider the consequences is customary, despite the awful consequences that keep occurring. The combination of impulsiveness and failure to appreciate danger results in accidents and mishaps.

Their lives seem barren and empty, without much forethought. Spontaneous to a fault, they seem never to plan ahead and have little concern or preparation for the future.

Although hyperactive children know the rules, they seem to lack the self-control to follow those rules. There seems to be a general weakness in the ability to self-regulate and to resist temptations for acting improperly.

Perceptual Difficulties. These children can become confused about common opposites. Differentiating up-side-down and inside-out may be difficult—for example, putting on clothing inside-out without realizing it. Transpositions in reading and writing are common to all children, but for many ADHD children the problem remains and creates frustration and embarrassment long after other children have overcome it. They may use letters like *W* and *M,* *d* and *b,* and *p* and *q* interchangeably. Sometimes the reversals occur within words, as when *dog* is seen as *god*, or *was* as *saw.*

Understanding position, such as vertical and horizontal or backward and forward, and recognizing relationships like over, under, beside, and between cause confusion. Skills such as telling time, reading maps, and doing math problems require spatial awareness and are especially difficult for some ADHD children.

Right-left discrimination, which is a combination of positioning awareness and opposition, can also be difficult for these children. Some are poor readers, partly because of problems with left-to-right progression, and some try to read from right to left and from the bottom to the top of the page. They might put their shoes on the wrong feet or simply have trouble remembering which hand is left and which is right.

Accurate visual perception requires seeing things as a whole. Instead, these children break down a picture or design into parts and do not perceive the parts as connected to each other. Their reading is disjointed, only one word at a time with no flow between words and incorrect pauses for punctuation. They might not be able to fill in missing parts of what they see or hear.

Handwriting is notoriously poor among ADHD children, and they might be unable to draw what they see. They might be looking at a five-pointed star but draw one with six points, or draw a square instead of a slanted parallelogram.

They may perceive corners of objects as protruding farther than they do, or not as far. This poor depth perception results in clumsiness and awkwardness and occasional stumbling and running into things.

Perceptual problems can also affect their sense of hearing. Many of the reading problems these children have stem from problems hearing and remembering the separate sounds made by the individual letters and common letter combinations. They omit words and letters when reading and have weak rhyme perception. Analyzing words into sound units may be troublesome: "ing" may be pronounced as "in" plus "g." Their ability to hear harmony, melody, and rhythm in music is also often impaired, and they may have trouble singing on key.

Inattention to Body States. Many ADHD children have an incorrect perception of their internal and external body states. They seem to be somewhat insensitive to pain; they might injure themselves severely, then fail to report the injury until much later. They might not feel hunger even though not having eaten for an entire day.

From 40 to 50% of hyperactive children have problems with bowel and bladder control. Daytime wetting and soiling occur because they are underresponsive to their internal body signals, thinking their bladders are full when they are not, or that there is no need to go to the bathroom when in fact they are about to wet their pants. Daytime pants wetters and soilers may also be reluctant to interrupt their play to find a bathroom. Nighttime lack of control can be caused by sleep-related problems.

Physical Difficulties

Constant Movement. This trait is one of the two that define the syndrome in its narrowest sense. These children act as if driven by a giant mainspring that is wound too tightly. There is poor channeling of energy, with irrelevant and useless movements of various body parts. They jump, fidget, squirm, rock, wiggle, and run. Somehow, they hardly ever sit still or walk calmly from one place to another. They often run ahead, flit around, and need to be called back by supervising adults when in public. Sitting through an entire meal is an unusual event for some.

They need to be constantly busy and are unable to sit quietly and restfully. Even when focusing on a television program or computer screen, they change body position, make tapping noises, or move constantly. They tend to poke, touch, feel, and grab, especially in stores and in school hallways. Repetitive behaviors such as thumb sucking, nail biting, scratching and picking at sores and fingernails, teeth grinding, or pulling out hair one strand at a time are common.

These children also seem to be constantly moving their mouths. They are consistently noisy and loud at play, making clicks, whistles, and sounds and producing an endless stream of chatter. One mother summarized her 10-year-old's constant movement of the mouth: "He goes from loud to louder. He said his first word at eight months and hasn't stopped talking since."

Variable Rates of Development. During infancy and toddlerhood some ADHD children develop faster than their peers—for example, learning to walk and talk earlier than other infants. Occasionally, they skip a stage, the most common being learning to walk without first learning to crawl.

More often, however, these children are slow in passing the developmental milestones. They might not start crawling until after ten months or walking until after eighteen months. Some show delayed development of speech skills and a small vocabulary.

Food Cravings. ADHD children may try to satisfy a profound craving for sweets by eating powdered gelatin straight from the box, huge quantities of dessert at one sitting, and sugar by the spoonful. Many seem to have more liking for cheese than non-ADHD children.

Allergies and Sensitivities. Allergies are the immune system's response to "false alarms" triggered by allergens. Hyperactive children are among the most allergic, and they frequently show signs of allergy to offending substances such as animal bites and stings, chemicals, medicines, pet dander and feathers, dust, mold, and cosmetics. The most common food allergies among ADHD children are to chocolate, corn and corn products, eggs, milk, nuts, pork, sugar, and wheat products. These children also have allergies to pollens, resulting in a much higher than chance incidence of hay fever and asthma. Eczema and other skin rashes also occur often in ADHD individuals.

Sensitivities, on the other hand, don't involve the immune system, but reflect the body's mistaken attempt to incorporate foreign substances into normal biochemical processes. ADHD individuals tend to be sensitive to certain chemical compounds whose molecular structure is characterized by a donut-shaped ring of six carbon and six hydrogen atoms with an oxygen and hydrogen radical attached, called the phenol ring. When the molecules of such substances are small (have low molecular weight) and highly willing to break apart and combine with molecules from the body (unstable), they are especially liable to be picked up and misused by the nervous system in its ordinary manufacturing of its chemical products. The intended products don't occur because these unstable, lightweight phenol-based compounds are foreign to the body. The resulting chemical imbalance within the brain creates ADHD symptoms. Phenol-based unstable compounds are found in highly aromatic substances such as gasoline, paint, smoke, and perfume as well as in coal tar products such as dyes. Other sources of these compounds and their effects on ADHD individuals are discussed in Chapter 5.

Fair-featured children (blue or green eyes and blond or red hair) account for 40 to 50% of all ADHD children. These same features characterize the majority of patients of allergists, as there seems to be a genetic connection between being fair-featured and having a biochemically sensitive body.

Researchers have found little evidence supporting sugar as an instigator of ADHD symptoms. My experience is that a small percentage of ADHD children are reported by their parents as being especially liable to an increase in ADHD symptoms after ingesting a substantial amount of sugar. There is no need or advantage, however, in avoiding sugar or substituting honey for sugar.

One survey indicated that 45% of practicing pediatricians and family physicians in the early 1980s periodically recommended low-sugar diets for ADHD patients. Clearly part of the common lore is that sugar increases ADHD symptoms, though there is almost no research support for such a conclusion.

Sleep Problems. These children may not want to sleep and might oppose going to bed, even though they have been active throughout the day. It may be hard for them to get to sleep after going to bed. Some ADHD children have very shallow, short periods of sleep rather than an ordinary eight hours. The sleeping patterns of many of these children are quite irregular. Some ADHD children may sleep restlessly and others may experience sleep that is so deep they have nightmares, talk and walk in their sleep, or wet the bed.

Coordination Problems. Hyperactive children may have a poor sense of balance and problems with large muscle coordination. Riding a bicycle, a two-wheeled scooter, or skateboard, balancing on a trampoline, and skipping backward are especially difficult tasks for some of these children. Because of a general awkwardness of movement and a clumsy gait, they may find it hard to hop on one foot, jump rope, or play ball.

Small muscle coordination problems appear when they try to draw, write, or color. If there is a coordination problem, ADHD children are usually not impaired in both the large and small muscle groups simultaneously.

Emotional Difficulties

Self-centeredness. ADHD children seem to lack awareness of their impact on others. These children appear not to pay sufficient attention to the ordinary social signals and cues most people use. Although their actions seem willful, ADHD children almost universally are surprised, alarmed, and confused about why others are so upset with them. They may do harmful acts without meaning to hurt others, then be surprised when others show anger or are displeased by their misbehavior. Because they do not feel personally connected to a situation in terms of having directly caused any of the problems occurring, they are quick to blame others for being angry at them and consequently for being unfair.

They tend to blame others and external circumstances for their difficulties rather than accepting responsibility. Everything is everyone else's fault. These children have difficulty identifying needed self-improvements, and they seldom admit to being wrong. They are unable to adapt their behavior to respond to the feedback they receive from others. As a result, group experiences often fail to improve their future behavior or interpersonal habits.

Their own wants, needs, and whims often appear to be their dominant concern. When denied what they want, they pester and harp until the parent, teacher, or other caregiver gives in. They have an "I don't care" attitude if threatened or punished. They want the rules changed to their own advantage.

ADHD children tend to relate poorly to other children, especially in group settings. Though at first they may attract friends, they are not able to keep them. They are incredibly bossy, dominate play situations and intimidate their playmates, are bullheaded and stubborn about getting their own way, and remain inflexible to the appeals of another child. They have difficulty contributing to truly cooperative endeavors because of their weak sensitivity to others' feelings and their propensity for intruding on others' boundaries.

Impatience. They are typically negative, contrary, oppositional, and hard to please. Parents report that their ADHD children almost always manage to find something to complain about and seem to need to tamper with every situation and every comment made by others.

Impatience can be reflected in impulsiveness and acting without first asking permission. They respond too quickly before understanding the entire instructions for a task, becoming impatient to get started and just as impatient to stop. While standing in line, these children poke, push, and shove to get ahead. Hyperactive children seem unable to wait for anything!

Recklessness. These children tend not to be diligent. They make many careless errors and take a slipshod approach to tasks. They act lighthearted and carefree as though they take nothing seriously. Their thoughts tend to be of the reflex variety, with little apparent mental effort. In their "I don't know and I don't care" attitude toward their experiences, they commit acts that disregard safety and health, with no concern for obvious dangers. The devil-may-care child may have no fear of heights, strangers, animals, traffic, traveling alone, or wandering away from home.

These children tend to be too rough at play, wearing out clothes and toys long before other children do. They are destructive, not only from recklessness but also from anger and inquisitiveness. Social inhibitions may be rare. These children tend to be assertive, intrusive, and without shyness. Curiosity may seem unbridled, and they may seem to pry and be nosy.

Their recklessness shows in their susceptibility to peer influence and temptations. They gravitate to peers who are uncritical and undemanding and who have their own difficulties getting along with authority figures. ADHD children seem to attract and find each other, and their parents complain of the many difficulties that occur whenever their child is in the company of another ADHD child in an unsupervised setting.

Extreme Emotionalism. A lack of restraint or cushioning of their emotions, rapid mood changes, and extreme excitability, which often are expressed in raw, overwhelming, and extreme form, are characteristic of hyperactive children. Compared with ADHD boys, ADHD girls have more difficulty with emotional control.

Low frustration tolerance is a hallmark trait. They are irritable, easily upset, and react angrily to being teased; vicious and extreme acts of violence are not uncommon. Spanking may worsen rather than improve a situation.

Their emotional highs and lows illustrate the compartmentalized and fragmented view of life of many hyperactive children. They are moody and unpredictable, quick to forgive and forget: angry one moment and happy the next. Anger control training is almost always a needed service when these children come to the attention of professionals.

Weak Conscience. Many ADHD children have poor respect for invisible boundaries such as

Property: borrowing without permission, stealing trinkets and candy from stores and money from family members, invading purses and drawers of parents and siblings, and failing to return items they have borrowed

Living space: entering without knocking, sneaking into siblings' bedrooms, and interrupting others in the bathroom

Privacy: intruding on private conversations, listening on extension telephones, being too curious, and probing with offensive questions

Limits: pounding on the door and repeatedly ringing the doorbell while waiting to enter, badgering and demanding explanations when given an undesired answer, unwilling to accept no, and defiantly refusing to do things when asked

Body space: speaking too loudly, standing too close, poking and grabbing, tickling or hitting, and taking things from others

INDICATORS OF THE ADHD SYNDROME

Here are some factors that seem to be associated with the occurrence of ADD or ADHD. Many are impressionistic and controversial, and much more research is needed to clarify their relevance. They can be interpreted somewhat like pieces of evidence—the more there are, the firmer the diagnosis becomes. Most of these characteristics are associated with a greater than chance likelihood of the syndrome, but no ADHD child has all these indicators, and many occur in non-ADHD children.

Fetal Indicators

1. Apparent hyperactivity in the womb. About one-third of ADHD children are hyperactive while still preborn. Mothers report the child kicks and turns and punches or bruises her ribs. This increased activity is especially pronounced when the expectant mother is sitting or lying quietly.

2. Poor maternal health.
3. Mother under 20 years of age.
4. First pregnancy.
5. Elevated blood pressure during pregnancy (pre-eclampsia).
6. Convulsions in the mother (eclampsia) during the latter stages of pregnancy or during childbirth.
7. Maternal alcohol abuse.
8. Heavy maternal smoking.
9. Drug abuse. Though sufficient research has not been done for drawing definite conclusions, it is highly likely that heavy maternal marijuana use and abuse of drugs such as cocaine also are associated with ADHD in the developing child.

Birth Indicators

(Many are somewhat controversial because of insufficient controlled scientific studies.)

1. Extreme prolonged lack of oxygen at birth.
2. Labor lasting longer than eighteen hours.
3. Birth injuries.
4. Congenital problems or physical malformations.
5. Fetal alcohol syndrome. This syndrome includes low birth weight, small head size, birth defects, withdrawal symptoms, and mental retardation. When the expectant mother consumes a large amount of ethyl alcohol, she can cause fetal damage. The actual amount needed to harm the nervous system and period of pregnancy in which the developing child is most sensitive to this insult are not yet known.
6. Prematurity. Studies of low birth weight babies suggest a relationship between perinatal factors and the syndrome. In one study, prematurity was found to be associated with hyperactivity at age

seven. In another study, the ADHD rate was 18% in low birth weight children and 6.5% in full birth weight children.

7. Low placental weight.
8. Breech presentation.
9. Inflammation of the outermost of the two membranes enveloping the preborn child (chorionitis).

Early Infancy Indicators (birth–6 months)

1. Inadequate sleep.
2. Irritability.
3. Excessive crying and colic.
4. Feeding problems such as difficulty nursing or accepting a formula and differing appetite levels.
5. Health problems such as allergies, colds, asthma, upper respiratory infections, and fluid in the ears.
6. Poor bonding. The baby is not cuddly and responsive and is restless and difficult to manage during such routine activities as bathing, diaper changing, or feeding.

Late Infancy Indicators (6–18 months)

1. Unusual crib behavior such as foot thumping, excessive rocking, head banging, and climbing out of the crib
2. Rapid or delayed development of physical skills such as crawling, sitting, standing, walking, and running
3. Delayed or rapid development of verbal skills, such as saying the first word prior to ten months or after sixteen months of age
4. Low adaptability to change

5. Sleep difficulties including getting to sleep, staying asleep, obtaining restful sleep, and arising refreshed and pleasant in the morning

Toddlerhood Indicators (18–36 months)

1. Aggressive: pushes, shoves, pinches, kicks, bites, and grabs toys and can't play cooperatively for a sustained period
2. Destructive: breaks, throws, and tears apart things, toys, and clothing because of anger, curiosity, or wear-and-tear from high activity level
3. Overactive: acts as if driven by a mainspring that is wound too tightly, resulting in nonstop movement and an inability to sit quietly for more than a few minutes
4. Incorrigible: underresponsive to parental correction, unconcerned when threatened with punishments, and requiring constant attention, reminding, and restraining
5. Reckless: accident prone, careless with common dangers such as traffic, and susceptible to accidental poisoning

Preschool Indicators (3–5 years)

1. Stomach problems. By the time they are five years old, hyperactive children on the average have had more serious gastrointestinal complaints resulting in contact with physicians than their peers.
2. Lack of coordination in large or small muscle group activities. The child tends to produce sloppy and messy seatwork at preschool or kindergarten.
3. Off-task behavior. These children wander away from their tables at school and do other than what the teacher is instructing the class to do, thus

requiring an excessive amount of attention and supervision.

4. Overactivity. They won't sit still and pay attention, won't sit for storytime, are out of their seats too often, talk out of turn, and make inappropriate and disrespectful comments to classmates and the teacher.
5. Intrusiveness. Hyperactive children are almost universally unpopular throughout their childhood and adolescence. They bother other children by talking to them, touching them, or intruding on their projects and play, as well as by inappropriately seeking attention, such as by clowning. This trend starts shortly after they learn to walk and begin interacting with other children and becomes a lifelong problem of getting along in groups and a secondary problem of self-esteem.
6. Aggressiveness. These children are aggressive toward classmates and can't play cooperatively. They take their classmates' toys and hit, kick, and make them cry.
7. Distractibility. These children appear to have too short an attention span when compared to other children of the same age.
8. Parent-child conflict. Patterns of family disruption, such as nag-yell-spank cycles, become established. The parents perceive the child as a negative influence on the family.

PREDICTORS OF THE ADHD SYNDROME

Psychological studies of families of ADHD children have uncovered a number of factors that indicate a higher than chance likelihood of ADHD. Like the indicators, these factors do not "prove" the existence of ADHD in any specific child, but their existence increases the statistical likelihood that any one child will have ADHD. The more of these factors that occur, the greater the chance of the child's having ADHD.

Familial Factors

- ADHD in near relatives. The occurrence of the disorder in blood relatives such as parents, grandparents, aunts, uncles, and siblings is a predictor. An increased prevalence of ADHD of about 25% is found in nontwin siblings and a much higher percentage is found in identical twins.
- Alcoholism in near relatives. Alcoholism is one of the most common major conditions associated with ADHD, with about one-third of male alcoholics having it.
- Sociopathy in near relatives. Criminal tendencies in parents, grandparents, aunts, and uncles have been found to be associated with ADHD in the children.
- Depression in near relatives. Along with alcoholism and sociopathy, depression in parents, grandparents, aunts, and uncles is also a predictor.
- Allergies and sensitivities in near relatives. Having close relatives who suffer from hay fever, asthma, sensitive skin, or allergies increases the likelihood of the presence of ADHD.
- Adoption. About one out of every five adopted children has ADHD.

Physiological Factors

- PKU. This inherited brain disorder results in a biochemical imbalance in the brain. Some studies suggest over one-half of PKU children have ADHD; at least they seem to be more at risk for ADHD than normal children. PKU children are invariably fair-featured also.

- Tourette's syndrome. Tourette's syndrome (TS) causes tics, which are jerking muscle movements starting in the face and spreading to the neck and shoulders, then finally to the trunk and limbs. These muscle movements are accompanied by an assortment of other symptoms such as uttering of odd sounds, making irrelevant comments, and a host of ADHD symptoms including distractibility and restlessness. TS is an elusive, hard-to-diagnose disorder. Its severity and type and location of symptoms vary greatly from one patient to another. The symptoms seem to phase in and out over extended periods, with nearly one-fourth of TS individuals experiencing total disappearance of symptoms for up to seven years. Significant ADHD symptoms occur in about one-half of TS patients. In fact, if one simply subtracts the tics and guttural noises, TS is remarkably similar to ADHD. A closer look provides an explanation: ADHD is a subset of TS and might be the first cluster of symptoms to become obvious in an individual who has TS. One research project found that hyperactivity and attention deficits started an average of two to three years prior to the beginning of motor or vocal tics. In rare cases, the two start simultaneously.

In the majority of TS cases, the natural course of the syndrome begins with ADHD, then develops into tics and vocal noises. It is even possible that a hyperactivity disorder is the only observable reflection of the presence of a TS gene. Sometimes TS has a late onset, so that ADHD symptoms don't appear until after the age of seven, and tics don't start until early or middle adolescence. Onset of ADHD symptoms after the age of seven indicates that the hyperactivity symptoms might be part of a TS disorder in the affected individual.

ADHD DURING ADOLESCENCE

Research now indicates that hyperactive children continue to have multiple problems as adolescents, though some have asserted the hyperactivity itself usually decreases. My experience has been that severely symptomatic youngsters are more likely than borderline and mildly symptomatic children to experience a continuation of symptoms during adolescence. Problems with aggression, poor self-concept, impaired peer relationships, and poor school performance become prominent. The ADHD adolescent is often sad and depressed, though the co-occurrence of depression with ADHD in younger children is quite low.

Children whose observable symptoms continue into adolescence have higher rates of delinquency and conduct disorders and lower IQs and academic achievement scores than those whose symptoms stop at early adolescence. Seventeen-year-old symptomatic adolescents use harmful and addictive substances more than those who have stopped showing most ADHD symptoms. They also are more likely to develop depression during adolescence.

Conduct Disorders

Children with a conduct disorder show repetitive, persistent actions that violate the rights and property of others and major societal norms and rules. They are verbally abusive, overly contentious and power-seeking, overly critical of others including those in authority, rarely make kind or helpful statements, must have the last word in conversations, almost never admit fault or weakness, blame external circumstances and other people for difficulties, and call people derogatory names and swear at them. They are clearly delinquent and precriminal in their actions and motives. ADHD-cd children rarely acknowledge their antisocial behavior; they admit to problems of overactivity and attention deficit much more readily than to conduct disorder behaviors. They steal, run away, become pathological liars, set fires, burglarize, deliberately destroy property of others, are cruel to animals, initiate fights and use weapons, molest small children, and commit similar acts of terrorism against any convenient target.

Compared to non-ADHD children and to hyperactive children who are not ADHD-cd, these children are prone to more firesetting, vandalism, lying, truancy, fighting, carrying of illegal weapons, blatant aggression, substance abuse of alcohol and drugs, assaults, and motor vehicle offenses and accidents. They are even more likely to display these behaviors if they are raised in poverty or abused, the parents have psychiatric disorders, or they belong to a conduct disorder friendship group.

A significant proportion of adolescents in the juvenile justice system and adults in the penal system have a history of ADHD. As many as 30 to 40% eventually get into trouble with authorities as adults, most being from the ADHD-cd subgroup. Of all ADHD children, this subgroup is at greatest risk for adult antisocial and criminal behavior. In one survey nearly 50% of ADHD-cd adults were found to have arrest records for a felony. Many adult sociopaths displayed antisocial tendencies and hyperactivity as children.

Most researchers find an overlap of hyperactivity and conduct disorder in from 30 to 65% of the cases they investigate. The remainder of those in their studies exhibit one or the other, but not both.

These traits tend to be relatively stable. ADHD-cd children who show aggressive tendencies, lie, or steal often continue to show antisocial tendencies in adolescence.

An unduly high incidence of alcoholism and character disorders is evident among fathers of ADHD-cd children, and ADHD-cd children have siblings who also have a high likelihood of conduct disorders. Antisocial parents are more likely to have an ADHD child with the overlapping condition of conduct disorder than psychiatrically healthier parents.

Aggression. Aggression is one of the most serious behavior patterns in the ADHD-cd subgroup. It can be divided into four types: (1) person-oriented—fighting, bullying, using weapons; (2) object-oriented—breaking, kicking, tearing, slamming, and throwing toys, objects, doors, and furniture; (3) verbal—cursing, name calling, teasing, criticizing, bossing, and harassing; and (4) symbolic—making aggressive, obscene, or otherwise offensive gestures or threatening with a fist.

Aggressiveness toward others is the predominant factor determining whether a hyperactive adolescent will be accepted by peers. The less aggressive are able to retain a semblance of social acceptance. Because aggressiveness is one of the most stable and least changeable of the ADHD personality traits, it is vitally important to provide the anger control and social skills training outlined in this book.

Drug Abuse. Having a romance with or being a close friend of an adolescent who abuses drugs greatly increases the chance that an ADHD-cd adolescent will abuse substances also. The usual lag time between the time the adolescent starts abusing drugs and the time parents realize it is approximately six months. If you suspect drug abuse, get help immediately. The adolescent's physician can perform simple blood and urine tests for indications of drug use.

Confronting the adolescent might not result in much improvement. Almost every drug abusing adolescent denies the problem when confronted. Even with an adolescent's admission of usage and a promise to discontinue, the possibility of repeated drug usage is quite high.

The following behavior changes may indicate drug

abuse by an adolescent; the greater the number, the more serious the problem.

1. Energy changes: fatigue, sleepiness, changes in hours of sleep, difficulty waking, too much or too little sleep, staying up all night, periods of unusual excitement and drivenness
2. Physical changes: reddened, watery eyes; drooping eyelids; colds, runny nose, infections; hacking cough, shortness of breath, peculiar breath odors; pale cheeks, sweating or chills; stomach or intestinal problems; clumsiness; coordination problems; food cravings; appetite change
3. Mental changes: slurred speech, lack of emotion, forgetfulness and absentmindedness, slurred words; talking in incomplete sentences, losing train of thought, nervousness, irritability, distorted sense of time, paranoia, depression, suicidal threats, strange and bizarre thoughts, hallucinations
4. Social changes: withdrawal from normal contacts; dropping friends; seeking out less desirable acquaintances; idolizing questionable, older adults; attraction to drug-lyric and Satanic-lyric rock music and performers
5. Attitude changes: "I don't care" attitude about school; avoiding homework; resentment of teachers, police, and other authorities; flagrant disregard for rules
6. Emotional changes: rapid mood swings, extreme irritability, angry outbursts, unexplained crying, intense worry, oversensitivity to criticism
7. Nighttime activity changes: frequent short visits from strangers, secretive phone calls from strangers, refusal to tell names of new acquaintances, traffic violations, possession of drug equipment and smoking devices, strange odor to clothing

ADHD DURING ADULTHOOD

One-third to one-half of ADHD children who are moderately or severely hyperactive continue to have so many symptoms that they become ADHD adults. Compared with the general population, ADHD adults are at greater risk for psychiatric hospitalization and for criminal behavior. Many of these adults wrestle with issues pertaining to low self-esteem.

The chief predictors of a poor adjustment in adulthood are insensitivity to approval from others; cruelty to others without feeling guilt and remorse; history of antisocial behavior; family history of mental illness, alcoholism, or antisocial behavior in parents or close blood relatives; and history of harsh physical discipline or abuse. In short, the classic accompaniments to a conduct disorder are the strongest indicators of the likelihood of problems adjusting as an adult: more frequent rates of job changes, marital instability, traffic accidents, minor legal infractions, broken or stressed friendships, and abrasive relationships with others.

Although ADHD adults don't necessarily complain of being unable to focus their attention on what they want to do, they do consistently complain about impulse control and restlessness. About one-fourth show wholesale maladaptation such as the inability to hold a job, habitual criminality, or delinquency, and many who are not in this subgroup tend to be lonely and unpopular even though sidestepping the more blatant maladaptations.

More than one-half of ADHD adults, however, do not come in contact with mental health or correctional systems; they lead normal, well-adjusted lives. Some are able to channel their energy into home improvement projects, hobbies demanding vigorous activity, and civic and community involvement.

Accepting a job that provides challenge is one of the most important acts of self-care a hyperactive adult can undertake. While some become workaholics, they are usually good ideas persons who can delegate tasks to people who are better at handling details; but to attain a supervisory position, they have to believe in their own ideas. Those who go into fields requiring independence and self-control can sometimes do well by compensating for their need for structure and constancy in their working environment. It would be foolish and naive, however, to point every ADHD young adult toward a particular career. As with any other person, the choice of career needs to be formulated on the basis of a host of individual factors. It is best to regard ADHD symptoms during adulthood as personality traits that help determine which settings and circumstances the person would enjoy most for employment, recreation, and social life.

One mother of an ADHD young adult summarized the gradual blossoming of good adjustment during late adolescence and early adulthood: "The very traits that used to work against him now work for him. He's so aware of how everybody else is doing and how they are feeling. He strikes up conversations and has an easy time making good friends."

Many hyperactive adolescents adjust better after high school, when their academic problems are finally over. As a group, their work status and employer ratings tend to be somewhat lower than the non-ADHD adults. One predictor of more positive adult adjustment that consistently appears in the research is a supportive authority figure, most often the mother, who expressed confidence and positive expectations about the young person's ability to be successful in life.

A small subgroup of ADHD adults have developed compulsive mechanisms to compensate for their symptoms. They make a concerted effort to be overly organized. To overcome their forgetfulness, they write everything down and carry notebooks and calendars. They try to allow extra time for any deadlines. Some of those who come to the attention of mental health professionals for compulsive disorders are actually ADHD adults who have found what amounts to a collection of compensatory maneuvers to make life better than it would be without such measures.

A SCREENING CHECKLIST

Most of the rating scales used for diagnosing ADHD are lengthy and complicated, and some of the items are of questionable relevance. There has been a definite need for a quick screening test that any parent, teacher, counselor, or physician can use to help diagnose this disorder. The Taylor Hyperactivity Screening Checklist has been developed for that purpose.

The checklist contains (in Column C) twenty-one of the most consistent traits among ADHD children. The opposites of these twenty-one traits are also rare among ADHD children. Experience with this scale over the years has indicated that it is accurate from age two through adulthood. The items lean rather significantly in the direction of the fidgetiness and hyperactivity component of the ADHD syndrome. For persons with attention deficits but without a hyperactivity component (ADD-noH), however, it is still useful. I have found the scores to range from 18 to 34 for that particular symptom cluster.

The Taylor Hyperactivity Screening Checklist

For each of the twenty-one behaviors, put an X in one of the three boxes to show the typical behavior. Rate the behavior when not being supervised, helped, or reminded; when not watching television or a computer screen; and when not receiving any kind of treatment to control behavior.

Indicate the trend. Try to avoid Column B ratings; a 51% trend in either direction should merit an A or C rating. Compared with others of approximately the same age, this child typically shows behavior:

A *Somewhat more like this* ↘ | *B* *Absolutely no trend* | ↙ *C* *Somewhat more like this*

A		B		C
	1. Quiet person		Noisy and talkative person	
	2. Voice volume is soft or average		Voice is generally too loud for the situation	
	3. Few mouth or body noises		Makes lots of clicks, whistles, and sounds with mouth or body	
	4. Walks at appropriate times		Flits around, runs ahead, needs to be called back, jumpy	
	5. Keeps hands to self		Pokes, touches, feels, and grabs	
	6. Appears calm, can be still		Always has a body part moving; fidgets with hands or feet; squirmy	
	7. Can just sit		Has to be doing something to occupy self when sitting; quickly bored	
	8. Slow to react, deliberate; not impulsive		Too quick to react, impulsive, engages mouth and muscles before brain	

	A *Somewhat more like this*	B *Absolutely no trend*	C *Somewhat more like this*	
	9. Understands why parents/teacher/ others are displeased after misbehavior		Feels picked on, is surprised and confused about why others are displeased; doesn't connect own actions to others' reactions	
	10. Planful; thinks ahead to consequences before acting		Does things without considering consequences ahead of time; careless; not planful	
	11. Avoids other children's mischief		Gets involved in mischief; attracted or curious about it, or starts it	
	12. Concerned about punishments and consequences; submissive		Pretends to have an "I don't care" attitude if threatened or punished; defiant	
	13. Obeys directions and follows orders		Disobeys; needs supervision or reminding; forgetful	
	14. Constant mood with mild or slow mood changes; a calm person		Moody; unpredictable; quick to anger or tears	
	15. Easygoing; handles frustration without much anger; patient; can be teased		Irritable, impatient, easily frustrated	

A *Somewhat more like this*		B *Absolutely no trend*		C *Somewhat more like this*
	16. Emotions are reasonably controlled, are not extreme, and don't disrupt relationships		Emotions are extreme and poorly controlled; no "damper pedal" on emotion; explosive, tantrumy	
	17. Cooperates with, obeys, and enforces the rules of work and play		Argues and gripes about the rules; wants to be the exception; oppositional	
	18. Gives up when denied a requested privilege, item, or activity		Badgers, pesters, pushes, won't give up or take no for an answer	
	19. Concentrates and blocks out distractions when working on something of medium interest		Easily distracted by noises and people nearby; short attention span	
	20. Follows through, has an organized approach to activities, finishes projects		Flits from activity to activity; starts things without finishing them; gets sidetracked	
	21. Doesn't try to bother or hurt others with words		Needles, teases, mouthy; has to have the last word	

The score is the total number of items in Column B plus twice the number of items in Column C. The range of possible scores is 0 to 42. An individual (age two through adult) scoring 24 or less is probably not hyperactive; 25 to 27: borderline hyperactive; 28 to 32: mildly hyperactive; 33 to 37: moderately hyperactive; 38 to 42: severely hyperactive. Development and validity data for the original form, which had slightly different wording on some of the items but assessed the same traits on all items, appear in Appendix B.

No single checklist is final proof of the existence of ADHD. This instrument makes a crude division between ADHD and other behaviors. It is not a comprehensive list of all symptoms but lists the most *differentiating* symptoms—those likely to occur in ADHD individuals and unlikely to occur in non-ADHD individuals. As time passes, research will undoubtedly lead to more refined diagnostic methods. Meanwhile, screening checklists, behavioral history, and observation remain the best diagnostic tools.

SEVERITY OF ADHD

Borderline and mildly hyperactive children, scoring 25 to 32 on the Taylor Hyperactivity Screening Checklist, tend as a group to show somewhat different behavior from moderately and severely symptomatic children who score 33 to 42. In general, the *more severe* the hyperactivity and the *higher* the score on the THSC, the more likely the child is to

- consistently show symptoms of ADHD from setting to setting.
- require high dosage levels of prescribed medication.
- show sensitivities to many environmental irritants and chemicals.

- be allergic to foods, pollens, animal dander, mold, dust, or medicines.
- have noticeable symptoms before the age of two.
- have increasing or consistent ADHD symptoms throughout childhood and adolescence.
- experience little or no decrease in symptoms during adolescence.
- have many symptoms as an adult.
- have many cognitive impairments.
- show severe behavior disturbance.
- benefit little from counseling.
- be aggressive toward others.
- be enrolled in special education programs.

The *less severe* the hyperactivity and the *lower* the score, the more likely the child is to

- show variation in displayed ADHD symptoms from setting to setting.
- respond to lower dosage levels of medication.
- tolerate exposure to some environmental irritants and chemicals without showing ADHD symptoms.
- have no allergies.
- appear symptom-free until after the age of two.
- show symptoms at a constant level or decreasingly from age three to adolescence.
- experience decrease in many symptoms during adolescence.
- have few or no symptoms as an adult.
- have few cognitive impairments.
- show little behavior disturbance.
- benefit from counseling.
- get along well with other children.
- remain in regular classrooms without special academic help.

Once you understand that your child has ADHD, possibly with one or more overlapping conditions, you are ready to proceed with significant steps to improve your child's adjustment. Usually professional help is needed, partly to continue the diagnostic process and rule out ADHD imitator disorders, and partly to proceed with the various psychological, academic, and biochemical measures available to assist your child. Chapter 2 explains how to find the best professional help.

2

Getting the Best Professional Help

No single field of knowledge has all the answers about ADHD. Medical and mental health professionals can form the core, however, of a diagnostic and treatment team that has the potential for providing your child with the best possible help.

Because there are numerous ADHD imitator disorders, a medical diagnosis helps clarify the exact nature of the difficulties. Correct medical treatment for conditions causing apparent ADHD symptoms is crucial. If you choose medication, a physician will be needed to engineer the treatment and prescribe the proper medication and dosage. Clearly, the physician is a very important part of your child's diagnostic and treatment team.

Because ADHD is so pervasive and affects every aspect of your family's as well as your child's functioning, a mental health professional is also a potentially valuable helper.

Numerous other helping professionals can assist, depending on your child's specific needs and your resources for obtaining the most beneficial services. Especially when an overlapping condition is involved, an evaluation from members of several helping disciplines may be called for. Your child might see a psychologist, psychometrist, neurologist, speech and language therapist, counselor, allergist, audiologist, psychiatrist, occupational therapist, social worker, learning disabilities specialist, or a combination of these specialists.

GETTING HELP FROM A PHYSICIAN

Current training being given to students in the helping professions likely to become involved with ADHD children—medicine, mental health disciplines, nursing, nutrition, education, corrections—is inconsistent, haphazard, and sometimes quite inaccurate. The sense of uneasiness many physicians have about proceeding with diagnosis and treatment is well deserved. Most physician residency programs provide little or no training in diagnosing and treating those afflicted with attention deficit hyperactivity disorder. Some physicians rarely or never prescribe stimulants or antidepressants; others rely heavily on them. Some recommend the Feingold Program (see Chapter 5) while others avoid mentioning it. Some require lengthy series of unnecessary psychological testing beyond the customary teacher and parent reports and an interview of the child. Others rely on information from parents and observation of the child in the office. Some decide if the problem is or is not ADHD simply on the inaccurate and misleading basis of how the child acts during a ten-minute office visit. Fortunately, these trends are changing as increasing numbers of physicians gain direct experience with the families of these children and adolescents.

As a parent, you have valuable knowledge and information to share with the physician. You are directly involved in getting your child's cooperation, maintaining the medication regimen, and monitoring the results. It is important to stay informed and to be confident of your ability to learn whatever is necessary to find the best possible care and management measures to accompany the efforts of prescribed medication or the Feingold Program. Don't be afraid to keep asking questions until you understand your child's situation. An adequate information base increases your sense of personal control and effectiveness. It also maximizes the likelihood that any prescribed medications will be effective.

No single interview of the child or rating checklist can substitute for the combined observations of parents, caregivers, mental health professionals, and educators. Research has shown that in four out of five visits to their physicians, these children do not show any visible signs of the disorder. Be prepared for the first visit to the physician. Rate your child, and have the teacher do the same, with the Taylor Hyperactivity Screening Checklist. As a supplement to these observations take a copy of Chapter 1 with all applicable sections and symptoms highlighted. Bring a list of any known allergies and sensitivities, relevant information from school files, and a brief summary of any social skills problems. Give the physician target symptoms, particularly those that are most troublesome, rather than saying, "My child is hyperactive, so medicate him."

A crucial part of your physician's responsibility is to rule out the existence of imitator disorders and to confirm the diagnosis of ADHD. The following conditions produce symptoms similar to ADHD that are not usually helped by stimulants or the Feingold Program and can best be diagnosed by a physician.

- *Iron deficiency* can lead to difficulties focusing attention, problem solving, and controlling activity.

- *Lead intoxication* from consumption of lead-infested drinking water or lead-colored paint can lead to hyperactivity.
- *Direct physical or biochemical insult to brain tissue* as a result of encephalitis, chorea, a brain tumor or a skull fracture accompanied by unconsciousness, or Reye syndrome can cause forgetfulness, absent-mindedness, memory problems, distractibility, and weakened control over emotions.
- *Protein/calorie malnutrition* can interfere with an infant's normal development of brain chemical processes.
- *Diabetes* can cause temporary nervousness, hyperactivity, and short attention span.
- *Hypoglycemia* can cause shortened attention span, tremors, and inability to concentrate.
- *Wilson's disease,* a rare accumulation of copper in the body, can cause inattention, tremor, and loosened behavior control.
- *Thyroid dysfunction*—hypothyroidism and hyperthyroidism—can alter activity levels, sleeping patterns, and emotional control.
- *Physical discomfort,* such as breathing problems or an itchy skin rash due to allergies, can cause temporary irritability and decreased ability to concentrate.
- *Medications,* such as bronchial dilators, antihistamines, and anticonvulsants, can cause inattentiveness and temporary increases in activity levels.
- *Seizure disorders,* such as temporal lobe epilepsy, can cause temporary states of agitation and confusion.
- *Hearing loss* can appear as inattentiveness or refusal to cooperate.
- *Vision problems* can result in facial grimacing, squirming, poor school performance, and irritability.
- *Sleep debt* caused by sleep apnea or physical discomfort interfering with sleep can result in hyperactivity, irritability, difficulty concentrating, forgetfulness, listlessness, bedwetting, and school problems.

Maintaining a Good Relationship During Treatment

Your child should understand the functions of the physician and other helping professionals. Written materials, although never a substitute for personal guidance from a skilled professional acquainted with your child, can provide additional helpful information.

The primary physician's ability to relate to your child as an individual facilitates the use of prescribed medications. Your child's age and physiology, the pattern of symptoms associated with the ADHD syndrome, and the relationship between the physician and each family member change over time. A physician who has long-term familiarity with your family can understand these various factors and tailor the prescribed medications to fit your child's most current needs.

The physician should gather detailed information about the history and course of your child's ADHD and occasionally conduct a complete physical examination. The physician should also continue routine health care including well-child check-ups, supervision of general health, immunizations, and treatment of minor illnesses.

Do your best to facilitate a smooth working relationship between the physician and your child and between the physician and yourself. You want a physician who is skilled and knowledgeable or at least one who is willing to consult with others who may have more experience treating hyperactive children. The physician should inspire your confidence and earn your trust. Neither too optimistic nor too pessimistic, the physician should sustain realistic hopes while not arousing false ones about the effectiveness of the treatment or the course of your child's disorder.

The physician should be available on short notice if medications have been prescribed. Find out ahead of time the circumstances under which your physician should be contacted and make arrangements for vacation coverage. The physician should talk directly with your child about ADHD and the medication and should facilitate an exchange of ideas about treatment at any time. The physician should be sensitive to your child's capacity to accept medical information and should set aside a few moments to explain concepts and ideas or to explore options. For self-applied or home-applied programs, such as prescribed medication treatment, this aspect of professional care is important. The physician should give you anticipatory guidance, outlining the expected developments regarding the treatment.

You can encourage clear communication and establish an effective partnership with the physician. Expect to give a detailed picture of your child's routines. Take a notebook and a personal history, if needed. Be sure to mention any other medication your child is taking and report any outstanding emotional difficulties. During subsequent appointments bring notes, journal records, observations about your child's symptoms, a recent Taylor Medication Effectiveness Report (see Chapter 3), and a list of questions you may have. Don't camouflage stress. Be aware of the temptation to hide the negative impact of your child's disorder from the physician. The office of any helping professional is not the place to hide trouble.

Have your questions written down and be prepared to provide answers to the physician's questions. A list helps you provide orderly information and think ahead of time about the concerns you want to discuss. If your child accompanies you, your written notes are even more important as you juggle the distractions caused by your child's presence.

Take notes. You are receiving important information; be prepared to write it down. Because of the complicated and emotionally charged circumstances often surrounding conversations in a physician's office, you may not be able to absorb, understand, or use all that the physician has said in one conversation. If you have little opportunity to ask questions and are not able to formulate useful questions during the initial session, arrange for an additional session. Don't be afraid to reveal something you do not understand or your need for further explanation of some principle, idea, or procedure. From time to time check to make sure you and the physician have approximately the same understanding of your child's progress. You may want to ask for a written summary of what has been discussed in addition to the notes you have taken. This summary from the physician is especially helpful if the information you have discussed has been particularly complicated.

Ask what to expect from ingredients in prescription medications. If your child experiences any reactions, report them immediately. Inquire specifically about when your child should take the prescribed medication, rather than relying solely on the label instructions.

Your role as facilitator for sources of help for your child can be difficult, especially if the physician does not understand how knowledgeable you are. The physician needs to be aware of your skills as an observer and your accuracy as a reporter. You in turn need to learn how to monitor symptom flare-ups as an indication that the medication regimen may need adjustment or that your child may need some additional professional services. Learn to trust your own observations and judgments and understand the expectations of any helping professionals involved. Be assertive without being offensive, insistent without being pushy, confident without being overbearing, and informative without lecturing to the physician. The physician wants to exercise his or her skills for the benefit of your child and family, and you must give the physician the freedom to do just that. On the other hand, it is deeply important that a truly effective team helps your child. Use caution in selecting the physician and keep hunting until you find one with whom you feel comfortable. Don't endow physicians with magical or godlike powers.

Don't expect any physician to be universally knowledgeable, either about one specific area or many areas. Express your frustrations without questioning the physician's integrity or competence. Physicians understand misdirected anger dumped on them, yet might react with some anger in return. Focusing on the physician's limitations or expressing disenchantment with the physician's work does not help your child. Remember instead the intentions of the physician to help and the constraints on his or her time and energy. Remember that you and the physician have similar feelings when you are communicating with each other. Both of you may be just as frustrated, upset, unprepared, or burdened at the moment. Express empathy for the physician's frustrations now and then and be aware of your common feelings.

One of your functions is to use your expanding knowledge about your child to help prevent mistakes a physician or other helping professional might otherwise make. Persistent, assertive behavior gets the best results. Be straightforward, calm, and confident in your desire to help your child and in the knowledge you are gaining, but avoid a know-it-all attitude. Instead, maintain an "I know a lot and I'm learning more" attitude. Have faith in your ability to learn more about your child's ADHD and about prescription medications. If circumstances warrant your sharing information about aspects of medication treatment that do not seem sufficiently familiar to the physician, show relevant passages of this book to him or her.

Your physician has just as great a need for reliable help and information from you as you do from the physician. In dealing with the physician your honesty, courtesy, punctuality, treatment responsibility, financial responsibility, consistent feedback as to the effects of the medications, and other important aspects of being a partner in care are crucial in maintaining a consistent treatment approach for your child. Express appreciation for the care given your child, for specific acts your physician and the physician's staff have performed, and for suggestions that have worked well. Compliment the physician and staff for small courtesies. When they are exceptionally thoughtful, give prompt attention, provide a full explanation, require a minimum of paperwork, or are especially communicative toward your child, show your appreciation. This feedback not only strengthens your partnership with the physician but provides helpful information as to the office procedures and prescription recommendations that are most effective in helping other ADHD children.

In any established relationship, especially one in which people in different roles are mutually dependent, conflicts can arise. They occur naturally among families and among departments of medical organizations, and they can occur between you and your child's physician. It is difficult to change the habits of busy professionals when your child is under their care. If a continuing personality clash develops, say something like "I respect your knowledge and experience, but I am concerned that I don't understand why you are recommending this particular change in the prescription." This statement leads you either to a more understanding and a more successful partnership or a mutual decision to arrange for a different physician. If at any point you are not able to play out the correct balance between assertion and cooperativeness, learn from your error and improve your relationship with the next physician.

Getting Your Child's Cooperation

No emotionally healthy and deeply loving parent relishes the idea of having a child take prescribed medication for a long period of time. There is a natural tendency to be hesitant to embrace medication as the treatment method.

Most parents of successfully medicated ADHD children did not start out applauding the idea of using medication but became convinced of its helpfulness by direct experience and frank observation of the results. You must be objective in noting its results; underusing it, underreporting its results, and deviating from the physician's prescribed regimen are three frequent forms of balking at medication treatment. The project must have your wholehearted support.

The most productive attitude toward medication would be similar to that toward insulin for a diabetic child. If your child's physician were to tell you your child has diabetes and must take insulin daily or risk severe symptoms, what would you do? Few parents would respond, "You are trying to train my child to evade being responsible by hunting for chemical shortcuts," or "I prefer to use psychology to train my child not to have diabetes symptoms." A similar situation occurs on the question of medicating ADHD children.

GETTING HELP FROM A MENTAL HEALTH PROFESSIONAL

Not all ADHD children require biochemical treatment, particularly those with borderline or mild symptoms without overlapping conditions. Generally speaking, however, the more severe your child's symptoms, the greater the total impact on your child and family and the greater the need for help from a mental health professional. This person's role is neither to replace other forms of care nor to explain away your child's symptoms through social or psychological causes. The primary goals are to assist in diagnosis and to help your family counter the stresses ADHD poses to your child and your family. As with most services, those of a counselor or other mental health professional are more effective if sought early.

The counselor, who may be a psychologist, social worker, psychiatrist, or member of a similar profession, usually starts the diagnostic phase by gathering information about the nature of your child's behavior problems. Two or more interviews might be needed to gather sufficient information for a clear overview of the psychological stresses your child and family are experiencing. Most experienced mental health professionals cover these topics when ruling out ADHD-imitator disorders, confirming the diagnosis, and deciding about counseling or therapy interventions:

- Personal development: tasks of daily living accomplished by your child, muscle and coordination skills, emotional maturity, ages at which milestones of development have occurred
- Family relationships: key areas of conflict, power struggles, competitiveness, areas of appreciation and strength
- Activities outside the home: school performance, friendships, hobbies, talents, community involvement, church and civic involvement
- Insight and response to symptoms: understanding of ADHD, emotional reactions to symptoms, degree of awareness of the nature of the symptoms being shown
- Parent-child relationship: your views of and actions toward your child, your emotional reactions, your level of insight and acceptance of ADHD
- Other areas of parental functioning: how each parent functions as an individual, marital stresses and strengths, how each parent relates to each child in the family, outside stresses on the family
- Siblings' reactions: their overall adjustment, their feelings about the ADHD child, their potential to assist in biochemical treatment
- Support systems needed: community resources avail-

able to your family, ways in which helping professionals can provide additional support
- Previous diagnostic and treatment attempts: history of previous interviews or statements by other professionals, history of prior treatment efforts
- Review of symptoms and indicators: inventory of symptoms and indicators of ADHD (detailed in Chapter 1) and application of screening checklists such as the Taylor Hyperactivity Screening Checklist (THSC) and the Taylor S/E/A Adjustment Checklist (Appendix B).

In addition, those who are qualified to do so might want to administer some psychological tests to supplement the information gathered in the mental health interview. Psychological tests should be given only by persons who have sufficient training and experience in the complicated techniques of administering, scoring, profiling, and interpreting them; these skills are generally confined to psychologists and psychometrists. If the mental health professional helper is not qualified to provide these services, a psychologist can administer the tests and interpret the results. The tests most often used in evaluating suspected ADHD children include screening checklists and measures of intelligence; tests for eye-hand coordination, language ability, reading skill, and academic knowledge; and an analysis of personality traits. These formal tests usually compare the child's performance with norms obtained from the administration of the tests to other children.

After gathering these data, the mental health professional is in a position to assist in ruling out ADHD-imitator disorders. Numerous conditions produce symptoms overlapping those of ADHD. These symptoms are not usually helped by stimulants or the Feingold Program, and are best diagnosed by a mental health professional.

- *Profound conditions,* such as autism or childhood

schizophrenia, can cause extreme aggressiveness, difficulty relating to normal social signals, and profound distractibility and hyperactivity.

- *Distorted reports of misbehavior* by a parent, caregiver, or teacher can mislabel a normal emotional response by the child to an abnormally stressful situation, such as harsh punishment or rudeness shown by the adult toward the child. Hyperactivity becomes a convenient label to explain the child's rebelliousness and noncompliance.
- *Overburdening* of a child who is being pushed to grow up too fast by having to take care of too many needs results in agitated, impatient, aggressive, and distracted behavior.
- *Appeals for attention* by a child who spends a considerable portion of the day in a day-care center, for example, can take the form of hyperactive-appearing misbehavior.
- *Frustrations from non-ADHD learning disabilities* can lead to irritability, daydreaming to reduce the stress of facing difficult assignments, and refusals to cooperate at school.
- *Learning disabilities symptoms,* such as deficits in auditory processing or receptive language ability, can cause confusion, poor following of directions, and apparent attention-control problems. Some learning disabilities symptoms respond to the two biochemical treatment methods for ADHD and some apparently do not.
- *Conduct disorders* and oppositional defiant disorders without ADHD include aggressiveness, conscience deficits, impulsiveness, contrariness, and poor school performance.
- *Developmental delays,* with or without accompanying mental retardation, can cause restlessness, intellectual deficits, confusion, and shortened attention spans consistent with developmental age but not with real age.
- *Extreme emotional disturbance* because of a major

stress or traumatic conflict can result in restlessness, inattentiveness, aggressive behavior, bedwetting, and inability to focus on productive pursuits like schoolwork.

- *Situational stress* such as extreme hunger, poor teaching, an overcrowded classroom, or educational tasks far above or below the correct difficulty level can cause misbehavior, loss of interest in performing, or anger and aggression.
- *Normal exploratory zeal,* particularly in toddlers and preschoolers, and the normal uninhibitedness of that age group can mimic the drivenness of true hyperactivity.
- *Intense boredom* caused by long hours of unstructured time such as during vacation periods or loosely supervised classroom activities can lead to restlessness, inability to sustain attention, discontent, and irritability.
- *Depression* can interfere with any child's ability to concentrate or produce sustained effort and can cause daydreaming, discontent, irritability, and poor emotional control.
- *Anxiety,* one of the most common ADHD imitator states, causes irrelevant comments, attention deficits, drivenness, and difficulty staying on-task at school.

INTEGRATING MENTAL HEALTH AND BIOCHEMICAL TREATMENT

In spite of biochemical treatment, these children usually remain noticeably different from other children. The range of difficulties some families experience often requires the services of mental health professionals as well as of a physician. ADHD children with overlapping conditions seem to have more severe difficulties than those without overlapping conditions. In general, ADHD children who receive no special assistance beyond biochemical treatment do not succeed as well in school, in their relationships, in their overall emotional health and adjustment, and in their feelings of self-worth.

If problems remain, you should decide which resources would be most helpful. Think of your psychosocial assistance to your child as an aspect of your parenting that will continue for many years, along with the biochemical treatment program.

Mental health professionals can provide individual or family counseling or psychotherapy. Counseling explores options during face-to-face discussions. Group counseling is an option that may be particularly helpful for your child. With the assistance of the leader, participating children learn to better understand their feelings and thoughts. Reassured that they share challenges in common with other children, they gain emotional support from the group. Using the group format, a counselor can provide a safe arena for role-playing social skills and providing feedback from others.

Psychotherapy, a more intense approach, explores deeper difficulties expressed as angry outbursts, acute anxiety, or depression. Psychotherapy may also be indicated if your child has been abused, or if diagnosis comes after years of abrasive relationships at home or school. Psychotherapy attempts to relieve emotional pressures through procedures such as hitting a pillow, having make-believe conversations with family members, or using the powers of fantasy and imagination in play or art activities.

It is not always necessary for a mental health professional to be involved exclusively with the child. In general, mental health professionals can have as much impact working with parents as with children. If your child is enrolled in counseling sessions, stay abreast of what is happening and discuss his or her progress frequently. If you don't perceive sufficient progress, discuss your concerns with the counselor. The same principles apply for maintaining a close working relationship with a mental health professional as with a physician.

Although the training procedures given in this book involve sophisticated and effective forms of psychological intervention, you will probably be able to perform most of them without professional assistance. Many incorporate principles from cognitive behavioral training (CBT) to teach your child to develop self-control in particularly stressful situations or those likely to cause a deterioration in behavior. The basic approach is to provide self-reminder statements and mottos for use when your direct intervention or supervision is not available. Occasionally, you might want to ask for some additional ideas for a CBT approach from a mental health professional.

Regardless of the types and number of helping professionals involved with your child, never surrender your primary function as facilitator and coordinator. Develop a team spirit and urge a frequent exchange and updating of progress reports among those professionals. They are there to help you and your family. Take advantage of that availability whenever the need arises. Research and clinical experience consistently shows that better results occur when a multifaceted approach is used, including social and emotional factors, school adjustment, and biochemical treatment. Chapters 3, 4, and 5 detail the most effective forms of biochemical treatment for helping individuals with the ADHD syndrome.

3

Treating with Prescribed Medication

Of the biochemical approaches to treating ADHD, prescribed medication is the most popular, most researched, and best accepted within the medical profession. Most often, the medications prescribed for ADHD individuals are stimulants and antidepressants. Amphetamines (Dexedrine, for example), methylphenidate (Ritalin), and pemoline (Cylert) are the most frequently used stimulants. Antidepressants most commonly prescribed are the tricyclics amitriptyline (Elavil), nortriptyline (Aventyl), and imipramine (Tofranil).

You might wonder why stimulants would be used to create calmness in an overly aroused child. These medications strengthen the child's ability to block out irrelevant thoughts and impulses and to focus attention on what is most important. The net result is better self-control. These medications stimulate the child's "brake pedal," whereas without treatment, the child is all "gas pedal." They do not slow down everything the child does. Instead, they allow the child to do a more efficient job of choosing what to say or do. They also increase the ability to problem solve and to learn. They help the child become more alert and generally increase self-control.

Though the Feingold Program (discussed in Chapter 5) can sometimes be considered a viable alternative and there has been an increase in psychological (social skills training) and educational (modifications to the mainstream classroom) approaches, the most frequent treatment is prescribed medication. In a recent survey of nearly 300 ADHD children, for example, one-third were taking stimulant medication at the time of the survey and three-quarters had received a stimulant at one time or another.

Most surveys have estimated that between 2 and 3% of elementary school children are taking a stimulant. In about 40% of office visits to physicians by ADHD children, medication is prescribed.

Medicating adolescents occurs about half as often as medicating younger children. This lower incidence is the result of the physicians' reluctance to prescribe and adolescents' reluctance to take medication.

The ratio of medicated boys to medicated girls has been declining steadily, from about 8 to 1 in the early 1970s to about 5 to 1 in the late 1980s. This trend reflects an increasing awareness of ADHD's occurrence among girls.

Significant improvement occurs in about 70 to 75% of ADHD children treated with stimulants. Some treatment attempts are unsuccessful because of physician error—prescribing a medication, dosage, or time schedule poorly suited to a child's age, size, symptoms, or associated conditions—or because of purposeful deviation from the prescribed routine by the child, adolescent, or parent. Experienced physicians and those affiliated with specialized centers for treating ADHD individuals prescribe more accurately, with surveys indicating about a 90% success rate.

The search for an easy-to-identify indicator for knowing in advance whether a particular child will respond favorably to medication has been almost fruitless so far. The standard procedure is to try the medications one at a time until an effective treatment is established. Some general guidelines have emerged, but there are so many individual exceptions they cannot be rigorously applied. In general, highly anxious and highly aggressive children are less likely to show improvement from these medications than other ADHD children.

MEDICATIONS AND TOURETTE'S SYNDROME

There is great controversy about the use of stimulants with child and adult TS patients. Stimulants appear to worsen TS symptoms in one-fourth to one-half of TS individuals. In the vast majority of cases in which stimulants worsen tics, the administration of a major tranquilizer solves the problem. When stimulants are used together with the major tranquilizers, they counter some of the effects of the tranquilizers in addition to controlling the ADHD symptom cluster.

Because of the great variability from one person to another, much remains to be learned about the exact relationships among stimulant medication, tics, and TS. According to recent research, if symptoms like motor and vocal tics occur during stimulant treatment, the ADHD that occurred was probably the result of a TS gene.

The joint effectiveness of stimulants and tranquilizers points to the likelihood of two basic causes of TS through two chemical pathways. One is an undersupply of neurotransmitters, roughly equivalent to the presumed cause of most ADHD. The other is an oversupply of these same neurotransmitters in a different part of the brain. Stimulants correct the undersupply but also worsen the oversupply while tranquilizers have the reverse effect.

For an ADHD individual with Tourette's, clonidine hydrochloride (Catapres) and haloperidol (Haldol) are the two most recommended medications. Both give relief from most of the symptoms except some of the ADHD component. About one-third of TS patients improve if not treated, one-third get worse, and one-third remain unchanged. There are no generally agreed upon guidelines for the use of medications with children with TS-related ADHD who simultaneously have tic disorders.

HOW MEDICATIONS WORK

Although it is an oversimplification, the mechanisms by which these medications affect behavior relate to the manufacture of four key substances in the brain. These chemicals, called neurotransmitters, are among forty or so similar chemicals that help the nerve cells store and relay information and send out billions of messages to all parts of the body to control thought and movement. Tyrosine is an amino acid transported by the blood and concentrated within the nerve cells of the brain. It transforms into dopa, then dopamine (DOPE-uh-meen). After it migrates to the next nerve cell (at about 240 miles per hour) dopamine transforms into norepinephrine (nor-epi-NEF-rin).

When they have accomplished their purpose and assisted a nerve cell in sending its signal, dopamine and norepinephrine molecules are disassembled for reuse in the brain. During this process they release certain products, including the distinctive chemicals homovanillic acid and MHPG.

The limited research available at the present time indicates that the brain of an ADHD individual does not manufacture these four neurotransmitters in sufficient quantity, particularly dopamine and norepinephrine.

Researchers have discovered, for example, that MHPG and homovanillic acid are consistently undersupplied in the bodies of ADHD children. Serotonin, a chemical building block of the four neurotransmitters, has been found to parallel behavior in ADHD children. The lower the blood's serotonin level, the more hyperactive and symptomatic the child's behavior.

Relying heavily on a large supply of dopamine and norepinephrine, one cluster of nerve connections determines various aspects of inhibition, or self-control. The fact that ADHD children are especially weak in this aspect of their mental functioning adds further evidence in support of the neurotransmitter theory.

Brain chemistry is incredibly complex, and the exact mechanisms by which these medications work is the subject of considerable debate. They apparently increase the supply of the four key neurotransmitters. The molecules of stimulants such as methylphenidate and the amphetamines are structurally similar to naturally occurring dopamine and seem to work by specifically increasing dopamine and norepinephrine.

These medications probably produce several clusters of effects by affecting many chemical connections—called pathways—within the brain. Some, the expected clinical effects, are very desirable; others are unwanted side effects; still others are so adverse they indicate allergy or unusual sensitivity to the medication.

MEDICATION CHOICES

When dosage is correctly adjusted, Ritalin and Dexedrine (dextroamphetamine sulfate) start affecting behavior about one-half hour after ingestion and remain effective for four to five hours. Manufacturers claim sustained release forms (Ritalin SR, Dexedrine Spansule, and Cylert) of stimulants last twelve hours, but they are more predictably effective for a period of seven to eight hours.

The tricyclic antidepressants and the stimulants tend to magnify the effects of each other and can be used simultaneously. The tricyclic antidepressants smooth out the ups and downs created by the sharp wear-offs between dosages of short-acting stimulants. My experience is that the antidepressants are as effective as the stimulants and sometimes even more effective helping ADHD children become more aware of their internal body signals involved with bowel and bladder control during waking and sleeping hours. The antidepressants also help relieve depression, whether or not they successfully control other symptoms. Because they are measurable in the blood stream, blood level monitoring provides a convenient method for assisting the physician in adjusting the dosage. Antidepressants wear off more gradually and are less likely to create undesirable rebound effects. An additional advantage of antidepressants is that there are many more to choose from than there are stimulants. The physician, therefore, has more options if one particular type is ineffective. For these reasons, antidepressants are increasingly used with ADHD children, adolescents, and adults.

Neurotransmitter Building Blocks and Caffeine

There has been little research on giving the chemical building blocks of the neurotransmitters—called precursors—to ADHD children. Tyrosine, levodopa, and tryptophane have given encouraging results, however, in the few research attempts conducted so far.

Findings are controversial regarding caffeine, which was in widespread use prior to the development of

Ritalin. It seems to have an excitatory, stimulating effect on the central nervous system, and it tends to reduce the body's anxiety-relieving systems. A recent study using parents' ratings showed 600 mg per day (the amount in fifteen cans of cola or nine cups of instant coffee) brought about behavioral improvements in ADHD children. Some research indicates caffeine stimulates the production of dopamine and norepinephrine. Many studies, however, have failed to show significant gains from caffeine, and its chemical effects on the body seem to be broader than those of the customary medications for ADHD.

Though coffee is the second most widely consumed commercial beverage (behind soda pop) in North America and thus can conveniently and inconspicuously influence the central nervous system, there is little research support for caffeinated coffee as a way to assist the ADHD child. There is great variability from one cup of coffee to the next in the amount of caffeine, so the dosage is hard to control. For some ADHD individuals, however, caffeine seems to magnify the effects of stimulants, so some physicians advise an occasional cup of coffee as a supplementary measure.

Tranquilizers

The so-called minor tranquilizers, such as Valium (diazepam), Librium (chlordiazpoxide), and Vistaril (hydroxyzine pamoate) are used occasionally to control hyperactivity. Sometimes a physician prescribes a minor tranquilizer to help a young child get to sleep. Unfortunately, these medications are sometimes given in a mistaken attempt to slow down an ADHD child. If a child's apparent ADHD is actually a reflection of an imitator disorder such as temporary anxiety or emotional disturbance, however, the minor tranquilizers can produce some improvement.

Tranquilizers reduce the general activity level of ADHD children but further impair their thought processes. A minor tranquilizer given to an ADHD child who is not in a state of extreme anxiety merely worsens the ADHD symptoms and weakens the child's ability to control and organize thoughts and actions. The child becomes generally sluggish. The net result is a poorly controlled, attention disordered, impulsive child in slow motion. A hyperactive child who worsens when given a minor tranquilizer has some characteristics of the ADHD syndrome and is not hyperactive because of anxiety.

CONTRAINDICATIONS TO MEDICATION

Proper medical practice dictates extreme caution or complete avoidance of the use of these medications when certain conditions exist. You should discuss these possibilities with the physician, as there are many exceptions to these general guidelines.

Anxiety. Because these medications tend to increase nervousness and concern, those who are already overly "concerned" to the point of having an anxiety cluster of fear, nervousness, and intense anxiety can become even more anxious.

Cardiovascular Disease. Because these medications sometimes tend to increase heart rate and blood pressure, children who have cardiovascular disease should not take them.

High Blood Pressure. Children and adults who have high blood pressure or glaucoma should avoid these medications, not only because of the increase in blood pressure that sometimes accompanies them but also because these stimulants can weaken the action of blood pressure medication.

Hyperthyroidism. Primarily because of an elevated heart rate and blood pressure, persons with hyperthyroidism should avoid these stimulants and antidepressants.

Preexisting Tics. In about one-half of the children who have them, tics are made worse by these medications.

Allergy or Sensitivity. As with any potential allergic or sensitivity reaction, care should be taken to avoid giving these medicines when a child is acutely reactive in this fashion.

Pregnancy. The preborn child might be at risk for nervous system problems if exposed to these medications for extended periods.

Psychosis. These medications tend to make psychotic symptoms worse. If hallucinations—seeing or hearing things that are not present—occur, especially if the dosage is not high, the medication is probably triggering psychotic processes in a non-ADHD child. Hallucinations occurring in an ADHD child are an extreme overdosage indicator.

Medication Interactions. Medications whose action is impaired by amphetamines or whose action blocks the effects of amphetamines, such as MAO inhibitor antidepressants, Pressor agents, antihistamines, and blood pressure medications, should not be combined with tricyclic antidepressants or stimulants. Methylphenidate can interact with the pain reliever Talwin to produce an addiction.

HOW AGE AND OTHER FACTORS AFFECT MEDICATION TREATMENT

There is greater child-to-child variability before the age of six than afterward. Generally the effects of medications are less predictable in young children. Desired effects are achieved less often and side effects and slight overdosage effects occur more often than in those over the age of six. The developing brain apparently has special biochemical characteristics during its period of most rapid change—from the nine months in the womb through the first five years or so after birth. When your child loses those telltale two front teeth, the effects of medications become more predictable.

Children differ from one another internally as well as externally. Their biological systems responsible for absorbing, distributing, and using medications also differ. Predicting which side effects or clinical effects will occur is impossible prior to actually giving medication to your child. Be cautious and observant when your child starts taking any medication. The body is an extremely complicated system, and medications can create reactions along several chemical pathways simultaneously. Always consider the balance between the benefits and the risks when making decisions about biochemical treatment.

Factors a physician will consider when deciding what dosage level to use include your child's history of disease, current medical status, age, weight, severity of symptoms, and previous reactions to medication. Among the most important factors are contraindications. In general, the more severe the symptoms and the older and larger the child, the higher the required dosage.

The art in prescribing these medications is deciding which type to administer, how many times per day, the exact times, and what dosage level to create the desired effects with a minimum of side effects. Developing this skill takes considerable experience with ADHD patients and knowledge about the medications.

Because your child's social, emotional, and academic adjustment might pivot largely on your ability to obtain effective biochemical help, make sure the physician prescribes the most effective regimen. Show this chapter to the physician if there is any doubt about familiarity with this treatment approach for ADHD children. While maintaining a cordial working relationship as explained in Chapter 2, insist that an effective regimen be found. If the medication treatment is not working well, check to see that the physician is not making any of the following common errors in prescribing for ADHD:

1. Providing an insufficient dosage
2. Misdiagnosing as not ADHD because a too low dosage doesn't stop the symptoms
3. Misdiagnosing as not ADHD because behavior differs between home and school settings
4. Providing insufficient coverage for all waking hours
5. Providing medication for school hours only, leaving a lack of coverage during evenings and weekends
6. Accepting the parent's conclusion that medication doesn't work because the parent sees the child only after wear-off of effective medication from school hours
7. Providing insufficient early-morning medication
8. Not manipulating type and dosage sufficiently to eliminate troublesome side effects
9. Maintaining an arbitrary top limit of allowable dosage
10. Maintaining an arbitrary top age for medication
11. Failing to consider methods of enhancing the medication's effectiveness

12. Misinterpreting the normal slight increase in required dosage that accompanies brain growth as meaning the child has developed a tolerance that makes the medication ineffective.

ADJUSTING THE DOSAGE

Most physicians familiar with treating ADHD start the medication at a low dosage and increase it gradually until the desired effects occur; which safeguards against accidentally causing an overdosage or triggering an allergic or sensitivity response. It is important to allow three to five days at each dosage level to obtain an accurate and consistent measure of a medication's effectiveness. The medication should provide symptom control throughout all waking hours unless you and the physician prefer a different arrangement.

Desired Effects

When the dosage is properly adjusted, the desired changes occur during the medication's period of peak effectiveness—usually a four-hour period. If the effects wear off before the next dosage is given, symptoms rapidly reappear. These rebound states can be lessened or prevented by careful timing of subsequent dosages. When the dosage is at its proper level, a sudden and dramatic shift occurs in many aspects of behavior. These improvements can be summarized in seven traits—the A through G effects—beginning with the first seven letters of the alphabet.

1. Activity control. Inappropriate overactivity subsides and coordination improves in the large and

small muscle groups. Improved handwriting is, in fact, the most noticed academic feature of medication treatment at school. Verbally, the child stops chattering, making intrusive and irrelevant comments, shouting out, and interrupting.

2. Brain in gear. The child is alert, asks questions, discusses what is being taught, and expresses himself well in written compositions and sentences. Artwork becomes more creative, with a wider choice of colors and more attention to detail. The child is less impulsive, scatterbrained, and absentminded. He starts to use abstract reasoning, to understand cause-and-effect relationships, and to express ideas in a logical sequence.
3. Conscience. The child shows an improved sense of personal responsibility for mistakes or misbehavior, becomes better able to resist temptations and peer pressure, and is less attracted to mischief. The child respects boundaries and asks permission before doing things. Moral judgment improves, and the child becomes repentant and apologetic.
4. Diligence. The child becomes more earnest and serious about important matters; for example, volunteering to help, doing chores without coaxing, playing without breaking things, and working hard at school performance and grades. The child becomes concerned about neatness and tidiness.
5. Emotional control. Emotions have a normal range of expression; the child laughs and cries at appropriate moments. Irritability and impatience decrease markedly.
6. Focusing. The child pays attention to what is most important, is no longer easily distracted, and is able to follow through and complete tasks without supervision.
7. Gentleness. The child becomes generally more kind and cooperative toward adults and other children. Stubbornness decreases, and the child can be rea-

soned with, listens to alternatives, accepts guidance, and shows a genuinely caring attitude toward others reflected in politeness, generosity, forgiveness, kindness, empathy, and flexibility.

The mother of an 8-year-old ADHD boy described a typical blossoming of desired traits that indicates a correct dosage level after three weeks of medication:

> Mark's Sunday School teacher said he had been a real dream for the last two Sundays. His leaders for the evening program said they had been amazed at how he had been handling problems in their classes for the last couple of weeks. His English teacher at school said she had really started to see improvement in his behavior and work. My brother, who had not seen him for months, said he could hardly believe how good Mark had been at a recent family gathering—no arguing or shouting at the table and he sat through the whole meal without getting up. My sister-in-law saw him several days later and said she was amazed at how grown-up he had become since she last saw him two months ago. She had always had a hard time dealing with his noise and constant demanding chatter.

In the search for the correct dosage level, it is possible to encounter several different degrees of effectiveness as various dosages are tried. If there is no effect whatever from the initial low dosages, the physician is probably on the right track. As dosage increases, the desired effects are likely to start appearing. This process continues until the desired effects occur, side effects interfere, or an overdosage state occurs. There are two levels of overdosage states, one indicating a slight overdosage and the other indicating extreme overdosage.

Overdosage Conditions

If symptoms of slight overdosage occur, the physician should be consulted about reducing the dosage level or switching to a different medication. At the slight overdosage level, one or more of the following six side effects may be evident, and the condition can last up to four hours. Although some authorities include headaches, my experience has been that headaches usually indicate a more serious problem, an allergy to the medicine.

1. Narrowed mental focus. Alertness decreases and overall academic performance deteriorates to a level *lower* than when the child was not receiving medication. There is a lessening of problem-solving skills such as search strategies, flexible thinking, information processing, scanning visual patterns, and inspecting things. The child fixes attention too narrowly, resulting in decreased exploratory behavior, loss of creativity, and a tendency to repeat the same mistake on tasks that require creative solutions.
2. Loosened emotional control. The child experiences frequent and severe negative or unpleasant feelings and becomes fearful, sad, and tearful about insignificant events. Preschoolers show intense separation anxiety, clinging to parents and crying when separated from them.
3. Avoidance of contact. The child becomes withdrawn, avoids socializing with others, and acts aloof.
4. Apathy. The variety and frequency of positive or pleasant feelings decrease dramatically. The child is lethargic and apathetic and shows little surprise, curiosity, pleasure, or zeal.
5. Drugged appearance. The child appears overly docile, groggy, and drowsy; eyes are glassy, with lids half shut. The child might fall asleep for brief periods during the day.
6. Depression. Some ADHD children with family members who suffer depression may become depressed when initially treated with any of the stimulants. The combination of medication and genetic predisposition causes this side effect, which some-

times disappears without any need for lower dosage. Some depressed ADHD children can be helped with an antidepressant along with a stimulant; the former helps lift the depression while the latter helps control ADHD symptoms.

An extreme overdose reaction indicates that the body chemistry is not accommodating to the medication. This condition lasts up to four hours for the most intense symptoms, though milder symptoms can linger for many hours longer. As with a slight overdosage, the occurrence of even one of the following is a serious matter. The physician should consider switching to a different medication or discontinuing medication treatment.

1. Physical symptoms. Trembling, grimacing, spasms and twitching of facial muscles, darting movements of face muscles and limbs, or twisting of head and neck may occur. Eyes are glassy with dilated pupils. Nausea can lead to vomiting, accompanied sometimes by a severe lingering headache.
2. Psychotic symptoms. Hallucinations, severe confusion, or disorientation occur. Euphoria or elation can occur in adults.
3. Extreme hyperactivity. Indications include talking in a rambling, nonstop, incoherent fashion; frenzied movement; or inability to sit still or sleep. Twirling, rotating, and grinding of teeth sometimes accompany the constant, driven movement.
4. Extreme anxiety. Intense excitement, concern, and tension are evident. The child works furiously at a simple task, displaying extreme frustration and anger if interfered with.

Sensitivities / Allergies

During the first three months of treatment—sometimes at the very beginning of treatment—an allergy or sensitivity can be triggered by a particular medication. If allergy indicators appear or if the desired effects are weak while side effects are prominent, ask the physician to consider switching to a different medication. About 2 to 3% of ADHD individuals are considered highly allergic or sensitive to stimulants or antidepressants, resulting in headaches, hives, convulsions, or other complaints. The occurrence of these symptoms is usually not related to dosage level but to an intolerance to the medication itself. For this reason, it is wise to begin with low dosages. (See Chapter 5 for a further discussion of sensitivities and allergies.)

Tolerance

Tolerance occurs when the same dosage of medication no longer has its characteristic effects. Some ADHD children are helped with a certain dosage level for only a few weeks; then a higher dosage level is needed for a few weeks, then a higher dosage, and so forth. If an increased dosage results in a blossoming of desired effects in a series of plateaus of two- to three-week duration, the physician should try a different medication because tolerance is developing.

Though the behavior-affecting properties of a medication remain intact, tolerance of a side effect can increase after a few months.

A tolerance-like phenomenon as a child approaches adolescence is sometimes misinterpreted as being tolerance itself. Brain growth, which causes an apparent increased demand for the neurotransmitters, may require an increased total daily dosage for most ADHD children.

If an older child no longer seems to benefit from medication, check first to make sure it is being taken as prescribed. Second, consider the brain-growth phenomenon as a potential explanation.

The Taylor Medication Effectiveness Report

The Taylor Medication Effectiveness Report (TMER) can help you and the physician determine the effectiveness of medication. Designed specifically for that purpose, the form provides a simple, quick rating on the seven desired A to G effects. The medications are having their full effect when all seven effects receive an A or B. Until such a rating occurs, there is probably a need for some adjustment in the regimen. The form also lists side effects, so you and the physician can take into account all relevant factors in deciding on needed adjustments. A parallel form for use by teachers (TSMER) has a slightly different wording in the instructions and a different heading and requests information on side effects observable at school.

Another way to determine if the medication is correctly adjusted is to decide whether you would have sought professional help if your child had always behaved as he or she does on the current regimen. If the grades on the TMER are all A's and B's and the answer to the professional help question is no, the correct dosage level has been reached.

SIDE EFFECTS

Although they are considered among the least toxic, the prescription medications used for treating ADHD are associated with some side effects. Estimates of how often these side effects occur with successfully treated ADHD children range from 10 to 50%, and many occur only very rarely. Changing the dosage, type of medication,

The Taylor Medication Effectiveness Report

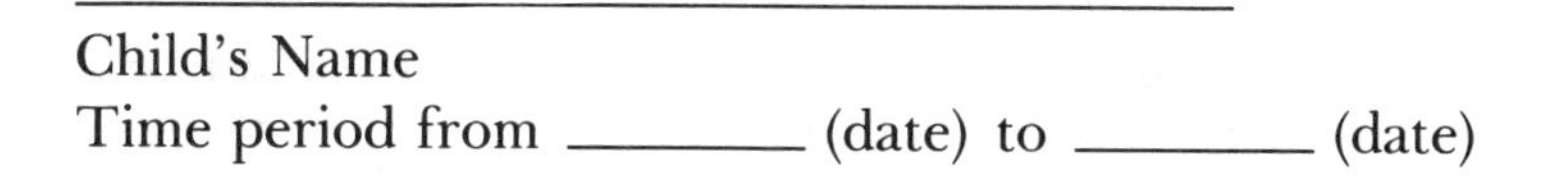
____

Child's Name
Time period from ________ (date) to ________ (date)

1. DESIRED EFFECTS

Give an up-to-date report on the effects of your child's current medication. If there is a difference from one time of day to another, give separate grades for each time of day. Supplying only one grade for each effect means the grade would be the same throughout the period during which the medication is having its effects. Use the following grades:

Grade	*Rating*	*Percentage of time trait is shown, from among all opportunities*
A	Excellent—very pleasant	80–100% of the time
B	Good—Okay, livable	60–80%
C	Fair—barely tolerable	40–60%
D	Poor—very unpleasant	20–40%
F	Failure—not tolerable	less than 20%

100%	___	80%	___	60%	___	40%	___	20%	___	0%
	A		B		C		D		F	

Grade	*Trait*
____	*Activity control:* Mouth, hands, and feet well controlled; sits for normal length of time; not fidgety or squirmy; doesn't poke, touch, and grab
____	*Brain in gear:* Asks thoughtful questions; understands and remembers clearly; not impulsive or absentminded, seems "tuned in"
____	*Conscience:* Considers moral aspects of decisions; doesn't lie, cheat, or steal; respects boundaries; asks permission before doing things; is repentant and apologetic if caught in a misdeed
____	*Diligence:* Does things without being reminded or

nagged; faces tasks and responsibilities head-on; wants to do a good and thorough job; earnest and serious-minded rather than flippant; careful rather than careless; volunteers to help; wants things to be orderly

_____ *Emotional control:* Shows patience, is not easily upset; can take frustrations in stride; doesn't have tantrums

_____ *Focusing:* Has normal attention span, pursues a goal without getting sidetracked, completes activities, is not overly distractible, doesn't flit from activity to activity

_____ *Gentleness:* Is polite, generous, courteous, kind-hearted, sentimental; doesn't demand own way or argue; is obedient and cooperative; respects authority

2. UNDESIRED EFFECTS

Indicate the occurrence levels:

0 = *Not occurring* or is so small that adapting to it requires no effort

1 = *Mild* and manageable with just a small effort that is not inconvenient

2 = *Moderate,* causing some inconvenience but still acceptable

3 = *Severe,* causing great inconvenience and cannot be allowed to continue

Rating *Effect*

_____ Groggy, overly tired

_____ Irritable, weepy shortly after taking pills

_____ Headaches

_____ Tics, jerking muscle movements

_____ Appetite decrease

_____ Stomach complaints

_____ Presleep agitation

_____ Other (describe):________________________________

____

____

3. OTHER CHANGES

Describe any other *negative* changes in behavior or performance.

____

____

____

Describe any other *positive* changes in behavior or performance.

____

____

____

4. OTHER CONCERNS OR MESSAGES

If you have any other concerns or messages, please indicate here and write them on the back of this page.

Yes ____ No ____

Signed ____

Mail to:

The Taylor School Medication Effectiveness Report

____

Child's Name

_____ ____________________________ _____

Grade Your Name Phone

Time period from _______ (date) to _______ (date)

1. DESIRED EFFECTS

Give an up-to-date report on the effects of the child's current medication. If there is a difference between mornings and afternoons, give separate grades for each half of the school day.

Supplying only one grade for each effect means that the grade would be the same throughout the entire school day.

Simply fill it out as you would a Grade Report, using the following grades:

Grade	*Rating*	*Percentage of time trait is shown, from among all opportunities*
A	Excellent—very pleasant	80–100%
B	Good—Okay, livable	60–80%
C	Fair—barely tolerable	40–60%
D	Poor—very unpleasant	20–40%
F	Failure—not tolerable	less than 20%

100% ___ 80% ___ 60% ___ 40% ___ 20% ___ 0%
A B C D F

Grade	*Trait*
____	*Activity control:* Mouth, hands, and feet well controlled; sits for normal length of time; not fidgety or squirmy; doesn't poke, touch, and grab
____	*Brain in gear:* Asks thoughtful questions; understands and remembers clearly; not absentminded; seems "tuned in"
____	*Conscience:* Considers moral aspects of decisions; doesn't lie, cheat, or steal; respects boundaries; asks permission before doing things; is repentant and apologetic if caught in a misdeed
____	*Diligence:* Does things without being reminded or nagged; faces tasks and responsibilities head-on; wants to do a good and thorough job; earnest and serious-minded rather than flippant; careful rather than careless; volunteers to help; wants things to be orderly
____	*Emotional control:* Shows patience; is not easily upset; can take frustrations in stride; doesn't have tantrums
____	*Focusing:* Has normal attention span, pursues a goal without getting sidetracked, completes activities, is not overly distractible, doesn't flit from activity to activity
____	*Gentleness:* Is polite, generous, courteous, kindhearted, sentimental; doesn't demand own way or argue; is obedient and cooperative; respects authority

2. UNDESIRED EFFECTS

Indicate the occurrence levels:

0 = *Not occurring* or is so small that adapting to it requires no effort

1 = *Mild* and manageable with just a small effort that is not inconvenient

2 = *Moderate,* causing some inconvenience but still acceptable

3 = *Severe,* causing great inconvenience and cannot be allowed to continue

Rating	*Effect*
____	Groggy, overly tired
____	Irritable, weepy shortly after taking pills
____	Headaches
____	Tics, jerking muscle movements
____	Appetite decrease
____	Stomach complaints
____	Other (describe):____________________

____

____

3. OTHER CHANGES

Describe any other *negative* changes in behavior or performance whether or not you think they might be directly related to medication.

____

____

____

Describe any other *positive* changes in behavior or performance.

____

____

____

4. OTHER CONCERNS OR MESSAGES

If you have any other concerns or messages, please indicate here and write them on the back of this page.

Yes ____ No ____

Signed ________________________________

Mail to:

or times of administration usually reduces or eliminates the side effects. When the medications are prescribed by a physician experienced with them, side effects remain unresolvable to the point of preventing or seriously impairing treatment in only about 5% of true ADHD individuals.

Three of the most common medication side effects during the first three months of treatment when the dosage level is monitored to prevent overdosage are presleep agitation, growth stunting, and decreased appetite. Weight loss, stomachaches, cardiovascular stimulation resulting in slight increase in heart rate and blood pressure, headaches (first five days *only*), nausea, weight gain, insomnia, nightmares, dizziness, dry mouth, skin rash, constipation, and hair loss also occur though very rarely and almost exclusively at high dosage levels, and should be discussed with the physician.

When side effects do occur, the following are basic alternatives available to the physician, in approximate order of increasing magnitude of change:

1. Ignore the side effects; they often decrease by themselves within the first three months.
2. Continue the medication without change and use psychological means to cope with the side effect.
3. Change the times of day and the amounts of medication taken at each time but maintain the same total daily dosage level.

4. Lower the total daily dosage level.
5. Give an additional medication to control the side effect.
6. Discontinue the medication temporarily, then reintroduce it (for imipramine rash but few other side effects).
7. Switch to a different medication.
8. Discontinue all medication if the child is very young and wait until the child is older.
9. Completely discontinue the medication.

In addition, there are numerous methods of compensating for side effects that go beyond manipulating medication. The following sections detail how to counteract the three most common side effects.

Presleep Agitation

Presleep agitation is a significant lengthening of the time spent trying to get to sleep. It involves many ADHD symptoms, usually because of a rebound effect from the wear-off of medication at bedtime. The average unmedicated ADHD child takes forty minutes to get to sleep, which is twice the time non-ADHD children take. During presleep agitation, the child takes a much longer time to fall asleep. This is one of the most common side effects of medication treatment, though its occurrence usually reflects the temporary reduction of medication within the brain. As many as one-half the ADHD children on medications report some presleep agitation, though in the majority of these cases its severity decreases as time goes on, and it does not represent a major stumbling block to treatment.

Here are suggestions for overcoming the presleep agitation (P-A) side effect.

Regular Bedtime. Create and maintain a regular schedule for bedtime and tuck-ins. Have a set routine for bedtime preparations—bathing, brushing teeth, putting on pajamas, or getting a drink. Let the clock do the enforcing, and have your bedtime companionship and services contingent on your child's accomplishing the necessary rituals by the time deadline. "It's 8:00 now" is all the reminder your child needs.

Timing of Meals and Snacks. Significant hunger can keep your child awake, particularly if there is an appetite-loss side effect and the medication wear-off period occurs shortly before bedtime. Suddenly your child feels very hungry when it is time for bed. The best solution is to honor the body signals and help your child satisfy the hunger with a wholesome snack.

Bedtime Medication. Ask the physician to allow a small amount of stimulant medication thirty minutes before bedtime or an antidepressant a few hours before bedtime.

Mental Focusing. Help your child channel thoughts by playing a tape recording of a bedtime story or music that the child enjoys. Some children prefer to read; others like to watch television or listen to the radio. The channeling of their thoughts and attention provides comforting, relaxing experience. Even though not falling asleep quickly, the child is not bothering anyone else at bedtime.

Noise Insulation. Create a constant background noise that does not vary, such as from an air conditioner, humidifier, or dehumidifier, or have your child listen to tapes or music with earphones. SOUNDSCREEN, a "white noise" machine, also blocks out all other sounds. (See Selected Readings and Resources for ordering information.)

An Active Day. Encourage your child to be vigorously active until about an hour before bedtime, so fatigue builds up. A nap during the day can worsen the P-A side effect, especially in very young children. Mild activity before sleep tends to extend and deepen sleep, while strenuous activity too near bedtime has the reverse effect.

Gentle Stimulation. It is important that your child be calm and not overly stimulated during the last thirty minutes before bedtime. A warm shower, a warm bath, or a bubble bath are helpful, as are washing and combing hair and sitting for a while in a rocking chair.

Pleasant Room. The ideal sleeping room temperature for most children is 64°–66°F. Arrange the physical aspects of the room to provide comfort, calmness, and an assurance of safety. Adjust night-light, window blinds or curtains, position of the door, and bedding in accord with your child's wishes.

Elaborate Tuck-in. Especially for the young child, an elaborate tuck-in procedure is well worth the effort and develops a calm and reassured state. Rubbing and touching affectionately, praying together, playing simple games such as writing letters or numbers on your child's back, telling a bedtime story, or playing quiz show with questions your child is capable of answering can provide rich and rewarding moments of togetherness. Bedtime tuck-in should be pleasant but brief, coming to an end at a reasonable time without frustrating you. The entire procedure shouldn't consume more than fifteen minutes. When tuck-in is over, give a good-night kiss or hug and depart quickly. Generally speaking, the more elaborate the bedtime procedures, the more completely your child's mind-set is on getting to sleep.

Adjustment of Daytime Medications. Some adjustment of the times of day during which your child takes medication or the type and dosage of medication can usually reduce the P-A side effect. The longer lasting forms of medication taken during the afternoon are less likely than the short-acting forms to cause P-A.

Day's Review. Bedtime affords an excellent opportunity to express love and talk tenderly with your child. Review the day's events with a focus on those that were pleasant and fulfilling. During this moment, express your love in a frank and honest way. This exchange at the close of the day is especially effective for a preadolescent or an adolescent.

Tough It Out. Until one or more of the other recommendations given here leads to a solution for P-A problems, work out a temporary arrangement that allows your child to avoid disturbing other family members despite the P-A side effect. Provide entertainment such as reading, coloring, writing, or watching TV, which will encourage staying in the room and being quiet.

Bright Ideas Notebook. Give your child a notebook for writing down thoughts and ideas that are contributing to wakefulness during the P-A period. Getting the ideas on paper allows your child to stop juggling them mentally and aids in preparing for sleep.

Growth Stunting

Probably because of an interaction with growth hormones, this side effect occurs in ADHD children with moderate to severe symptoms who take moderate to high dosages for several years. When the medication is discontinued for a few weeks, growth rebounds rapidly, so the net result is little or no difference in final attained height and weight as an adult. My experience is that about one-half the children on high dosage over a period of several months experience a noticeable suppression of the rate of height and weight gain for that period.

Some physicians try to compensate for this side effect by

taking the child off medication whenever possible; vacation periods provide the best opportunity. Most parents of children who discontinue medication for a two-month period during the summer report that the growth rebounds completely, and the child returns to a normal height and weight growth curve. Because this effect occurs only in some ADHD children on high dosages, I recommend close monitoring of height and weight before making any decision about medication-free periods. As in so many other circumstances with these children, the choice is between two difficult options.

The crucial question is whether your child's behavior can be tolerated if he or she is unmedicated (or undermedicated) during the summer months. Several adjustments are available. Your child can play outdoors more, attend camps, participate in athletic programs or other vigorous play activities, or even be sent to live with a relative. There is little or no requirement for intense academic pursuits, there is no need to sit still for hours as is required in school, and summer entertainments can take advantage of your child's interests to prevent boredom. If, however, self-esteem, social relationships, and family relationships suffer terribly because of the removal of medication during the summer, I would advise maintaining the momentum gained during the other nine months of the year. The child's self-concept and overall functioning are more important than height and weight.

Among those who are not given any medication-free periods and who experience the stunting effect, the average amount is less than two inches. If stunting occurs and becomes an important psychological issue, choice of hair style and footwear can compensate.

Decreased Appetite

The decreased appetite side effect varies from a slight decrease in appetite to severe nausea, with most cases involving a minor but noticeable drop in appetite during periods in which the medication is being taken. Appetite returns after wear-off of the medication and usually recovers after a few weeks. Stimulants and antidepressants tend to create this side effect in one-quarter to one-third of those taking them. Appetite decrease is less of a concern when the child is already somewhat overweight. The basic approach for countering this side effect is to allow your child to eat whenever hungry, in order to compensate for any nutritional losses.

Overly large portions may discourage your child. One method of compensating is modular feeding; provide only a small amount of food, such as half a sandwich. If your child is still hungry, offer additional food. This plan avoids food waste and irritation about fixing food only to have it rejected.

The choice of which food to offer can sometimes mean the difference between cooperation and conflict at mealtime. Avoid serving meals when your child is overly fatigued. A short nap before a meal or a readjusted mealtime might better accommodate your child's natural cycles. Exercise that gently stimulates without tiring your child before a meal can sometimes help. Offering a smaller meal or snack during the day when appetite seems to recover somewhat can also be a useful maneuver. On the other hand, the child who snacks too often is likely to lose interest and appetite at mealtime. Limit snacks prior to meals. Avoid foods with high fat content and encourage slow eating. Save liquids for after the meal, because they tend to fill up the stomach.

Mentally and physically prepare your child for the upcoming meal. Give a brief notice that the meal is about to be served so your child can complete activities and arrive at the table ready to eat. During those few moments prior to a meal, the shift of attention away from other activities encourages your child to anticipate the meal and respond to appetite or hunger.

Use your child's favorite placemat, novelty drinking

straw, personalized cup or mug, or other aspects of the table setting to encourage participation in the meal. Cutting or shaping food into interesting designs also helps. If slight nausea occurs when the medication is taken on an empty stomach, consider accompanying the tablet with some food.

Be willing to negotiate, but give your child's nutritional needs high priority. If you arrange a separate mealtime for your child, you do not have to prepare a separate meal. Simply put the child's portions of the regular meal into glassware containers and store them in the refrigerator. The meal can be conveniently reheated whenever appetite returns.

If nutrition is a concern because of severely depressed appetite, make sure that what your child is able to eat is highly nutritious. Cut down on less wholesome foods and snacks. Get your child to drink a nutritious beverage of the "instant meal" variety. Consider supplementing with a multivitamin and mineral tablet along with enough fiber to allow normal digestive processes.

Consider giving the tablet during or after rather than before meals, or switching to a different medication. Because this side effect varies from one medication and dosage level to another, of course, consult your child's physician or a dietitian if you have serious concerns.

BAD DAYS: DAILY VARIATIONS

Every child's brain chemistry varies from day to day and from situation to situation, and the effects of the medication are noticeably different also. Hyperactive children tend to be less symptomatic when they are ill, when they visit a new place such as a professional office, when they watch TV, and when they are operating a personal computer. Since the brain chemistry varies from one child to the next, the response of any two individuals to the same dosage level of the identical medication also differs.

During a bad day, your child's brain is using up the medication at an unusually high rate. Seven factors are the most likely contributors to these bad days:

1. Extreme emotional distress: a family crisis, a visit to a noncustodial parent, abuse, or other emotionally draining experiences
2. Inadequate sleep: a lack of sufficient sleep during the preceding twenty-four hours (probably the most common cause of bad days)
3. Inadequate nutrition: little or no protein intake or insufficient nutrients for day-to-day functioning
4. Extreme emotional excitement: a trip to an amusement park, a vacation, the birth of a sibling, a visit with playful cousins, or a similar event
5. Vigorous mental work: having a battery of academic tests throughout the entire school day
6. Vigorous play: a three-hour soccer or football game, for example
7. Chemical exposure: ingestion or exposure to a substance to which the child is highly reactive, especially with a sensitive-allergic ADHD child

Don't forget that your child has normal fluctuations in mood, likes and dislikes, and energy level and is just as likely as anyone else to become temporarily irritated, bored, excited, exuberant, obstinate, inquisitive, or pushy. Medication treatment won't eliminate the normal range and variability of mood, energy level, and self-control that occurs in all children.

While prescribed medication is the most commonly used form of treatment, its complicated nature tends to confuse and intimidate most parents of ADHD children initially. As you sift through the information—some of it false and some accurate—that you receive about medication treatment, you might feel somewhat overwhelmed and frustrated about the lack of consistency shown by helping professionals in their opinions about this form of treatment. Don't become sidetracked by that confusion. As the training of helping professionals becomes more consistent and as research advances our understanding of these medications, this form of treatment will become more refined.

Stay in close contact with the physician and provide consistent, detailed information on the effects you are noticing. You can make medication treatment work for your child, but like any other important project, you will need to keep monitoring and make adjustments from time to time for maximum effect and minimum complications.

Even though you may be quite pleased with the results, you face another set of challenges having to do with the attitudes of your child and others toward biochemical treatment in general and medication treatment in particular. Chapter 4 prepares you to meet those challenges head-on.

4

Sustaining Cooperation During Treatment

The information and techniques presented in Chapter 3 prepare you to deal strongly, confidently, and effectively with the issue of using prescribed medication to assist your child. This chapter details the various types of resistance you are likely to encounter, not only from your child, but from others who express their concerns to you. Many of these principles apply also to the Feingold Program, the other major biochemical method, which is discussed in Chapter 5.

CONCERNS ABOUT MEDICATION TREATMENT

On many occasions, you are going to receive raised eyebrows, frowns of disapproval, doubts, and even outright criticism regarding medication treatment. Others will be reflecting a combination of their own biases, knowledge or lack of it, emotional needs, and affection. Your child might even raise some of these issues as a way of opposing treatment during the first few weeks. Here are some common concerns you may be confronted with, and suggested responses to them.

Objections from Family and Outsiders

Medications develop craving and addiction. Physiological addiction usually occurs after the body is forced to accept an abnormally high amount of foreign chemicals. The body then adjusts by erecting chemical imbalances of its own. When the foreign substances are withdrawn, the body tries to readjust but finds the resulting state very unpleasant.

When medicating ADHD children, however, the physician prescribes a dosage that replaces a shortage of neurotransmitter chemicals, so the resulting level is more nearly normal. There is no forcing of an abnormally high amount of neurotransmitters, and therefore no basis for addiction. At proper dosage level, these medications do not addict. Headaches and a brief depressive state are the most noticeable reactions to suddenly discontinuing a high dosage level.

These medications are not hallucinogens; they do not result in overstimulation, euphoria, a chemical "high," or loss of reality contact. In fact, as this chapter details, many ADHD children gradually oppose taking the medication or simply tolerate the regimen, rather than relishing the process. When children or adolescents tamper with the dosage without their parents' and physicians' knowledge, they almost always take less medication, not more. Surely any chemically addictive component would result in quite the opposite tendency.

Even if purposely trying to become addicted to these

medications, an ADHD child or adolescent would most likely experience only the mental and physical sluggishness due to a slight overdose. This state is quite unpleasant, and hyperactive children resist reentering it once they have ever experienced it.

Medications teach irresponsibility. Taking the medication is an act of self-care and an exercise in increased personal responsibility. The effects—including increased diligence and conscience—tend to increase rather than decrease the child's sense of personal responsibility.

Though a useful assistance, a crutch cannot do the walking for a crippled person. These medications for your child assist, but do not substitute for, effort. The child must work hard to improve behavior and academic performance while taking medication. The medication strengthens their determination to adjust.

Medications are a prelude to drug abuse. Appropriately given, medication helps prevent the problems that would otherwise propel a person into the drug-abusing subculture. Hyperactive children who have taken correctly prescribed medication are less likely, not more likely, to become involved in drug abuse or violence than untreated ADHD children because their goal is to eventually discontinue the treatment. There is no evidence that formerly medicated ADHD children develop any kind of craving that bursts forth in late adolescence or adulthood.

Proper management also prevents psychological dependency. The child often notices improved behavior and enjoys life more, but the appreciation of the changes is the result of realizing the natural consequences of behavior improvements.

Medications involve mind control and zombielike states. At proper dosage level, there is no slowing down of mental processes. Properly prescribed medications strengthen independent and creative thought and help ADHD sufferers become more concerned, more serious, and more thoughtful persons than they were without the aid of medications. They do not tranquilize, sedate, subdue, or act as a chemical straitjacket.

Medications cover up the "real" child. Treated children don't suddenly lose their personalities; instead, they become better able to follow through on their decisions. Their personalities become more expressive, not more hidden. The untreated child is the incomplete child, functioning poorly because of an undersupply of chemicals needed by the nervous system. When these chemicals are contributed by the treatment program, the result is a different-behaving, different-feeling, and different-thinking person who gets along much better in all phases of life. Prior to treatment, neither the child nor anyone else had the benefit of becoming acquainted with the "real" person.

Objections from Your Child

Though you might obtain cooperation at first based simply on your leadership or disciplinary position, present a realistic expectation of results from the treatment. Be specific and concrete rather than making vague references to acting better or shaping up. Focus on the strong benefits of the treatment program. The most important aspect of winning your child over is to show the strong contrast between life before treatment and life after treatment. I call this the pre- and post-treatment contrast, or pre-post contrast. Don't make such exaggerated promises as that your child will feel or act perfectly, get straight A's, never forget anything, and hit nothing but home runs in Little League. Indicate you expect improvement rather than cure. Avoid giving the impression that medication can change something difficult into something wonderful.

The most common observations by ADHD children who are on successful biochemical treatment programs are that their schoolwork improves, they get along better with other children, they feel calmer and more in control of themselves, and they get into trouble less often; those with coordination difficulties notice improved coordination. Modify the wording to fit your child's age and circumstances:

> You'll be calm and less easily bugged or bothered by things. You'll feel more in control of yourself, as if you can stop and think and choose what you want to do, rather than saying or doing something first without thinking about it then being sorry and wishing you hadn't done it. Your memory might improve so that it would be easier for you to understand and remember what your teacher talks about. When these things happen, you should notice that I (parent) am not so aggravated at you and your brothers and sisters aren't so mad at you. Basically, life will go better for you. The medication won't control you or make you do anything; it will only help you do whatever you want and try to do.

Usually the reasons for the child's opposition have little to do with the side effects of the medication. Instead, they stem from psychological issues: denial of a need for special help, rebellion against parental control, fear about loss of "self," fear of being different, or an impression of unfairness. Your goal is to help your child surmount these issues and accept the reality of ADHD.

Denial is the most common reason for refusing to cooperate. The child staunchly maintains nothing is wrong and she can pay attention, get better grades, and stop arguing at home whenever she wants to. One response to denial is to take a survey. Keep an accurate record of all instances of symptoms during the survey period, usually two to four weeks. At the end of the survey period, confront your child with the list; if ADHD symptoms abound, your child has lost the denial line of defense and will be more willing to negotiate, at least for an experimental start of a treatment program.

Another response is to have the child do a self-rating

on the Taylor Hyperactivity Screening Checklist (see Chapter 1 and Appendix B), then compare those ratings with your and the teacher's ratings. If all three ratings are similar, then the evidence is unanimous that hyperactive behavior is occurring. If the child's ratings reflect denial, the evidence is at least two to one in favor of the existence of ADHD, which supports the need for at least an experimental treatment period.

Another reason for refusing to cooperate is part of a larger issue of power, a *rebellion* against parental control. The greater your effort to force cooperation, the more resistance your child shows. Some ADHD children are stubborn and argumentative, with a "you can't make me" attitude about biochemical treatment. To prevent this attitude from developing further, encourage opportunities for the exercise of free will and self-expression. Allow choices, such as hobbies, sports, participation in family meetings and discussions, and the development of skills and talents.

Reinforce the idea of free agency, which is your child's ability to be the ultimate determiner of behavior:

> This treatment isn't making you do anything. It allows you to control your actions better. You get the credit for these changes. You are making very wise choices about how to act now that it is easier for you to stop and think about what to say or what to do. And you are choosing to be the New Calm Matt—playing nicely with your brother, doing your homework eagerly. Thank you for being the New Calm Matt.

Hyperactive children are often concerned that they will no longer be their real selves: that biochemical treatment will change them into sedate, goody-goody individuals. The slowing of their formerly rapid and chaotic behavior is so strange that they feel a *loss of "self"* and wish for a full return to the untreated state. I have talked with ADHD children who have complaints like "I can't be me . . . Everything's too dull now . . . I'm boring . . . Nothing excites me any more."

It is important to prevent any feeling in your child of being robbed of control over self by becoming dependent on pill taking. Offer reassurance that the effect of the treatment is to provide chemicals to create a more normally functioning nervous system, and the consequent ability to stop and choose behavior rather than reacting on impulse. The treatment decreases your child's sense of drivenness and allows more time and alertness for making more reasonable choices.

If these concerns are interfering with your child's cooperativeness, find peer support. Locate another ADHD child who is on a successful treatment program and arrange an interview of the child and one or both of the child's parents. This other child might even become a new friend and form a "buddy system" for escorting your child through the treatment program.

Emphasize the benefits of treatment and point out that the feeling of loss of excitement is only a temporary illusion. Life will become exciting again, but in a new and better way involving more social, personal, and academic successes.

Indicate that the untreated "self" is neither the "real" nor the "whole" person. For illustration, ask what she would think if she ordered a hamburger but received only a bun with ketchup and a pickle slice. That item is not a "real" hamburger until it has all of its proper ingredients, including the meat. In the same way, the "real" person has all the chemicals the nervous system is supposed to have, with the aid of the treatment program.

A *fear of being different* is another reason for balking at medication treatment. The child is embarrassed and self-conscious about having to take medication. If the child's opposition is based on feeling different from other children, point out that she is already different, in a negative way. Being different in terms of being calmer and better controlled may be novel and strange, but the rewards are plentiful. When people first put on a new pair of glasses, everything looks different, yet the glasses help them see more clearly than before.

Helping your child thoroughly understand the benefits and necessity of the treatment program will lessen her worries about peer pressure. Also, strengthening your child's refusal skills will help insulate her from the effects of temptations to deviate from it.

Some ADHD children oppose medication treatment because of its supposed *unfairness.* Teach your child to accept the fact that not all things in life are fair and that everyone has burdens. Point out the strengths and advantages she has experienced in contrast with less fortunate children in other families. Many ADHD children never receive treatment and remain unhappy and unsuccessful in school, in society, and within their families. In fact, untreated hyperactive children and adolescents run a much greater risk of delinquency and substance abuse than their treated counterparts. Help your child realize that complete fairness in all aspects of life is unrealistic.

> Unfairness is a part of life, and everyone has a share of unfairnesses that accompany almost everything he does. You have a choice. You can either gripe about every unfairness every time it occurs throughout your life, or you can make the best of it and put your effort into making your situation work the best that it can. You can't eliminate the unfairnesses, but you can choose to adjust to them.

Emphasize that the assistance provided by biochemical treatment is limited and that she must provide her own efforts to accomplish genuine improvement in life at home and at school.

Use the pencil-and-paper explanation:

> Whenever you write something with a pencil, the pencil helps you do the writing but can't write all by itself. It can write only when you want to write and try to write. Your treatment acts the same way. It helps you do things, but you must decide what you want to do and try hard to do

> them. Your pills will help you focus your mind on your work at school as long as you want to and try to. If you don't want to do your homework, the pills won't grab your hand and force you to start writing out your assignments against your will!

As in any other area of self-care, the goal is gradually to increase your child's share of personal responsibility for taking the medication and using proper medicine etiquette. Gradually decrease your supervision while increasing your child's participation until a comfortable level of supervision is achieved for both of you as the medication is integrated into her daily life. You have a greater responsibility for maintaining the treatment regimen than your child, but you must determine the increasingly larger share to be given to her as time goes on.

Sometimes a hesitant ADHD child will accept the idea of an experiment with treatment. Explain that you would like cooperation for at least the six weeks necessary to adjust the dosage level and to experience positive results. At the end of the six-week period, if things have not improved, you will agree to discontinue treatment and not bring up the topic again for a year. For the very stubborn and resistant child or adolescent, this arrangement sometimes does the trick.

YOUR CHILD'S RESPONSIBILITIES

Make it clear that there are unknowns about which type and amount of medication is best, or even whether a particular medication will bring about the anticipated results. State your need for cooperation in taking the medication until you determine whether the desired changes are happening. Here are the several key responsibilities for practicing self-control after treatment has started.

Ask your child to:

- cooperate with all biochemical and psychological treatment
- not argue about taking the medication
- watch for side effects and report them to you
- hunt for the desired effects and report those to you also
- not deny the ADHD symptoms and the problems they cause
- be alert for potential troublesome moments (yellow-light situations in Chapter 6) that may result in a weakening of self-control or yielding to temptations
- find ways to prevent trouble at those moments, such as by practicing the problem-solving and anger control skills in this book
- develop and rely on strengths and pursue activities where the ADHD symptoms are irrelevant and won't represent a stumbling block
- work at rebuilding his reputation when treatments are successful
- compensate for symptom-reactive (S-R) states by suspending family contact until able to interact appropriately
- not share medications with others
- avoid discussing medication with those who don't have a need to know
- cooperate with your efforts to reduce undesirable side effects and increase desirable clinical effects.

These duties are paramount; they form the framework for all other responsibilities in your child's daily life until the treatment ends. Help your child meet these responsibilities by referring to them periodically. Try to obtain a once-and-for-all commitment from your child to cooperate with treatment.

MAINTAINING THE TREATMENT PROGRAM

After dosage is established, schedule an office visit every six months. The physician should note height, weight, blood pressure, and heart rate. Tell the physician the dosage that you have been giving and describe the desired and undesired effects. The TMER form (see Chapter 3) will help. Give updated information from the teacher, in addition to having the teacher submit a TSMER form. Discuss your child's attitude about treatment and any concerns you might have. Indicate anything you want the physician to help explain to your child.

Because the taste might be unpleasant, you need to supervise the ingestion of the first few doses. Hand the pill to your child and watch him swallow it. If you are concerned that he will try to sell the medicine, either out of choice or under pressure from other children, keep it locked and under your direct control. Medicine at school or a child-care center should, of course, be safely stored and dispensed under adult supervision.

If your child must take medication unsupervised, place the needed dosage, not the whole bottle, in a prearranged location where it will be safe from other children. Leave a reminder note if necessary. Give the child a reminder phone call at the time the medication is to be taken. Have your child take the medication, then return to the phone to tell you that she has just taken it.

When ADHD children forget to take medicine, the forgetting is usually the result of memory problems and has nothing to do with motivation or lack of desire to cooperate. Supervision and structure can prevent forgetting. If a pill is accidentally skipped, the physician may authorize you to administer it as soon as the error is noted, or prefer instead that you wait until the next regularly scheduled administration time.

Try to avoid confrontations that appear to be challenges or power struggles when you remind your child to take medication. For example, "It is time for your pill now" is preferable to "Take your pill now." The first statement addresses the flow of time, while the second is a direct confrontation that might invite rebellion. By careful wording and timing, keep your reminder impersonal. Don't let your child maintain, however, that any forgetting to take medication is your fault because you didn't give a reminder on time. If needed, provide more than one reminder—for example, a chart indicating when the pills are to be taken, a check-off sheet showing they have been taken, and a note taped to the child's door.

During times away from home, such as camp, visits to the noncustodial parent, extended travel, and overnight visits, there are three basic choices: (1) your child self-applies medication without mentioning that fact to the caregivers; (2) you advise the caregivers to supervise the taking of the medication; (3) your child goes off the treatment program while away from home. Each of these options has its advantages and drawbacks, so your decision should be based on the specific circumstance. Generally, the second method is preferred.

DEMONSTRATING THE BENEFITS OF TREATMENT

There are going to be times when your child will need to explain and perhaps defend the treatment program, struggle with temptations to skip or stop the medication, or face ridicule about the treatment. To bolster against those moments, help your child develop a deep conviction that the treatment works. Don't just let your child participate from the mouth down; involve your child's brain and explain why you want him to try medication. To the extent that you increase his familiarity with the treatment program, your child will be less intimidated by its rigors.

When you notice a particularly distinct difference between the medicated, symptom-controlled (S-C) state and the unmedicated symptom-reactive (S-R) state, use the moment for alerting your child to the benefits of the treatment program. The goal is that your child recognize every symptom-reactive state, wear-off times of medications, and the effects of the treatment in bringing about symptom-controlled times.

If an S-R state is occurring, help your child understand the effectiveness of the medication. Position yourself for close eye contact and use short sentences: "This is one of those times when you are showing the Old Wild Jeanette. You need to go to your room for a few minutes to calm down. The pill is starting to wear off."

After your child has become calm (minutes to hours later, depending on the circumstance) explain your reasons for intervening and once again draw the contrast between S-R and S-C behavior under the influence of the medication.

It is much more effective to make these contrasts when your child is mentally alert and not hyperactive. When you notice very controlled behavior, clearly compare it with S-R behavior that would have occurred without the benefit of treatment: "Usually at a time like this, you'd be unable to sit still so long, complaining that you are bored, or teasing Andrew. It seems easier for you to control how you are behaving now, and your pills are probably helping you do that."

ADHD children usually express their awareness of the pre-post contrast in terms such as these, which reflect the kinds of insights that are important for sustaining your child's continued cooperation: "The pills help me not fight with my sister . . . calm me down . . . make me behave better . . . help me pay attention at school . . . make Mom happier with me . . . help me stop being a nuisance . . . make it so I don't talk as much." The majority of ADHD children who violate their prescribed medication regimens are aware that others can tell they have not taken their medications.

To help your child monitor the effects of medications, use a tape recorder to demonstrate the difference in how your child acts during wear-off periods. The goal is that your child understand and agree with the need for medication. As far as possible, keep your child's role that of an informed partner in the treatment.

Though it may sound unusual to point out your child's behavior in terms of training in pre-post awareness, do it anyway: "You just sat down and answered all ten homework questions without stopping." "You did both of your chores right away, and I didn't even have to remind you about them." "You stayed calm and didn't lose your temper with Julie tonight, even though she acted up the way she did."

There is no need to draw the pre-post contrast each time you comment favorably on your child's changed behavior. Give compliments for a few days, then summarize them as reflecting the impact of the treatment program.

After the effective dosage level is reached, help your child make comparisons between his own and others' behavior: "Did you notice the way that child acted at the park today—yelling all the time, bothering his sister, being rude to those other children? I'm glad you're not acting like that any more since your treatment started, and I'll bet you are too!"

Of course, keep such comparisons in a light vein, never appearing critical and making sure your child understands you are not gossiping or making fun of others.

Find opportunities to portray what your child would have done prior to medication: "Before your treatment started, you would have never been able to sit still for the ninety minutes this program took tonight. I'm so glad you can do that now. You can enjoy these programs more now!"

The goal is that your child celebrate the joy of victory over the Old Wild Self, and part of the celebration is noticing the differences between the two selves. Your examples need to be specific and undeniable, because the pre-post contrast must not stay at a generalized level such as "I was bad; now I'm good." You want your child to avoid thinking in such self-condemning terms as being a bad person, or a person who might accidentally become bad again.

The social impact—changes in behavior of friends, teachers, siblings, and you—might be difficult for your child to perceive, even when quite obvious to you. You should point them out in clear, simple terms whenever they occur.

With biochemical treatment ADHD children gain better self-esteem and a new measure of success. The cycle of continuous frustration and discouragement is interrupted and replaced by a cycle of encouragement. They become aware of their increased academic efficiency and productivity and generally become more responsive to the educational process as a whole.

According to numerous research findings, after successful treatment of the ADHD child, adults improve their style of relating. Teachers become less intense and less controlling, talk slower, smile more, give more encouragement, and raise their voices less often. Parents become less directive and more likely to give affirmations and do favors for the child. These domino effects contribute to the encouragement cycle.

One parent of a 10-year-old ADHD boy summarized the first four months of medication treatment: "We are so encouraged by the changes in behavior in Jared. It is like night and day. Just knowing that the problem was ADHD and that it can be helped by medication has alleviated half the stress."

Encouragement Cycle

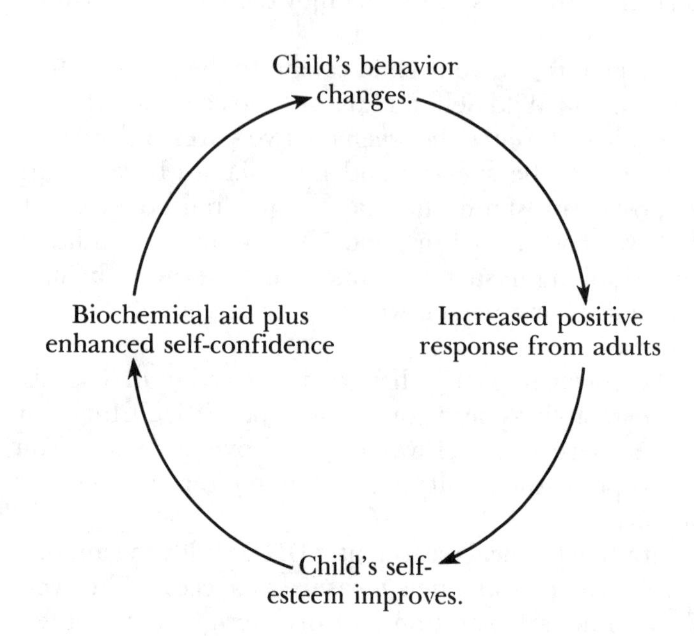

PREVENTING COMPLACENCY

Typically, when a dramatic improvement occurs because of biochemical treatment, parents describe the changes in superlatives, for example:

> This can't be real . . . I'm waiting for the other foot to drop . . . I have to pinch myself to be sure this isn't just some wonderful dream . . . this child can't be the same child of two weeks ago . . . I can't believe how different this child is . . . I wouldn't have believed this much change was ever possible . . . for the first time ever, he actually accomplished . . .

When your child becomes less demanding and less disruptive with medications, teachers tend to be less alert to learning problems that might still remain. It is doubly important to monitor carefully your child's schoolwork and academic performance. Learning problems can remain even though behavior problems have decreased with treatment.

Another response to watch for, but to prevent rather than welcome in yourself and your child, occurs after your child cooperates with the treatment regimen and symptoms are controlled. Self-confidence increases and leads to complacency and decreased diligence about following the regimen. Feeling better and starting to attend to other aspects of life, the child eases up on diligence and eventually finds excuses for skipping medication. Symptoms and difficulties suddenly increase, and your child is once again urged or forced to take the medication on a regular schedule. In this complacency cycle, your child weaves in and out of the prescribed regimen, first obeying it, then disobeying it. Prevent this cycle by urging constant diligence and by frequently monitoring and checking that your child is upholding the responsibilities for treatment. Help your child understand that the chief error occurs when things are going smoothly. Teach this self-reminder statement: "When I start to improve in my behavior, I need to be even more careful about taking my pills on schedule."

Make sure your child understands that the improvements are due to diligent adherence to the treatment program. Sometimes a complacency cycle is brought on by a parent. One ADHD child told me "When I'm acting good, Mom doesn't give me the pills so many times. She says I don't need them."

Your child should be concerned about any self-harm generated by skipping medication, but excessive wallowing in guilt won't be helpful. Build on the positive. Encourage self-forgiveness. Strengthen refusal skills and investigate how to eliminate temptation moments. Provide reminder notes and show your confidence that the deviations will decrease.

An important disciplinary tool if your child violates the treatment program is that the family should not have to experience the result—a chaotic and out-of-sorts hyperactive child. When your child starts showing disruptive symptoms at the beginning of an S-R state, your child should be sent to her room and should remain there until she attains an S-C state. This should be done calmly, not harshly. Do not try to explain the procedure to your child when she doesn't have the full benefit of the medication.

During your adjustment to successful biochemical treatment, try to be more flexible and relaxed toward the child's requests. One of the best ways to accomplish this is to get into the habit of saying, "Just a minute," or a similar statement giving you license to delay your response. Use the delay to be doubly sure you are not being too harsh and are not reacting from leftover feelings about how things were prior to the treatment program.

TERMINATION AND OFF-MEDICATION TRIALS

Sometimes physicians will want a medication-free period to test whether medication is still needed. The best time is after school has started and the child seems reasonably well managed. The off-medication trial period should last only long enough for the teacher and you to observe the presence or absence of ADHD symptoms. A variation of the off-medication trial involves making the child and teacher think the medication is still being given but instead substituting a placebo, a harmless false pill. Medication holidays, which are periods of one or two days during which the child does not take any medication, also provide an opportunity to assess the need for continuing the medication.

Some physicians prefer that the teacher not be informed until the trial period is over. Denying the teacher the place of an informed ally, however, is an unnecessarily secretive approach. Left without knowledge of the off-medication period, the teacher might conclude the sudden reappearance of ADHD symptoms indicates the medication isn't working or is toxic. My experience is that it is better to keep the teacher informed, ask for close monitoring and objective judgment of the behavior, and have the teacher submit the TSMER form weekly during the trial period.

If a good blossoming of the A through G effects appears without medication, do not restart it. If your child's adjustment seems satisfactory without medications, continue to monitor how things are going but await deterioration in behavior before resuming medications. If stopping the medication caused deterioration in behavior, restart it. If the trial resulted in no appreciable change in your child but there is not a full blossoming of the desired effects, the medication dosage was probably too low and may need to be adjusted upward. All these events need to be discussed with the physician; discontinuing or restarting the medication should not be a decision made independently by you or your child.

There should not be an arbitrary age after which medications are no longer prescribed. The only way to know for sure how long a given individual will need to take medication is through consistent and thorough monitoring. Termination should be based on a biochemical change that results in a disappearance of symptoms, so that the medication is simply no longer needed. When high dosage levels are suddenly stopped, severe rebound effects can occur, including headaches, depression, and suicidal thoughts. One of the safest ways to terminate medication is to lower the dosages by one-half for three to five days, then half again for an additional three to five days, then give no further medication. The termination period for antidepressants should be somewhat longer, preferably around two weeks. But, again, the physician should be consulted.

The most common reasons given by adolescents for terminating their medication without their physician's knowledge or consent are

1. a belief they would no longer have S-R states if medications were discontinued;
2. unpleasant, poorly controlled side effects, such as stomach complaints, appetite loss, and presleep agitation;
3. a changed perception of the self, including feeling different from peers, feeling strange and unlike the "real" self, and feeling too juvenile;
4. improperly prescribed dosages resulting in a slight overdosage reflected by an inability to maintain control, such as feeling drugged, numbed, depressed, lethargic, or spacey.

Although embarrassment is one of the most common feelings noted by hyperactive adolescents who take medications, it is not one of the chief reasons for termination. To avoid having your adolescent stop taking medication against your better judgment, show him the fallacy of these four reasons. The best way to accomplish this is to carefully and regularly monitor the medication's effects, particularly its side effects, and to have the physician periodically make fine-tuning adjustments in the dosage level.

Compensating for the many difficulties of ADHD sufferers does not stop when biochemical treatment ends. Home-based as well as professional support should be integrated into a smooth, coordinated effort to increase functioning at home, in the neighborhood, and at school. The Feingold Program is a treatment option, whether or not medication is being used. Chapter 5 explains that method so you can make an informed decision about whether or not to use prescribed medication as the only form of biochemical treatment.

5

CONTROLLING FOR SENSITIVITIES

Few issues in this controversial field have aroused more contention and disagreement among professionals and parents than the proposal that controlling chemical exposure can reduce ADHD symptoms. Developed in the early 1970s by pediatrician-allergist Benjamin Feingold, M.D., the Feingold Program identifies the chemicals to which most ADHD children are sensitized. Virtually all are low molecular weight, unstable phenol-based compounds, and many have been found to be carcinogenic. ADHD children who are very sensitive to them usually reflect other sensitivities and allergies that render them in the sensitive-allergic (ADHD-sa) subgroup.

Exact data on the number of children being helped by the Feingold Program are not available. The National Science Foundation estimated 200,000 families were using it in the early 1980s. Comparisons of the total incidence of ADHD, the proportion being treated with prescribed medication, and estimates based on communications received by the Feingold Association of the U.S.

would indicate that about one-tenth of serious attempts at biochemical treatment of ADHD in the U.S. involve this method.

Estimates of success rates by those familiar with the program range from 50 to 70% for those children receiving a correctly enforced control of exposure to the suspected chemicals. Those estimates match well with recent scientific studies of its effectiveness. The desired A through G effects, summarized in Chapter 3, are the same for this method as for prescribed medication. In fact, a recent university-sponsored study involving 170 families using the program showed wide-ranging improvements in such diverse areas as more compliant response to parental discipline, decreased truancy, and better ability to get to sleep. In addition, use of this method resulted in unintended but beneficial health-related improvements seldom seen with medication treatment, such as decreased leg and joint pain, decreased diarrhea and constipation problems, and fewer skin rashes.

HOW THE FEINGOLD PROGRAM WORKS

The theory behind this method is that the brain of an ADHD child is experiencing a chemical sensitivity reaction—not an allergy—to the offending chemicals. My conclusion, based on years of assisting ADHD children and their parents with this method, is that the chemical exposure results in a lowering of the level of neurotransmitters. As long as numerous offending molecules are available to the nerve cells, the production of neurotransmitters is impaired and ADHD symptoms occur. When the offending molecules are no longer available, the correct level of neurotransmitters is produced and ADHD symptoms disappear.

The program requires eliminating contact with chemicals commonly added to food products, cosmetics, and medicines, as well as exposure to airborne or skin-contact sources of offending chemicals for some individuals. The ADHD-sa subgroup represents the extreme of those who are sensitive to these chemicals. Available data indicate the vast majority of ADHD individuals are probably sensitive to some of these chemicals, though their reactions are not as obvious as those of the ADHD-sa subgroup.

Because the same substances that consistently create problems for the sensitive-allergic subgroup also seem to worsen the symptoms in other ADHD individuals, a review of these sensitivities provides a convenient way to understand the chemical exposure that can be limited under the Feingold Program.

THE SENSITIVE-ALLERGIC ADHD CHILD

Research into why some ADHD children do not respond favorably to prescribed medications has unearthed a subgroup who have problems absorbing medications and various nutrients through the intestinal tract. Blood studies have indicated they have difficulty absorbing the medications into the bloodstream. The inability of the medication to work its intended effects for these children apparently has more to do with abnormal digestion than with any special neurological processes. These sensitive-allergic children (ADHD-sa) are also among the most chemically sensitive. Of all the organs, the brain is the most easily disturbed by a temporary overabundance or undersupply of any of its needed chemicals. Thus, we have the most precariously balanced organ system in persons with very precarious bodies in terms of biochemical status.

An ADHD-sa child usually has the following characteristics prior to the age of two: difficulty nursing or accepting a formula, prolonged colic with poor sleep and frequent crying, little smiling, frequent spitting or vomiting, reluctance to cuddling, prolonged and frequent tantrums, excessive perspiration, and excessive drooling.

The exact mechanisms by which allergens produce distinctive and dramatic increases in hyperactivity and other ADHD symptoms are not yet fully understood. Allergic responses mobilize the body's defenses against infection, namely the immune system; skin rashes and hives are common indicators of an allergic response. Sensitivity reactions involve the body's misuse of chemicals that enter it, without triggering a response from the immune system. Current knowledge about brain biochemical processes is insufficient to clarify further the differences between sensitivities and allergies that lead to flare-ups of ADHD symptoms. For most persons, the issue is academic. Behavioral deterioration occurs with exposure; whether the cause is labeled "allergy" or "sensitivity" makes no practical difference.

Approximately one-third of the children being treated for asthma are hyperactive, according to a recent survey. There is very possibly a genetic link between asthma, ADHD, and allergies.

Milk and dairy products can produce a milk allergy syndrome in some ADHD-sa children. This syndrome includes throat clearing, clucking throat sounds, fatigue, bad breath, leg and muscle aches, nasal congestion, constipation, diarrhea, and recurrent ear infections. Milk should be considered a possible culprit if your child has many nasal symptoms, especially when an infant or toddler suspected of having ADHD has colic and is treated for otitis. Bedwetting can also reflect an allergy to milk, dust, or mold. If your child wets the bed prior to midnight, suspect an allergy.

Most people know that pollen causes hay fever and asthma, but for some ADHD children, behavior also deteriorates on exposure to certain pollens. If your child's behavior or mental clarity seems to deteriorate seasonally, consider pollen allergy as a possible contributing factor.

Some key indicators of contact with an item causing an adverse sensitivity or allergic reaction include

- *Facial symptoms:* glassy or glazed eyes, circles under eyes, wrinkles or puffiness below eyes, itchy or watery eyes, swollen eyelids, swollen or cracked lips, reddened ear lobes, sudden facial paleness, red cheek patches, itchy nose
- *Head symptoms:* nasal stuffiness, sniffling, clucking sounds, frequent throat clearing, coughing and wheezing, frequent ear infections, frequent headaches, sudden ear pain, profound ringing in ears, excessive thirst, bad breath
- *Digestive symptoms:* nausea, bloating, passing of gas, diarrhea, constipation
- *Skin and muscle symptoms:* itchy rashes (especially in arm or leg creases), frequent muscle and leg aches
- *ADHD symptoms:* irritability, belligerence, depression, silly behavior, tantrums, sleep disturbances, bedwetting, sudden mental confusion and absentmindedness, daytime bowel and bladder control problems, overactivity

An extreme and sudden shift in behavior is typical of the ADHD-sa child. Whether the offending substance enters the body by being eaten, by skin contact, or by being inhaled, an extreme and sudden shift in behavior is not unusual for the ADHD-sa child. Here is how one parent described to me her discovery that her 4-year-old child was in this subgroup:

When we first went on the Feingold Program we saw a huge change in Merri's behavior. For the first time she showed remorse for misbehavior, she helped pick up after herself, and she showed us lots of affection. After four days of discovering our "real" Merri, we discovered a whole new problem.

My husband was out shopping one evening and Merri and I were home alone. She had a sore on her upper lip and I playfully suggested an adhesive bandage that would look like a moustache. After only a minute or two our "new" child began to fall apart. She suddenly had to touch all the furniture, would not stop making mouth noises, twisted herself in the curtains, significantly stuttered, repeatedly ran into me, and would not obey. In addition, her cheeks suddenly became bright red.

That night Merri could not get to sleep for a long time and was up screaming several times with nightmares about spiders. She wet the bed for the first time since she'd been potty trained. At that point we began to realize that Merri's problems included some chemical sensitivities.

TESTING FOR FOOD ALLERGY

ADHD-sa children sometimes have intense cravings or aversions toward a food or ingredient to which they are sensitive. If ADHD symptoms flare up every time a certain product is eaten, your child is reacting to the product's ingredients or additives; reacting to something else that coincidentally accompanies the eating of the food item, including psychological factors; or experiencing a digestive disorder. You can conclude that a specific food is not contributing to ADHD symptoms if your child (1) is in a symptom-controlled state, (2) is not taking medication, (3) shows no sudden behavior deterioration after receiving a single suspect food, and (4) continues to repeat the same result at least two more times on different days.

Blood studies easily detect which ADHD-sa children are allergic to dust, mold, pollen, and some foods. However, some chemically sensitive ADHD children produce a negative test to a food that can trigger temporary hyperactivity. These children test positive to some foods that cause dramatic deterioration in their behavior, but test negative to some other foods that can also cause behavioral deterioration. Though it helps to confirm a food allergy, the typical blood test is not a 100% accurate indicator of culprit substances for the very sensitive ADHD-sa child.

Routine allergy testing is a common method to verify a dust, pollen, or mold allergy. The typical scratch or needle tests of many foods at one time are not entirely accurate. A particular allergy usually exists if the food causes a strong positive skin reaction, but an allergy still might exist in foods with a lesser reaction. A totally negative skin reaction suggests that a food allergy is not present, although either a true food sensitivity or a food allergy is still possible.

The best method is under-the-tongue testing with one potential allergen introduced at a time, under objective testing conditions such that neither the parent nor the child knows which item is being tested. By careful observation of the child during the testing procedure, relationships between the ingestion of an offending chemical (see Appendix E) and physical and behavioral deterioration become quite evident.

Most physicians who have experience with ADHD children with hay fever or asthma recommend routine allergy extract therapy, though many are not aware that such treatment has a direct effect on ADHD symptoms. If your child is sensitive to several major foods such as milk, corn, wheat, and sugar, allergy extract treatment might be helpful.

USING THE FEINGOLD PROGRAM

The first phase of the Feingold Program involves eliminating exposure to many of the chemicals commonly added to foods and beverages for cosmetic purposes. For most ADHD children and especially the sensitive-allergic ADHD child, major offenders are synthetic food dyes (petroleum- or coal tar-based); artificial flavors; flavor enhancers such as MSG; and preservatives such as BHA, BHT, and TBHQ. Salicylates, a naturally occurring group of low molecular weight phenol-based compounds that seem to interfere with neurotransmitter production, are temporarily removed during the first few weeks of the treatment program. They are found in aspirin and in almonds, apples, apricots, all berries, cherries, chili powder, cider and cider vinegar, cloves, coffee, cucumbers, currants, grapes, mint, nectarines, oranges, peaches, bell and chili peppers, pickles, plums, prunes, raisins, tangerines, tea, tomatoes, and wine.

In addition, the substances from the categories listed in Appendix E are minor offenders for the typical ADHD child but can represent serious problems for an ADHD-sa child. Contact with these substances must usually be limited somewhat, depending on the child's overall sensitivity to them, which is reflected in the severity of ADHD symptoms.

Sometimes there is difficulty accomplishing the necessary first step of controlling the ADHD symptoms and obtaining the blossoming of the A through G effects. Label reading of food products, while helpful, is not sufficient to guarantee elimination of the offending chemicals from your child's food. For maximum success, follow the procedures given in the grocery shopping guide, handbook, and other materials available from the Feingold Association (see Appendix C).

After contact with the offending chemicals is eliminated, ADHD symptoms decline or disappear. Because most hyperactive children are sensitive to only some of the salicylates, the next step involves gradually replacing the salicylate-containing food in the child's normal diet. The foods are replaced one at a time, so any sudden flare-up in symptoms can be traced to a specific food.

To assist in this process, the Taylor-Latta Diet Diary provides a method of double-checking the ups and downs of symptoms in response to the reintroduction of potentially offending salicylates. To use the diary, enter the types and amounts of food, beverages, and ingredients consumed during each time period. Then rate your child's behavior at the end of each time period. The association between particular food items and sudden behavior improvement or deterioration will be much more apparent than if you kept no such record.

MAINTAINING THE TREATMENT

My experience is that one accidental exposure can trigger a dramatic return of ADHD symptoms for a period lasting from two hours to three days. In general, the more severe the child's hyperactivity, the longer the symptom-reactive state. Children who are ADHD-sa almost always have extended S-R states.

The Feingold Program is a viable alternative to prescribed medication for the majority of ADHD individuals; it tends to work especially well with small children, whose intake of food chemicals and exposure to airborne chemicals are easy to control. Snack and convenience foods are permitted, and there is no prohibition of sweets. Alert label reading and a grocery shopping list help prevent accidental exposure to synthetic additives.

Monitoring and supervision are vital. It is necessary to make advance preparations for extended visits away from home, car travel, camping, and school lunches. The

Student	Grade	School
Rater	Class	Date

ONLY ONE (✔) IN EACH SUBCATEGORY!

1. Academic Expression

Achievement concern

- ☐ Works near capacity; is concerned with quality; enthusiastic
- ☐ Usually tries; sometimes needs reminding
- ☐ Underachieves; does slipshod work
- ☐ Ignores assignments; doesn't bring materials

Creative initiative

- ☐ Contributes ideas; brings in outside materials; is curious
- ☐ Occasionally uses new ideas or materials
- ☐ Has little imagination; doesn't question; plods
- ☐ Copies others' ideas; follows; is apathetic

Independence

- ☐ Seeks only necessary help
- ☐ Is fairly self-sufficient
- ☐ Too frequently demands help
- ☐ Needs one-on-one help; doesn't function alone

2. Academic Response

Alertness

- ☐ Pays attention; is "tuned in"
- ☐ Follows most of class work
- ☐ Daydreams; often needs prompting
- ☐ Is oblivious; often not reachable

Attendance

- ☐ Nearly always present
- ☐ Recurring legitimate absences
- ☐ Excessive unexcused absences
- ☐ Rarely in attendance

Comprehension

- ☐ Retains and applies new ideas
- ☐ Knows enough to get by
- ☐ Understands little
- ☐ Rarely or never understands

Attention span

- ☐ Sustains concentration; is organized
- ☐ Is generally attentive
- ☐ Doesn't stay with tasks; needs reminding
- ☐ Is restless; has short attention span; is disorganized

earlier discussion (Chapter 4) about gaining your child's cooperation, encouraging increasing responsibility for maintaining the treatment program, and making a strong pre-post contrast applies equally to this program.

CONCERNS ABOUT THE FEINGOLD PROGRAM

Although nobody sounds any alarms about potential addiction, side effects, mind control, or the teaching of irresponsibility, a number of criticisms have been leveled against the program. By far its most ardent opposers have been from outside the helping professions. The concerns have no more validity than those that have been leveled against medication treatment. They fall into two categories: claims that it doesn't work, and excuses for why it does.

Those who maintain a firmly anti-Feingold stance usually have the following characteristics:

- Little or no direct experience guiding or applying it
- Knowledge based on reading anti-Feingold material published by the food and food chemical industries
- Knowledge based on reading summaries of research heavily slanted toward the food industry
- No familiarity with the studies in Appendix D or other studies substantiating the method.
- An advocate of one or more of the criticisms listed below

Claims That It Doesn't Work

The Feingold Program is simply another health food fad that necessitates shopping at exotic locations to unearth unusual food items and that denies the child the pleasures of "ordinary" convenience food. This criticism is that these chemicals must be safe for everyone, including ADHD individuals, because the Food and Drug Administration scrutinizes the safety of additives and "certifies" the petroleum-based dyes in food and beverages.

Whereas about 80% of the food products in the average supermarket contain synthetic chemical additives, the primary limitation on food purchases has to do with brand choice rather than the type of food. When you shop for mayonnaise, you don't buy one jar of each of five different brands; instead, you buy just one brand. The grocery shopping guide available from the Feingold Association lists products by brand name that don't contain the offending chemicals and can be purchased in ordinary markets.

The Feingold Program creates resentment and division in the family. Another claim is that the method involves wholesale disruption in routines and burdensome, expensive, and elaborate changes in shopping, food preparation, and meal habits. The result is that the other family members resent the ADHD child, who then will assuredly become worse, not better, as a result.

The changes in food-related routines needn't be elaborate or burdensome. In fact, shopping is simplified. The parent knows what to purchase, has a shopping list, and goes straight to the desired food items. The food expenses decrease rather than increase, because there is no susceptibility to impulse buying of overpriced and overprocessed items, empty-calorie snacks, or gimmicky sales tactics by the grocer. When used in place of medication, there are no expenses for drugs or physician visits.

Scientific studies have proved the Feingold Program ineffective. This is by far the most damaging criticism launched by the anti-Feingold groups, which consistently and frequently aim their attacks at physicians, mental health professionals, and educators. The food and food chemical industries are intimidated and frightened by the Feingold Program's success at curbing ADHD symptoms. They actually perceive the Feingold Program as the forerunner of a movement that would have every parent blame Crispy Crunchy Yummies eaten for breakfast as the cause for every school problem, temper tantrum, and refusal to do chores. The food industry wants those Crispy Crunchy Yummies to stay crispy, crunchy, bursting with flavor, and brightly colored during storage, shipment, and shelf life. They want the synthetic chemical additives left in, and they want no connection drawn between those additives and children's problems.

With promotion from their public relations organizations (the Nutrition Foundation and the American Council on Science and Health) they have sponsored and publicized a series of investigations of the wolves-guarding-the-sheep variety. These studies had many of the superficial appearances of scientific objectivity, including a double-blind format, the accepted procedure for assuring impartial results. These "experiments" always used one small part of the Feingold Program, misapplied it, then drew the conclusion that the results "proved" the Feingold Program invalid. Often a "modified Feingold" approach was used in which ADHD children continued to receive artificial flavorings and preservatives while being "tested" for the effects of artificial colors. Of course, the children usually remained symptomatic.

Despite this thinly disguised effort to discredit the method, symptom control in many children improved. Unable to hide that aspect of the findings, the researchers almost invariably excused those changes as the result of increased attention or the power of suggestion. Articles describing these studies have appeared in journals read by the members of the relevant helping professions, and a book has been published by one of the chief perpetrators of this line of "research," ostensibly to settle the matter by summarizing the findings and reiterating the conclusions the food industry wanted.

In the early 1980s, the National Institutes of Health held a conference on defined diets and childhood hyperactivity. One of the conclusions from this panel of experts was that "controlled challenge studies have primarily involved the administration of food dyes to children, but have not included other food flavors or preservatives that are allegedly implicated in the causation of hyperactivity. Therefore, these controlled challenge studies do not appear to have addressed adequately the role of diet in hyperactivity." With this gentle and understated slap on the wrist, the Concensus Development Conference acknowledged the transparent motives and structure behind this line of research.

As incredible as it may seem, few research investigations have compared a group of hyperactive children using the Feingold Program with a group not using it or with themselves when they were not using it. In the late 1980s a startling study compared the behavior ratings of a group of hyperactive boys during a period of stringent control of chemical exposure as contrasted with a period of no such control. An article describing this research, which was done under the auspices of the University of Calgary/Alberta Children's Hospital and is the most scientific investigation ever done on the effects of food additives on hyperactive children, appeared in the journal *Pediatrics* (see Appendix D). Although not an exact test of the full Feingold Program, this carefully researched project showed improvement in 58% of treated children, without including the elimination of salicylates. It was engineered to rule out such things as power of suggestion and extra attention for the children during the dietary changes. If salicylates had been included, the results would, in my opinion, have been even more conclusive.

A number of other studies have reported favorable findings, including a study in the British medical journal *Lancet,* which found that 79% of a large group of ADHD children (ages 2 to 15) experienced marked symptoms when exposed to food coloring and preservatives (see Appendix D). In general, the more scientific the research study, the more the results reflect a relationship between chemical exposure and ADHD symptoms.

The Feingold Program involves an imbalanced diet. This criticism centers around the temporary elimination of some salicylate-containing fruits that are also sources of vitamin C. The salicylate fruits are customarily reintroduced and seldom are entirely eliminated.

Fruits that can be eaten include avocado, banana, breadfruit, cantaloupe, casaba and other muskmelons, coconut, date, fig, grapefruit, guava, honeydew melon, kiwi, kumquat, lemon, lime, loquat, mango, papaya, pear, persimmon, pineapple, and watermelon.

There is no imbalance and certainly no shortage of vitamin C in this program, and parents are urged to use the four basic food groups.

Excuses Why It Does Work

The Feingold Program works by the power of suggestion. In an attempt to account for the success of the program in controlling ADHD symptoms, some have concluded that because the parents expect it to work, the child conforms to their expectations.

From what source do the thousands of parents successfully using this method obtain their expectation of success? Physicians, teachers, mental health professionals, nurses, dietitians, or other helping professionals superficially acquainted with the program are likely to have been influenced by the massive efforts of the food and additive manufacturers. Unless they ask for impressions of others who happen to be successfully using the program, parents are likely to receive neutral or negative reactions, not positive ones.

Most parents have tried discipline techniques, behavior modification programs, counseling, special education, or other methods before attempting the Feingold Program. Parents have already "expected" more stringent discipline to stop the child's problems. Then they "expected" academic alterations to do the trick. If expectation causes a reversal of ADHD symptoms, there would be no need to go beyond whatever the parents tried earlier. Many times the Feingold Program is a last resort, and often the parents have the opposite expectation—that it will be one more failure.

Many parents have used this method successfully for many years—far too long for a suggestion or placebo effect to be operative. Many preschoolers are unaware of any change in their eating habits so have no basis for perceiving any new expectations from parents.

The Feingold Program works by giving the child extra attention since the Feingold Program involves food-related changes, and the child gets a sense of being the center of it all. The result is that the child conforms and stops all ADHD symptoms because of the naturally rewarding qualities of receiving attention from adults.

If getting attention were the cure for ADHD, most hyperactive children would be cured by the time they reach first grade. Anyone familiar with these children knows that they already are claiming more attention than most other children. When they are successfully treated, they receive less attention, not more. Interestingly, we don't hear claims that this method works by decreasing the amount of attention shown to ADHD children, yet that is exactly what happens.

When children accidentally contact an offending chemical and experience a rapid display of symptoms, there is often no adult around to increase or decrease attention. When the opposite situation occurs and ADHD symptoms are well controlled, the children usually prefer to go about their lives more independently. They work harder on homework and chores and they play harder. There is no clinging or demand for more attention.

The Feingold Program works because of increased order and structure in the home. Just a fraction more plausible than some of the other concerns, this one acknowledges there is less chaos in the kitchen and more order around meal-times in Feingold households. Order in the environment is a well-known aid in controlling ADHD symptoms.

When a child has an infraction and a sudden flare-up of symptoms occurs, changes in the level of orderliness of family processes don't necessarily precede or accompany the S-R state. Contact with an offending substance brings quick and dramatic deterioration in behavior, whether or not mealtime, food preparation, or other family routines were orderly at that moment. Children on the Feingold Program also have good symptom control in poorly structured and constantly changing situations, such as extended travel. For many children, there is no change in household order at all, merely in the brands of food purchased.

The Feingold Program works because it eliminates sugar. The contention is that success is due to the elimination of empty calorie foods and sugar, not because of any effect of the stated chemicals on the central nervous system.

Much to the surprise of critics and new Feingold parents, the grocery shopping guide has sections for candy, baked goods, cookies, crackers, chips, and other snacks. Of course, good, balanced nutrition is encouraged. But a child on the Feingold Program also needs to feel as minimally different as possible from other children. Fun foods are an important part of life, and although sweets are not particularly advocated, they certainly aren't eliminated. Because only about one in ten hyperactive children is especially reactive to sugar, specifically prohibiting it would probably help only a small fraction of the children using the program.

Advantages and Disadvantages

My experience has been that the Feingold Program reduces the amount of, or entirely eliminates the need for, medication. It works for all age levels, including babies.

This aspect is especially important because antidepressants and stimulants are much less effective with children below the age of five than they are with older children. For the very young child, the Feingold Program may be the most practical choice. It involves no deviation from a standard wholesome and balanced food selection, keeps parents alert to good nutrition, and teaches the child good self-care habits. There is no worry about side effects or the unknowns that accompany the use of medication. A commonly reported observation from parents is that if they also follow the program, their own allergy- and sensitivity-related problems decrease. This finding is particularly striking because most parents don't expect or look for such changes, but find to their surprise that they do occur. Such things as skin rashes and frequent headaches are consistently reported as decreasing or disappearing in family members who eat the same food brands as the ADHD child.

One accidental exposure to an offending chemical can trigger an S-R state within minutes. Two or three such contacts per week can keep some ADHD children in a constant S-R state. Monitoring the child is important, as is winning the child's cooperation for self-monitoring when you are not available to supervise. The fact that minor alterations of chemical exposure through additives in food can switch the ADHD symptoms on and off is reassuring and proves the accuracy of this approach. The challenge is to inoffensively provide the needed structure. A thorough winning over of the child to a commitment to self-care is increasingly important as the child grows older.

If the parents are following the program stringently and ADHD symptoms are still occurring, there is a strong likelihood the child is in the ADHD-sa subgroup and is still frequently contacting substances to which she is allergic. The search for allergens must then overlap the effort to avoid chemical exposure.

Identifying environmental irritants can become an exercise for a detective. Suddenly the child has ADHD symptoms, and the parent must retrace the child's activities during the preceding hour or so to uncover the source of exposure. The situations that can occur are illustrated in this typical example, reported by the mother of a 2-year-old ADHD-sa boy on the Feingold Program.

> A guest used Brian's bed for a rest. She remembered afterward that she had hair spray on, and I said I'd change the pillowcase but forgot all about it. That night, Brian had trouble falling asleep and woke several times saying, "I'm sick; I'm sick." Then I remembered the hair spray. I changed the pillowcase and he slept soundly the remainder of the night.

Cooperation from the entire family is important. Though some of the child's food items might need to be different from what the rest of the family is eating, there is usually opportunity for considerable overlap so that the child does not feel isolated or uncomfortably different. It helps if the entire family can make some switch in food brand choices. Rebellious adolescents are poor choices as candidates for this program, because they too often and too easily allow chemical exposure when not supervised.

I have found that some parents, particularly those near emotional bankruptcy (described in Chapter 8), simply do not have the necessary energy to provide the occasional home cooking and relatively constant dietary supervision needed. The elimination of salicylates, even when simplified and streamlined by using the Diet Diary, represents too large a project for some distraught parents of ADHD children. The replacement foods are introduced during symptom-controlled times, and the repeated flare-up of symptoms that accompanies the testing of substitute foods is too stressful an accommodation. For these parents, the rapid resolution of symptoms that can occur with medication is preferable to the two- to three-month trial period of testing foods for their effect on the ADHD symptoms. An alternative is to start the child on medications, then slowly switch to food brands without the indicated chemical additives and gradually integrate them into the family's menus. The medication gives the family and the child quick relief from ADHD symptoms, and the resulting boost renews the parents' energy for beginning a more stringent observance of the Feingold Program.

Using the Feingold Program tends to decrease the amount of medication needed, or to eliminate the need for medication entirely. It is impossible, however, to assess for specific sensitivity to individual chemicals while the child is successfully being treated with medication. The determination of which salicylates to avoid must be accomplished during medication-free periods.

PREVENTING CHEMICAL EXPOSURE WHEN OTHERS ARE IN CHARGE

Some attention needs to be given to persons outside the family who may mistakenly offer off-limit food brands to the child. Explain the program to the child's friends and playmates, caregivers, relatives, or others who are in charge.

Some adults are not able to respond maturely to your child's situation and, in an attempt to show kindness, might encourage your child to eat food containing chemicals that will bring on an S-R state. It is common for grandparents or other compassionate caregivers to be indulgent. This tendency is more likely to occur if the off-limit items are commonly regarded as healthful, as when the caregiver exclaims: "How can milk or an apple possibly hurt a child?"

Some adults might express doubts about the diagnosis or the need for the Feingold Program, might disagree with some aspects of how you are administering the program, or might simply lack sufficient knowledge. Parents using this method frequently discover that symptoms flare up because caregivers did not know that an ingredient in a juice or treat would cause an S-R state.

To prevent these difficulties when your child must be temporarily under the care of other adults, be clear and firm in stating the importance of following the exact guidelines. People usually respect firmness, a positive attitude, and determination cushioned with courtesy. Explain that the program involves certain absolute standards, including prohibition of certain chemical exposures in any quantity.

Give easy-to-follow guidelines. Lists of acceptable foods and beverages are better than lists of restricted items.

PREVENTING CHEMICAL EXPOSURE WHEN TRAVELING

For extended travel, keep at least two days' supply of approved foods, with an emergency snack always available. Use the snack whenever the eating schedule is disrupted or unexpected events interfere with meals. This simple precaution prevents embarrassment and spares everyone from a hungry, hyperactive, and out-of-sorts child.

Restaurant dining can be tricky. The Feingold Association provides information about food ingredients in addition to a description of which approved items are on the menus of major fast-food restaurants. One way to select the best restaurants is by advance planning through local support groups and Feingold Association representatives in the geographic area of your travels.

Cafeteria-style restaurants have the advantage of allowing inspection of each item prior to its purchase. Menu items that are closest to their natural state have the most predictable content and least likelihood of chemical additives. To maintain the best control, choose simple, individual dishes instead of casseroles, meat loaves, chef salads, creamed foods, sauces, gravies, condiments, and food with coatings. Fried food often contains additional additives or ingredients. Whole cuts of meat are usually better than chopped or ground meat, which may contain fillers or breadings. A bit of fresh lemon juice squeezed on salads avoids all questions about ingredients in the salad dressing. It is best to order a plain food item, using acceptable condiments and other foods from your own supply to round out the meal.

Obtaining efficient and understanding service is an important part of restaurant dining. Ask about ingredients used or methods of preparation of specific menu items if you need more information. Restaurant personnel are likely to cooperate if you don't put them on the defensive. Show by your attitude, statements, and actions that you intend to patronize the restaurant, plan to enjoy the meal, and assume the meal suits your family's needs. Make it clear, however, that you must double-check certain aspects of the menu because of important medical considerations.

State that your child is considering a certain item but you need information about its ingredients before you can place your order. If you need to give a brief explanation, use discretion and don't let the necessity for scrutiny become a spectacle. Use a statement such as "My child has some allergies and can't eat food that contains certain chemicals." Then follow up with the request, "Can you please tell me whether this item happens to have . . . in it?"

ENLISTING A TOTAL EFFORT

A child's involvement in the Feingold Program, like any other project, goes more smoothly when the parent-child relationship is solid and the child perceives the program as desirable. You will need to teach your child some refusal skills for moments when off-limit food with chemicals in it is offered. A suitable standard statement that works for most ADHD children on the Feingold Program is "Thanks, but I'm not allowed to have that type of food. Do you have any . . . [permitted chemical-free item]?"

Avoiding chemical exposure involves more than label reading at the supermarket. If a product lists "spices, seasoning, or flavoring," for example, the substances could include salicylates. "Natural flavorings" can mean pits and leaves of salicylate fruits as well as MSG. Some foods labeled "artificial colors" are acceptable when the source of color is annatto or turmeric, but unacceptable if synthetic dyes. Many substances used in food processing remain in the product but are not listed on the label.

Many parents briefly attempt the program but give up when no noticeable behavior changes seem to occur within a week or so. They usually have tried to prevent chemical exposure merely by label reading and have overlooked nonfood chemical exposures or have experienced allergies that create confusion because the allergen is on the "approved" Feingold list. It is imperative to obtain the Feingold Association's reference materials, including the shopping guide and newsletter giving updated food chemical information. These materials are crucial in assisting you with limiting your child's chemical exposure, training your child to self-monitor to avoid such exposure, and adapting to away-from-home situations.

Just as with prescribed medication, there are those who will judge you negatively for choosing this method. You may need to fend off the remarks of some helping professionals who are unfamiliar with its validity or biased as a result of the well-orchestrated maneuvers of the food manufacturing and food chemical industries. The summaries of the dietary studies appear in Appendix D for that purpose.

As with any other aspect of helping your hyperactive child, the keys to success with the Feingold Program are arrangements that prevent problems from occurring and supervision along the way. Parents experienced with the program generally find it reasonable, powerful, and practical; they don't complain of difficulties shopping, and they typically persist in preferring it to medication.

Whether you choose the Feingold Program or prescribed medication, there are limitations and drawbacks as well as benefits. Only you can weigh those factors to determine the best option for your child. The following chapters detail the major facets of a total support program to assist your hyperactive child and your family. These efforts should continue to be applied even if medication treatment or the Feingold Program has been terminated.

6

UPLIFTING SELF-ESTEEM

One of the most common concerns I have heard parents express is that their ADHD child's self-esteem is not only low, but "horrible . . . dragging on the floor behind him . . . abominable . . . as if he is an absolute nothing . . . as if she can't do anything right . . . nonexistent." This tragic loss of the most basic sense of self-worth results from the child's sense of being driven, confused, victimized, rejected, uncontrolled, angry at others, and angry at self. You can help your child overcome these feelings of low self-worth and then nurture self-esteem by offering encouragement, developing time management skills, and teaching how to learn from mistakes.

OVERCOMING ADHD TRAITS

Being Driven

The most common wish of ADHD children is that they stop misbehaving. They want to do better. I have asked this question of hundreds of hyperactive children: "If you had a magic wand and could wave it and change something about yourself, what would you change to make life go better for you?" The most common answers all have the same general theme—to stop misbehaving: "I'd wish for being able to stop acting up . . . not be so bad . . . stop bugging my sister . . . control my temper better . . . stop making Mom and Dad mad at me . . . stop getting into trouble."

Stuttering is a useful analogy for ADHD symptoms. The stutterer is familiar with the language, knows the disadvantages and difficulties that result from stuttering, wants to correct the problem, and tries not to stutter. Nobody accuses a stuttering child of not knowing or caring about others' inconvenience when the stuttering occurs. Despite the child's best efforts to prevent it, the stuttering continues. The difficulty is the control of self-expression—not a lack of knowledge or caring. Similarly, the ADHD child has difficulty controlling self-expression even though aware of the problems that keep happening because of hyperactivity.

ADHD children's drivenness makes them appear senseless, excessive, automatic, and intrusive. They have a genuine fear of being out of control and feel helpless to prevent their impulsive acts, even though they know better than to commit them. Sometimes they think of themselves as being two people—a calm self and a wild self. I often use this awareness in therapy as part of self-control training after medication treatment or the Feingold Program. It becomes the starting point for rebuilding a sense of control over drivenness. The child can, often for the first time ever, actually choose whether to act like the Old Wild Self or the New Calm Self.

For many people, trying harder means working faster on a task. For the hyperactive child, however, the best way to improve performance is to slow down and think about each step. Tell your child: "When you want to try hard at something, that means slow down so you are sure to do it correctly."

Two general-purpose, self-reminding statements for decreasing drivenness and helping ADHD children feel more in control of themselves are "Stop and think: what do I need to do next?" and "Sit on my hands and think."

ADHD children tend to make two errors when facing problem situations. The first is to make the decision too rapidly without stopping to consider how to recognize an effective solution. Though they have the necessary information to solve a problem, their impulsivity gets in the way. They react so quickly the result is more like a series of chance guesses than reasoned judgment. This error represents the drivenness aspect of self. The second is to become sidetracked by unimportant aspects and neglect the major factors needed for an effective solution. You can prevent both errors by teaching your child the four-step procedure given here. The goal is to get your child to react more slowly and less intensely. Slowing down the action-decision process long enough to consider alternatives is the key element in this type of impulse control.

As a general guide for all decision making and problem solving, teach your child to break down tasks into these simple steps:

1. Understand the task. Examine the problem, determine what needs to be done, and break the task into parts.
2. Generate possible approaches. Be creative and search for various possibilities. Use similar experiences with other problems as a starting point. This step involves noncritical consideration of alternatives. When your child generates an idea you think would not be helpful, don't argue or criticize the solution. Say "That is one thing you could do; what are some other ideas that might also work?"
3. Try one of the approaches. Use critical judgment to filter the possible approaches. Decide which of the

various strategies would probably be the best to try. Use cause-and-effect thinking: "If this happens . . . then that will result."

4. Monitor progress. Put the plan into action as an experiment. Devise a timetable of expected results. Decide what to hunt for as indicators of progress. Evaluate results at the end of the time period. Modify the approach until the situation has been resolved or the goal accomplished.

Any self-reminding statement should be general rather than specific, so your child will not have trouble deciding whether or not to apply it. Don't expect self-reminding statements to be as powerful an assistance as biochemical treatment. The best improvement occurs when both methods are used simultaneously. Don't rely on elaborate discussion, abstract thought, or analysis of each situation on its own merits. Challenge your child to apply the two general-purpose, self-reminding statements in various settings and to use experience from one situation as a basis for choosing how to act in another.

Being Confused

ADHD children and adolescents vary greatly in their degree of insight and awareness into how they act, how well they are doing in school, and why they act as they do. I have often experienced a marked contrast between their ratings by parents on the Taylor Hyperactivity Screening Checklist (THSC) and their own self-ratings. Occasionally, I have had ADHD children rate themselves as extremely nonhyperactive, when teachers' and parents' ratings were quite the opposite and the child's history and interview behavior clearly confirmed severe hyperactivity. This contrast is an interesting measure of the degree to which the child feels confused and unaware about what is happening from day to day at home and at school.

To help the child understand his behavior, two ingredients are needed. First, the child must have convincing and undeniable feedback that problem behaviors are occurring at home or at school. Second, an explanation of ADHD must be given in a way the child can understand and accept, at least to the point of partially agreeing that it applies.

The best way to accomplish the first step is to point out instances of symptomatic misbehavior or performance problems when they occur, as explained in Chapter 3. The best way to accomplish the second step is to help your child recognize her ADHD syndrome. Without such an awareness, your child is left with bizarre and terrifying explanations: she is crazy, mentally retarded, sick, a "bad" person, or possessed by the devil, as well as a giant disappointment to you. Help your child understand the connection between hyperactive behavior and negative responses from other children and supervising adults.

Insist on explaining the diagnosis and its biochemical causes to your child. Refer to the fact that everybody has special challenges, and your child's particular symptoms represent her cluster of challenges. Acquaint your child with the correct words: *attention deficit* and *hyperactivity*. There is nothing wrong with using proper terms to describe the symptoms. The danger of labeling comes from its abuse, as when others use it for name calling or teasing.

Your child's awareness of her unique difficulties as well as strengths helps with self-understanding and self-acceptance. One of the most persuasive ways to explain ADHD is to have your child rate herself on the THSC. Then give this explanation, modifying the wording to fit your child's age and circumstance: "You know your body makes its own liquids—tears, blood, and saliva, for example. Your body isn't making enough of certain liquids (chemicals). Because of that, you . . . [give examples of ADHD symptoms your child agreed to from the THSC]."

Refer to the fact that most other children's natural tendency is to act like Column A on the THSC, whereas her natural tendency is to act like Columns B and C. Explain the reason for this difference as the presence of ADHD symptoms.

If your child wants to know the location of the liquids, acknowledge that they are in the brain. Refer to ADHD as a uniqueness or a disorder rather than a disease. Explain that problems with brain chemicals do not mean mental retardation, mental illness, or infection or germs in the brain. Give only as much information as your child seems ready to accept.

Being Victimized

Untreated children and adolescents believe much of what happens to them is unfair, in part because they do not perceive or understand their own contribution to the social difficulties that engulf them. Because they perceive themselves as unable to control their behavior, they consider it unfair when others react negatively toward them. They think others are out to get them, dislike them personally, or are picking on them. ADHD children often learn to assume the role of a victim.

Whether or not child abuse has occurred (see discussion in Chapter 8), the hyperactive child develops problems with self-control and social relationships to the extent that he assumes a victim's perspective. This factor greatly increases the likelihood for delinquency as an adolescent and criminality as an adult. It is imperative to obtain skilled mental health counseling if your child appears to have developed this outlook, and the sooner the better.

To the extent your child is unaware of the presence of ADHD and its contribution to her problematic behavior, the feeling of being attacked and abused by others will be more prominent. Your child is likely to interpret others' negative reactions as malicious, unfounded, and cruel, even though those reactions are in direct response to hyperactive behavior. She often feels in trouble, picked on, and blamed for things. The attacks are perceived as coming from everyone: siblings, friends, teachers, parents, other family members, school principal or counselor, and people in the community.

If the child doesn't understand the validity of the criticisms, he simply becomes bent on revenge for what he perceives as an unfair attack. When correctly accused of stealing, for example, the hyperactive child often is more concerned about getting revenge on the tattler than about the moral issues.

The key to overcoming these negative feelings is to recognize and accept the existence of ADHD. When the impulsive poor decisions and feelings of being victimized decrease, so will the negative responses from others. Only then can he deal with the criticism realistically and experience personal growth. As clearly as you can, describe the domino effects of your child's actions on others, so he can begin to perceive the relatedness of others' negative responses to his own actions.

Being Rejected

A hyperactive child sometimes lacks a clear sense of the passage of time. For example, he may be unaware of the amount of time you have just spent with him. When you announce you must turn to something else, the child feels neglected and abandoned. The sense of rejection may be the same as it would have been had you not spent any time with him at all.

Your child might conclude that you and others are purposely not paying attention to him. Even though he is bossy, impatient, or critical, he does not perceive the relationship between the hyperactive behavior and being left to play alone. Your child might eventually feel quite unwanted, unloved, or hated. A common reaction is to reject most other children and claim exclusive friendship rights on one or two other children. Sometimes hyperactive children even run away from home as a testimony to their intense feelings of isolation and displacement from the social arena.

Whenever a genuine rejection occurs, determine the cause and be realistic in judging your child's contribution. Teach your child exactly what to do in a situation where there is a risk of rejection. Rehearse proper behavior to prepare your child for the possibility of rejection and encourage broadening social contacts and experiences. Additional suggestions and detailed instructions appear in Chapter 7 for helping improve social awareness and friendship skills.

Being Uncontrolled

Faced with a constant stream of negative reactions from others, your child might take the path of least resistance and decide those who criticize are correct. The result is the adoption of a troublemaker or brat role in the classroom, family, and play group. Prevented from being the best, your child may elect to become the best worst in the group. This role is hard to stop once it has started.

Numbed by the constant negative responses from others, your child may adopt an "I don't care what you think" attitude. As time goes on, he may convince himself that he truly does not care what others think about how he acts. When he stops caring about others' feelings, he loses an important motivation for remaining socialized.

When competition is carried to an extreme, children tend to become opposites or to be in vivid contrast to each other. Motivated by an intense underlying rivalry toward the hyperactive child, and seeing an opportunity to exploit the inappropriateness of the hyperactive child's behavior, other children can go to great lengths to appear very obedient, cooperative, and innocent. At the same time, they try to make sure parents and other adults see the marked contrast between their seemingly angelic traits and the uncontrolled behavior of the hyperactive child.

The angel is very much concerned with maintaining her image and an equally one-sided image of devilishness for the hyperactive child. Whenever your hyperactive child is in a weak or vulnerable position, the angel may be quick to point out that she does not do the same kinds of things. The more determined angel may goad, urge, dare, or trick the hyperactive child into misbehaving, then quickly tattle. The angel's ultimate goal is to gain special status with parents and to prove herself better than the troublemaker. The angel's manipulations are attention-getting misbehavior, which is every bit as destructive and inappropriate as the misbehavior of the supposedly devilish hyperactive child.

The angel-brat syndrome can eventually result in your child's becoming the black sheep of the family, classroom, or neighborhood. The hyperactive child can become a scapegoat, the dumping ground for all of the group's or family's stresses, and the whipping boy for frustrated adults.

Sometimes your child may be afraid to stop being a brat. She may fear others will expect her to continue good behavior. At the same time, she may be afraid of losing control. She purposely misbehaves to make sure others do not begin to expect her to maintain good behavior for an extended length of time. A hyperactive child can be as terror-stricken at having to meet others' expectations as a normally well-behaved child would if she were expected to misbehave.

Where there's a brat, there's usually an angel nearby. Be aware of the total situation whenever your child seems to be receiving a negative reaction from other children. Notice their special interest in tattling on, or comparing themselves favorably with, him.

Notice others' reactions to your child based on his reputation and urge them to react instead to the current, improved behavior. Watch for any tendency of your own to jump to conclusions about who did it. If your child must go on trial, let the trial be conducted on evidence, not on reputation! Detailed instructions for freeing your child from the yoke of bad reputation are given in Chapter 7.

Help your child find better avenues for fulfilling attention and belonging needs. Channeling his boundless energy is half the battle of turning the child away from the role of troublemaker.

Being Angry at Others

Hyperactive children often are angry because of the combined effects of the self-awareness traits discussed thus far. Unable to stop themselves from misbehaving, they feel persecuted and rejected, sometimes surrender the fight, and settle into unacceptable roles.

Their emotions tend to be extreme and poorly filtered: they are very affectionate or very hostile, and changes between these extremes are rapid. A complicating factor is that ADHD children have trouble expressing their emotions verbally, so their feelings build up before being discharged in violence. Typically, these children are irritable, short-fused, and volatile.

They punch holes in doors and walls, tear curtains from their mountings, break windows, throw things, yank drawers out of dressers, and toss dressers over. They attack adults as well as children with fists or kicks, and they sometimes threaten with blunt objects or knives. Verbally, their anger takes the form of needling, harassing, name calling, cussing, and picking on other children and adults.

Like most highly competitive persons, they are poor winners and poor losers. If they win, they make fun of the loser and flaunt the victory. If they lose, they demand a rule change, quit the activity, accuse the opponent of cheating, or attack the victor.

These wholesale problems with anger control are generally much more pronounced in those who have an overlapping conduct disorder (ADHD-cd subgroup). Even for those not in that subgroup, anger control training is one of their most consistent needs.

Help your child control anger by using the I CARE method described in Chapter 13. Don't expect to have a calm discussion about anger control when your child is out-of-sorts; talk after your child has calmed down. Decide together what can be done next time to prevent a similar outcome.

Train your child to become aware of the early signs of the buildup of anger. What happens first—does he clench his fist? Does he tell himself something is unfair? Does he tell himself he is not going to let someone get away with something?

Because dealing aggressively with others is unacceptable, your child must learn how to problem solve and get wants and needs met through cooperative relationships. The suggestions given here are effective for teaching anger control. The specific methods you use should be carefully suited to your child's readiness.

Keep It a Little Anger. Teach your child to separate the notion of the "little anger" of frustration from the "big anger" of rage. Little anger doesn't cause problems and unhappiness, but big anger does. Your child tells himself "I'm not going to turn over the control of my happiness to you [the person or situation angering your child]." Teach your child how to keep the anger "little" by labeling situations according to their potential to stimulate him to become angry. For example, a green-light situation is one in which he is unlikely to become angry; a yellow-light situation is one in which he might become angry, and it calls for extra alertness and self-control; and a red-light situation is an anger emergency that requires your immediate intervention.

The code words are used for three purposes: (1) to self-monitor and provide a convenient label for what your child is experiencing at the moment; (2) to communicate his feelings to you, and (3) to communicate his feelings to others who are aware of the labels. Teach your child to use appropriate self-reminding phrases, such as "I need to be super careful and control myself now" during yellow-light situations, and "I need to turn around and leave" (or one of the other anger control measures listed here) during red-light situations. Also teach how your child can best avoid yellow-light situations.

When you intervene, ask "Is this a yellow-light time, or is it a red-light time for you?" "Yellow light—I'm starting to get angry" or "Red light—I'm really getting angry" alert others to stop any irritating actions. Used for these purposes, these code words are emergency substitutes for a more graceful expression of concerns. Your child should not use them to threaten or bully people.

Check In. A daily check-in on frustrations often helps ADHD children who are extremely volatile and short-tempered. The child has a Concerns Notebook (see Chapter 13) but, instead of waiting for a PPI meeting, discusses the concerns at the end of each day. Keep making the point that addressing all concerns quickly helps her to be less irritated. Tell her that in exchange for such attention from you, she owes the family a reasonable effort at controlling anger.

Tell an Adult. An instant version of the daily check-in, this technique allows your child to come to you for advice in resolving the situation whenever anger starts to develop. Introduce the "magic words" to obtain help during conflict moments: "Just come to me and say, 'I'm starting to feel angry.' I will stop doing whatever I'm doing, listen to your concerns, and give you advice about what you can do so you won't stay angry."

Blow Off Steam Safely. Throwing stones at a row of empty soft drink cans in a safe location and pounding a sturdy punching bag are additional ways to vent anger safely. Your child can also go to his room, lie on his bed, scream into a pillow, and pound the mattress with his fists. Give him a safe place for jumping, such as a mattress and pillows to throw on the mattress. Although these methods do not decrease the anger, they provide a temporary detour to prevent attacks on others, tantrums, or other harmful acts.

Leave the Scene and Breathe. Your child can leave and take ten long, slow, deep breaths. While breathing, your child can use the self-reminders "Stay in control" and "Relax." Your child should break off visual contact with the anger-arousing situation, turn around, and depart. Leaving the scene allows for cooling off and regaining self-control. Teach your child that leaving is not cowardly but instead shows assertiveness and self-control.

Cool Off and Calm Down. Your child can calm down after leaving a scene of conflict by listening to music or finding some other worthwhile distraction, such as locating an object to stare at.

Say "Stop." Announcing clearly and honestly the need for the other person to stop irritating actions is an important part of learning how to confront others. A three-part message defines her personal needs: she states how she feels, asks for what she needs to feel better, and makes a win-win deal with the other person. For example: "When you do that, I feel frustrated and confused. Please don't do that; do this instead. If you do it that way, I'll do what you want in a few minutes."

If your child has trouble with the entire three-part

message, substitute a basic assertion statement: "That bothers me; please stop it"; "Please don't do that to me"; or "Please stop doing that." Introduce the statement as a special "trick" or "magic phrase" to use whenever she senses frustration building up.

Run. Have your child run around the outside of the house five times or some other equivalent distance to decrease the anger.

Get a Cool Drink. Your child can leave to get a drink of water, milk, or juice. This action provides distraction, forces organized thought by requiring a series of steps to obtain the drink, occupies her in purposeful activity, allows tempers to cool down during the delay, and supplies a refreshing and pleasing sensual experience of coolness.

Write It Down. Your child can write the incident in her Concerns Notebook. Later, you can have a calm discussion about the matter. This method gives your child an opportunity to express feelings in writing rather than displaying them physically.

Keep Hands in Pockets. Using the self-reminding phrase "Keep my hands in my pockets" makes your child less likely to strike out, grab, or get into a fight.

Stay in Control. Using the self-reminders "Stay calm" and "Stay in control," which are more helpful than "Don't get angry," transforms anger into a determination to remain self-controlled and trains your child to own responsibility for one-half of the confrontation. Even though the other child may have been partially to blame, it is important to get your child to assume at least a significant share of responsibility for making things different in the future.

Zip the Lip. This simple rhyme is also effective as a self-reminder to prevent volatile situations from exploding.

It can be combined with other methods, such as keeping hands in pockets and leaving the scene. "Zip my lip, turn around, and leave" is a useful self-reminder, especially if the other children do not respond well to the three-part message when asked to stop.

Count to Ten. Perhaps the most famous of the emergency anger control procedures, this ageless remedy also works with ADHD children.

Talk It Out. Teach your child to negotiate rather than have tantrums. Learning conflict-solving skills is a good long-term anger control method.

Each of these suggestions has its benefits and drawbacks. Teaching your child to leave the scene when angry doesn't permit practice using negotiation skills. It is, however, a starting point for a change in your child's behavior because it allows regaining composure. Venting anger also doesn't teach good social skills. The best long-range solution is to teach your child how to negotiate when potential conflict situations arise.

Being generally less bothered by things is a great help to the ADHD child with self-esteem problems. Feeling overwhelmed and out of control frequently results not only in broken relationships but in an attitude of "I don't care" or "I give up." Training your child how to react constructively to stress ensures better cooperation with treatment attempts, better harmony in the family, and much better symptom control, thus leading to increased self-esteem.

Stress is personal and situation-specific. What is stressful for one child might not be for the next. What is stressful at one time or circumstance might not be stressful under different conditions.

Pinpoint the pressures occurring in your child's life to aid understanding. Inventory your child's feelings, paying special attention to unpleasant ones. If you suspect your child is having a particularly difficult day, suggest possible sources of stress. Once specific stressors are identified, they can be dealt with more easily.

Rest breaks are very important. Mental fatigue from a restrained situation or academic task decreases the ability to cope. Instruct your child to leave stressful situations temporarily if restlessness and tension seem to be building up.

Your child needs a convenient hideaway. Periods of rest and being alone are essential tools for good mental health to balance against intense activity and social interaction. Provide a location at home (not to be confused with a time-out place for discipline) where your child can have refuge from stressful events and situations. The time-away place should afford peace and should not be barren or unpleasantly sterile. A bedroom may be the best choice. Encourage a quiet activity your child enjoys from the Fun Idea List discussed in Chapter 13.

As an integral part of stress reduction, relaxation procedures can help some ADHD children. The greatest benefits of relaxation training lie in increased control of emotional expression, better tolerance of frustration, and decreased aggressiveness. Like other forms of training described in this book, however, these procedures should not be considered substitutes for effectively applied biochemical treatment.

The best relaxation procedures to teach your child are those that are usable on the spur of the moment in a wide variety of situations. Twenty minutes of meditation is not as helpful as a two-minute procedure. The suggestions given in Chapter 3 for counteracting the presleep agitation side effect of medication are usable at other times of day than bedtime.

Slowing the rate of breathing increases calmness. Your child should take ten long, slow, deep breaths for relaxation within a couple of minutes. As an added measure, instruct your child to think of relaxation words, such as *calm* when breathing in and *quiet* when breathing out.

Simple imagery, another relaxation method, requires a comfortable sitting or reclining position in a quiet place free from distraction. Instruct your child to tense various muscles, one at a time, then relax them to gain a total sense of relaxation. Encourage your child when relaxing to focus on some encouraging low-energy scenes such as a pleasant memory, a delightful fantasy, or a beautiful picture. Make or purchase a stress-reducing tape to use until the art of creating the needed imagery becomes natural. In controlling imagery, your child should focus on what *to* think about, not on what *not* to think about. Instructing "Don't think about . . ." only forces the thought of the very thing you mention.

Being Angry at Self

Most hyperactive children have terribly low self-esteem and are just as angry at themselves as they are at those who are dissatisfied with them. They gradually become adept at thwarting most positive messages, discounting and explaining away any "accidental" high grade or success. Wallowing in self-hatred, they can become bitterly pessimistic and unhappy about life.

Clues that your child might be depressed include:

1. Irritability, loss of emotional control
2. Decreased interest or pleasure in nearly all activities
3. Apathetic "I don't care" attitude about most things
4. Decrease in appetite and loss of interest in eating (not caused by medication)
5. Disturbed sleep (not caused by medication)
6. Fatigue and insufficient energy for normal activities
7. Feelings of worthlessness and talk of escape by running away or suicide
8. Marked indecisiveness and inability to concentrate or think
9. Frequent sobbing or crying

Estimates are that as many as one-third of ADHD children become depressed at one time or another. An especially consistent phenomenon is a minor preadolescent depressive phase occurring in 10- to 12-year-olds. Typically, the childhood depression fluctuates because of stresses such as a family move, school problems, or marital discord. During adolescence, the "up" periods become rarer, and the "down" periods become more common and longer lasting.

Research consistently shows that regular moderate exercise is one of the best guarantees against depression. Physical activity brings considerable pleasure to ADHD children and adolescents. The more hyperactive the child, the greater the need for structured movement, such as a regular exercise program. Regular exercise encourages grace, agility, and skill at coordinated body movement, and it increases strength and physical appearance by enhancing muscle firmness.

Exercise is not limited to team sports and competitive activities. Your child does not have to go to a recreation center, purchase expensive equipment, or take lessons. Most exercise can be self-initiated and pleasurable without bringing exhaustion. Good exercise does not have to be grueling to be effective.

In addition to its many health benefits, regular exercise provides mental distraction. Exercise done in a recreational frame of mind promotes relaxation and helps build endurance and self-confidence.

Most hyperactive children get enough exercise so they do not require a strictly regimented program. If you would like to arrange additional exercise, however, here are some general and specific questions to ask.

- *Is the exercise self-regulatory?* Can your child determine how long or how fast to exercise? Can your child avoid comparing performance with that of other children? Can the activity be done alone if desired? Can your child happily participate before building up high skill? Can the exercise be accomplished one step at a time?

- *Is it interesting?* Is it fun and will your child enjoy participating? Will it help avoid boredom? Will your child want to continue exercising in this way? Will your child be able to use this exercise to release tension? Will it have a stimulating effect and break up the monotony of day-to-day life? Can other types of exercise be performed simultaneously for variety?
- *Is it convenient?* Can your child do the activity at or near home? Can it be done at times of day and in locations that are not too restrictive? Can your child exercise regularly? Can it be conveniently rotated with other exercises? Can it be performed without the purchase of expensive equipment, uniforms, lessons, or memberships?
- *Is it appropriate to your child's needs?* Do the demands of the exercise parallel the frequency and the amount of exertion your child wishes to devote to it? Is the activity in concert with your child's age, state of health, physical condition, and activity preferences? Does the activity improve your child's physical appearance or overall physical condition? Is it physically invigorating to a pleasant degree without creating exhaustion?

Your child's physician, physical therapist, or other helping professional may be able to give guidance about the factors to consider when selecting exercises for your child. A sensible diet, sufficient rest and relaxation, stress control, and good personal hygiene are key ingredients to any successful physical fitness program.

A cardinal principle is to begin slowly. Even limited steps can be rewarding. The biggest danger is getting involved in complex exercises too early. Your child should stay loose and playful; the simpler the exercise, the better. Make sure your child is having fun. Gradually build up to more demanding activities. With a properly guided program of vigorous physical conditioning, a healthy but unconditioned child can significantly improve physical fitness in six to twelve weeks.

Hyperactive children have a way of overdoing almost everything they attempt. Train your child to identify and respect the fatigue point. Your child should stop immediately if there is pain in any body parts; labored breathing; extremely fast heartbeat; or discomfort from cold, cramps, or sore feet. The goals are to develop a positive attitude toward physical activity, to have fun, and to enjoy the vigor of the activity without extending beyond the fatigue point. A disadvantage of overdoing exercise is that stimulant and antidepressant medications are metabolized faster, so that wear-off and rebound effects can sometimes start to occur after the exercise period.

Avoid forcing your child or adolescent to join any regular group-exercise program. Your child might prefer calisthenics or weight lifting at first because they offer privacy. As confidence increases, your child might become interested in progressively more social or more public exercises. Concentrate on adding variations. Exposure to several options keeps interest high and gives your child a sense of decision-making power to compensate for the restrictiveness of biochemical treatment.

Sports such as soccer, swimming, and bicycling are especially suitable because of the movement involved, the changing array of possibilities, and the constant excitement. Athletics allow discharge of energy, often don't require high coordination, and provide opportunity for socialization and success in a completely different arena from the scholastic pressures of school. Find pursuits in which your child can succeed. Select a sport not requiring complex coordination, if coordination is a problem. One parent of an adolescent ADHD boy happily reported that her son had finally found a sport he could succeed in: "All his life, Erik was awkward and too poorly coordinated to participate in sports. Finally we found an answer. He got a new ten-speed and has joined a bicycling club. He's doing great! Take his feet off the ground and he's all right!"

NURTURING SELF-ESTEEM

Self-esteem is a key issue of paramount importance for personal change. Without a strong basic sense of self-esteem, the child has no reason to care whether a behavior is desirable. Cooperating with biochemical treatment is an example of a personal growth project requiring an awareness of self-benefit and personal worth. Your child needs to conclude he deserves the improvements that are expected from the treatment effort.

Help your child establish suitable goals. Those that are too simplistic and too easily attained offer no challenge; reaching them would be only hollow victories. On the other hand, goals that are too challenging are usually not accomplished and result in discouragement. The goals can be in various areas on which you and your child agree, such as social, educational, or athletic.

Offering Encouragement

Encouragement is the process through which a person becomes more aware of his capabilities and of his sense of belonging. Positive self-esteem develops when the child learns to feel good about what he does and about the favorable messages others give him.

Encouragement is love. The encouraged child, the loved child, feels good about herself and about others. In giving encouragement to your child, your ultimate goal is to help her learn to apply it. Children who feel and act unlovable need the most encouragement; those who feel and act lovable receive and accept encouragement most easily. The backbone of your ability to deliver love to your child is your ability to provide encouragement.

Encouragement manifests itself in your underlying attitude, which is shown in many ways—by your opinions, your level of trust, your tone of voice, your actions, and your words.

Encouragement is more like food than medicine: a steady diet of it over a long period of time will strengthen your child's self-esteem. It will also help prevent self-esteem from crumbling under stress. When your child is ready to stop trying, remind him of his strength and potential. Few gifts are more precious than your gift of encouragement. Here are some guidelines for establishing an encouraging atmosphere in your family.

Talk with, Not to, Your Child. Talking *to* your child gives him no choice. It is one-way communication in which you preach and demand unthinking obedience. You tell your child what to think, without exploring his logic. Your child receives no credit for his creativity. There is no exploring of his uniqueness, and you *insist* your child accept your point of view. With this approach, your child soon learns to keep his feelings and thoughts to himself.

Talking *with* your child means having a two-way conversation. It shows respect for your child's uniqueness. You discover your child's logic by asking leading questions instead of preaching. Your child expresses his opinion, and you learn his point of view. You can help him correct mistaken beliefs, and he receives credit for his creativity. There is a request, not an order, that he consider your point of view. Talking *with* the child promotes harmony and is encouraging. Talking *to* the child destroys harmony and is discouraging.

Teach Constant Choice. Teach your child to assert herself. She needs to learn to ask clearly for what she wants in relations with others. Your child must not expect others to magically know her desires. Ask "What do you think you could do now?" so she is reminded of her ability to take action to make things better.

Adjust Your Help. When you give assistance, do not give too much. There are two basic methods of adjusting the help you give your child.

1. Help is available but withheld. Your assistance is offered but is not forced on your child. Sample statements include: "I will help you if you think you need it, after you've tried"; "Go ahead and try; I'll be around later"; "Do it yourself and I'll watch"; and "You know where to find me in case you need me." Sometimes a kitchen timer can be used: "Do the best you can until the timer goes off; then I'll come and see how things are going."
2. Help during part of the activity. Your assistance is offered only during the beginning, or the middle, or the end of the task, but not throughout the entire task. Sample statements include: "Would you like some help to get started? . . . at this point? . . . to finish it up?"

Adjusting your help prevents you from becoming overinvolved. Your child can feel his strength while still not being overwhelmed by fears of being left too much on his own. Adjusted help sends the clear message that you have faith in your child's abilities; giving too much help does *not* convey that message. Without physically involving yourself, you can convey your deep interest in what your child is doing.

Show Faith in Your Child's Ability. Express faith in your child's ability to cope with stresses and challenges. When you let your child undertake a task with an element of challenge or difficulty, you show your trust in her. Expect her to be competent. The you-can-do-it philosophy is very helpful for strengthening a child's sagging self-confidence.

Help Your Child Over Hurdles. Sometimes your child may get stuck at a difficult part of a task. Help him over the hurdle by giving a supportive reminder to start or to continue the activity. A statement such as "Start now and we'll see how it goes" or "All beginnings are difficult" can boost your child's courage to begin a challenging task. "How will you know you can't do it unless you try?" is another helpful statement. Focusing on the challenge and expressing enthusiasm about it can also be reassuring: "This looks like quite a challenge; it's going to be fun to see how it turns out."

Understand Your Child's Concern. A sincere expression that tells your child you know how he feels is often comforting. Statements such as "I know this seems difficult to you" and "This is hard for you, isn't it?" let your child know you understand his feelings. Just knowing you do understand and care can be helpful and can often help your child become unstuck.

Emphasize Your Child's Gains. Point out to your child that her current performance is an improvement over past performance; for example: "Look how much your skill has improved since you first started" and "It's becoming easier for you, isn't it?"

Teach Satisfaction with Small Gains. Teach your child to notice how far she has come and to enjoy the progress that she has made. Point out that even the longest journey starts with just a single step. Mountain climbers never run up the mountain; they always take one small step at a time, and they always walk slowly. Many tasks will be beyond your child's abilities until she learns to break them into manageable parts she can cope with one at a time.

You can build stopping places into the task, with an instruction such as "Let me know when you have this much done; then I'll check to see how things are going for you." This allows you to help her stay on the right track, so she won't have to redo parts of it. It also assures her you will be there in case of difficulty and you will be ready to admire her progress at each step along the way.

Show Casual Appreciation of Quality. Train your child away from perfectionism. Appreciate high skill, but don't put excessive emphasis on it. Although the quality of your child's performance is appreciated, it is not the primary concern. The amount of effort and degree of enjoyment your child shows are the important aspects. Quality of performance is a secondary concern. For the highly discouraged child, it is important to comment on the completion of some of the task, without mentioning the quality level. Quality will take care of itself as long as your child is showing serious effort and enjoys the activity.

You can refer to your child's effort with statements such as "I'm glad it's getting easier for you" and "I can see how hard you are working on this." You can put emphasis on your child's enjoyment of the task with statements such as "It will become more enjoyable as time goes on" and "You will learn to like this as you keep trying."

Emphasize Your Child's Strengths. Say "I like the way this part was done" when commenting on your child's performance, rather than drawing attention to the errors. Trying to build self-confidence by focusing on weakness is like trying to build a house on quicksand.

Encourage Identification with Others. Your child might enjoy reading about successful ADHD individuals. Thomas Edison had rather severe symptoms throughout his childhood and adult life. He had trouble as a student and as an employee. He created a work environment where he was free to develop his own hours and work at his own pace. He slept four hours per night and developed 1200 patents, including the phonograph, mimeograph, and electric light bulb.

Other prominent people suspected of having ADHD and/or learning disabilities include Winston Churchill, Eleanor Roosevelt, Albert Einstein, Bruce Jenner, Nelson Rockefeller, and Louis Pasteur.

Developing Time Management Skills

To give your child a further boost, teach better use of time for constructive purposes. As your child learns to accomplish things, confidence and self-esteem will increase. Help your child develop a list of the tasks to be done. Put them in the intended order of accomplishment, taking into account their importance and difficulty. Some children need to have the difficult tasks high on the list because they have more zeal for diving in and accomplishing things early. Others seem to need a buildup of confidence from conquering little tasks before facing larger responsibilities later. Estimate how much time each task will take, build in an extra 10% for all time allotments, and insert the resulting approximate timetable next to the tasks on the list.

A simple time chart can help your child gain better control of carelessly invested time. Develop a large chart with twenty-four one-hour segments on the left side. Put the major categories of daily activities across the top; for example, family, school, recreation/TV, chores, social, study, hobby/personal, lessons, clubs/athletics, church, sleep. The chart should contain 264 rectangles (24 down times 11 across). At the end of each day, have your child color in a portion of each rectangle to illustrate the time spent. Make several copies and use one chart per day for about two weeks. The pattern of your child's use of time will become quite apparent and you will have a helpful basis for making adjustments in your child's daily routines.

Using Mistakes Wisely

Mistakes confront your child in a never-ending parade, but they need not cause lower self-esteem. They are an opportunity to strengthen self-esteem and to grow psychologically from struggling to make fewer errors and to achieve a greater degree of competence.

Nobody behaves perfectly. Mistakes and imperfections are a natural part of life. It is not true that mistakes must be the focus of criticism and the destroyers of your child's self-esteem. Teach your child to learn from mistakes.

It is important to accept the imperfections in yourself and in those around you. It is also important to handle mistakes constructively so your child can imitate your maturity. When your child is losing self-confidence because of his mistakes, reassure him briefly by teaching him these truths.

Mistakes Indicate Temporary Unreadiness. Mistakes indicate he was not ready to do the activity. Mistakes are not proof of permanent incompetence or inability to do the task. Encouraging statements are "Mistakes sometimes mean that we aren't ready yet" or "It looks as if you weren't quite ready for that part yet."

Mistakes Have Causes. Mistakes are not intentional. They are excusable and justifiable. Be willing to trace the roots of the mistake. In this way, you will teach your child how to use mistakes to improve her abilities. Your child needs the courage to be imperfect, and you need to be courageous enough to allow that imperfection.

Mistakes Are Sometimes Laughable. Look for humor and irony in situations, and laugh at your own mistakes whenever possible. This approach sets the tone for treating mistakes with the right degree of lightness. An appeal to your child to look on the bright side of her errors expresses your refreshingly encouraging attitude.

Mistakes Are Expected. You should provide materials and procedures for helping your child bounce back from mistakes. Build some safety nets into your activities and into your child's activities. Telling your child there is no possibility of mistakes overemphasizes the importance of mistakes. Even though it may appear at first as though expecting mistakes is discouraging, it isn't at all discouraging when done in the proper spirit; for example, "That's why pencils have erasers"; "Of course, there will be mistakes"; and "You only proved that you're human!"

Mistakes Are Accidental. Tell your child you know he did not make a mistake on purpose. Treat mistakes like any other accident. They happened, they need to be corrected, and life must move on with as little wasted effort as possible. Sample statements include "Accidents can happen, and mistakes can happen" and "I know you didn't do it on purpose."

Sometimes a child may use a mistake such as spilled milk, dropped pencils, or bumping into other children as a means of getting undue attention. These situations call for discipline rather than pure encouragement. Disciplinary techniques are discussed in Chapter 13.

Mistakes Are Proof of Effort. Mistakes are a necessary and natural by-product of earnest effort. The only sure guarantee for not making any mistakes is not to try to do the task at all. Remind your child that even the greatest baseball stars strike out often throughout their careers. Emphasize that mistakes indicate your child is trying. Avoid emphasizing the number or severity of mistakes. Examples of encouraging statements include "Mistakes only prove you are trying" and "If you weren't making any mistakes, I wouldn't know that you were working at this task."

Mistakes Are Incompletions, Not Failures. Mistakes are not reasons to stop; they are reasons to continue. Teach your child to interpret errors as unfinished work. Expect your child to continue with tasks not only until they are completed, but until they are done with reasonable accuracy. Being careful not to overemphasize quality of performance, encourage your child to correct errors in his work. A famous football coach once said after his team lost, "We didn't lose; we just ran out of time!" Your child can well use the same philosophy.

Mistakes Are Unfortunate, Not Catastrophic. The less commotion and fuss made over a mistake, the better. When your child makes errors, stay calm, quiet, and reassuring. This is sometimes hard to do, especially when your child makes the same mistake repeatedly, but patience is vital. Encouraging statements include "The world isn't going to come to an end over this" and "Nothing is so bad that it can't be overcome."

Mistakes Are Profitable. Teach your child that profit and improvement can come from mistakes. Challenge your child to avoid wasting the experience. Encourage him to modify his actions so that the mistake leads to improved performance. Examples of encouraging statements you might make to an older child include "We need mistakes to show us the blind alleys so we can go back on the right course" and "The only difference between a stumbling block and a stepping stone is how you use it."

It is important not to preach at your child about how to use mistakes wisely. Instead, discuss and display your own constructive attitude toward your own mistakes. When you notice your child is starting to be bothered by his mistakes, reassure her briefly and lovingly. By word and deed, provide a convincing demonstration of the encouraging ideas presented here about using mistakes wisely.

Your child's self-esteem needs constant attention and nurturance because it is the basis for all your child accomplishes now and in the future. A universal need is to belong, to feel a part of the group. Chapter 7 details how to improve social skills and assist in normalizing what for many ADHD children is a very difficult aspect of day-to-day life.

7

Developing Better Interpersonal Relationships

Hyperactive children are less alert than others to the subtle signals children and adults use when expressing their needs and wants, such as facial expression and body position. They are apparently poor at reading body language and unable to notice others are annoyed, tired, offended, bored, or hurt. They talk too much, carry a joke too far, speak too loudly, act too critically, insist on continuing an activity too long or giving it up too soon, laugh at the wrong times, tease in hurtful ways, argue and debate about trivia, make tactless remarks, and talk back to authorities.

Researchers have observed that ADHD children engage in high rates of aggressive and annoying behaviors toward their agemates in play situations, earning extreme ratings of dislike and rejection. The most commonly reported complaints from classmates are that hyperactive children get in trouble and get other children in trouble, are rude, are difficult to get along with, insist on having their own way, and are bullies.

The emotional reactions of other children to a hyperactive child are, of course, extremely varied, depending greatly on the personality of the hyperactive child in relation to the personalities of the other children. The situation in which the children interact also influences each child's reaction to the other. There can be many positive emotional reactions to hyperactive children: other children may enjoy their optimism, high energy level, willingness to try new approaches to tasks, or sense of humor. These positive reactions pose little or no difficulty for parents and other caregivers and are generally helpful to the hyperactive child's self-esteem.

Many hyperactive children, however, have a hard time establishing smooth and cooperative relations, because other children resent the intrusion on their time, their activities, their personal space, and their property. This chapter highlights the most common stresses that occur in hyperactive children's relations with those who live, study, and play with them.

SIBLING RIVALRY

Siblings often complain that the hyperactive child won't stay out of their rooms and won't leave their belongings alone, or that the hyperactive child has stolen things from them or has taken things from their rooms without permission. The hyperactive child may not be reliable about returning these borrowed items and may be careless about the use of the objects. The hyperactive child may be accused of interrupting and pestering. Siblings sometimes feel as if their time is being monopolized by the hyperactive child; they may feel helpless to improve the situation and are confused by the ineffectiveness of their parents to control the misbehavior.

Often the hyperactive child's intrusion is an attempt to get attention. Instruct the sibling in a few basic disciplinary techniques as responses to attention-getting misbehavior. For instance, have the other child leave the company of the hyperactive child when she starts being inappropriately intrusive or use this simple technique to alleviate the behavior:

1. Stop whatever you are doing and look directly into her eyes.
2. Ask her what she wants.
3. If possible, make a deal in which you let her have her way, to some extent, in exchange for no longer interrupting you.
4. End the conversation with a firm statement of exactly what you want; for example, that she not pester you.

This procedure should be used early in the interchange between the two children. This technique will gradually train the hyperactive child to ask directly and honestly for what she wants rather than misbehaving to have her own way.

Changing certain situations at home can help. Locks can be put on bedroom doors, if necessary. The hyperactive child's bedroom can be located somewhat distant from a sibling's bedroom.

If violation of others' property rights by the hyperactive child becomes an issue, the most frequently taken objects can be put in secret locations or locked away. Arrangements can be made for the hyperactive child to earn his own belongings so there will be no more need to borrow them from siblings. In some cases you may want to search the hyperactive child's room if there is reasonable suspicion that he has been taking other persons' things. Such a search should be done as a demonstration of your firmness in not tolerating violation of property rights within your family. This intrusion on the hyperactive child's personal space must be done with an awareness of his right to privacy. Routine searches of the hyperactive child's room without specific evidence to justify them are more destructive than helpful.

In hundreds of subtle ways, adults treat hyperactive children differently from the ways they treat their siblings. Often the hyperactive child gets a great deal of attention and seems to monopolize the time and energy of adults. Other children may become resentful and jealous of all the excitement that accompanies the hyperactive child. In their desire to receive equal treatment, they may misbehave or start to imitate the hyperactive child.

Even before the parents realize what is happening, siblings can often see a pattern of overinvolvement developing. They consider the adults too supportive of the hyperactive child and become angry at their apparently biased total absorption with the hyperactive child. They sense that the hyperactive child continually demands special exemption from rules, refuses to cooperate with established routines, and in other ways tries to claim special privileges.

Equally destructive is the hyperactive child's tendency to violate restrictions, limits, and guidelines. Somehow the hyperactive child may seem to get away with lots of misbehavior and rule violations that are forbidden to the other children, which may result in the other children's demanding an equal right to misbehave in the same way.

Make sure each child senses your unique and special concern. Try to help siblings understand the plight of the hyperactive child. Jealousy will be reduced when they realize the hyperactive child's apparent privileges come at great cost and are evidence of difficulties rather than success in life.

It may be helpful to point out the various emotional stresses the hyperactive child is experiencing. Assure the other children you deeply appreciate their willingness to cooperate and their agreement not to demand similar exemptions. The other children must be able to use this appeal wisely for their own benefit and must not hurt the hyperactive child by repeating what you have told them.

Helping them understand both the hyperactive child's and your feelings allows siblings a meaningful part in the total situation. Let them know of your frustrations and assure them of your desire that the hyperactive child not continue to violate routines, disobey rules, or demand further exemptions. When the other children understand you are aware and concerned about the exemptions and are doing your best to keep them under control, they will be less inclined to stay angry toward you and to demand special privileges for themselves. Explain you are aware of how difficult it must be for them to do chores or obey rules while the hyperactive child refuses to be cooperative.

Managing Inconsistency

Suppose you promise a trip to a favorite store in the evening, but your child misbehaves during the day. Which type of consistency do you show? Do you follow through on promises, treat all children with the same consequences for misbehavior, or reflect your true feelings by your actions? In your attempt to avoid favoritism, you might be tempted to pursue any of these but by doing so, you frustrate yourself and confuse your children.

The persons, the relationships, and the situations within your family are in a state of constant flux. Beware of a rigid adherence to consistency, which can cause disharmony and competition. The following are some consistency misconceptions:

Evenness of Mood, Moment-to-Moment and Day-to-Day. *"I will always smile and be pleasant to all of my children"* (even though my sleep, nutrition, and stresses vary greatly and the children's behavior fluctuates).

Values and Beliefs About Right and Wrong. What is unacceptable behavior in one child is also unacceptable in any other: *"If it is wrong for Billy to do it, then it is wrong for Amy to do it"* (even though Billy and Amy handle responsibilities entirely differently).

Follow-Through and Determination. *"Because I promised that I would do this favor for Sheila, I'll do it"* (even though I don't feel like it anymore because of the way she acted after I made the promise).

Universality of Rules and Their Enforcement. The same rules and consequences apply for all of the children: *"Since I won't let Matt climb on it, I won't let James climb on it either"* (even though James uses great care and won't hurt it).

Maintaining Order and Routine. *"We don't do what Candi is asking for. We've never done it before so she can't do it now"* (even though this circumstance is a unique opportunity for Candi).

Pairing Certain Actions with Certain Consequences. *"Every time Tyrone does that, this will happen to him as a consequence"* (even though the circumstances and his intentions are different).

Equivalence. *"What I do for one child, I will do for all"* (even though some may not want it done and others are desperately seeking it).

Parental Agreement. *"We must always agree on every aspect of raising our children"* (even though we differ in hundreds of other ways and seldom have the same understanding of a situation).

In contrast to the consistency misconceptions listed above, two types are worth striving for.

Congruence. Matching feelings and actions. Parents act according to how they feel, giving a direct and honest indication of their response to the child's behavior or to their own circumstance: *"This is how I feel, so this is what I am going to do. I feel this way in part because you acted the way you did." "I know I promised to take you shopping, but I'm just too tired right now. I'll rest a bit and try to arrange to take you later today or tomorrow. I'm sorry."*

Contemporaneous Treatment. Treating according to readiness. Parents provide whatever guidance appears to be needed by a specific child at the moment, regardless of whether a similar action would have been taken with a different child: *"I'll let you go over to Sam's house because you have been so helpful to me with Sara, even though we don't usually let anyone from our family visit Sam at this time of day."*

Managing consistency with congruent and contemporaneous treatment is generally the most useful day in and day out. If your actions are an honest reflection of your response to how the children have acted, then your children are receiving useful feedback about the impact of their behavior on others. Discourage demands by others for equal privileges. Substitute instead the concept of *equally special* privileges that are uniquely suited to each child. The safest, most reliable consistency is to provide whatever each child needs and is ready for, without having to give a parallel privilege or expectation to other children at the same time.

Decreasing Competition

Most siblings of ADHD children who respond to biochemical treatment are pleased with the improvements that occur and quickly forgive the ADHD child for past misdeeds. They launch a close, loving, mutually appreciative relationship with the treated child.

Some, however, react negatively to the positive changes that occur in the hyperactive child. The two children then become like two animals on a carousel, such that as one rises, the other lowers. Self-esteem of children in your family is in part based on their comparison of themselves with the ADHD child. The carousel effect involves sudden deterioration in the behavior of a sibling when the child's behavior improves. The sibling who was formerly in a favored position suddenly no longer seems so angelic, because the ADHD child is no longer so devilish. The children trade roles, and a new family brat emerges.

People gather in groups naturally, not to show how much better they are than each other, but to cooperate and to enjoy each other's acceptance, affirmation, and company. Children's love for others cannot blossom in a competitive atmosphere, which always brings with it a tendency to be rude and critical. Sibling harmony can flourish only in an atmosphere of cooperation and mutual respect.

To decrease sibling rivalry, decrease competition in your family. Interpersonal competition—one person against another—is very destructive. Intensely competitive children usually believe that competition is necessary and that they are preparing themselves for the cold, cruel, competitive world. Such thinking can lead to tragic consequences.

Competition may be needed in a free market economy, but only at the corporate level of businesses competing for goods, services, and markets. The majority of economic trade activities are based on cooperation. There is an exchange of interdependent services. The division of labor allows each person to contribute a skill or service and receive other services or goods in return. Large groups—such as nations—trade their goods back and forth in a system of mutual trust and cooperation.

Even the most vigorous of corporate competition requires that the involved individuals remain intensely *co-*

operative with their co-workers, not competitive with them. Interpersonal competitiveness makes a person unpopular and alienated rather than an effective group member. Competitive persons are simply not enjoyable to be with. Their activities, particularly their play and recreation, have a joyless, driven quality that ruins the experience for everyone. The emotionally well-balanced person with no great desire to compete with or outdo others is much more likely than the discouraged, overly competitive person to produce high-quality work and be successful in the long run.

Competition and sibling rivalry go hand in hand. Children who are jealous of each other quickly become competitive. One child might have a boastful "I'm better than you" or "I'm the best" attitude, which invites an answer. The desire to compete might be coupled with a desire to dominate or defeat, and thus, symbolically at least, to destroy each other. This intense competitiveness is terribly destructive in a family.

Although your intentions may be good, urging one child to do as well as a brother or sister in some activity or skill is insulting and discouraging rather than helpful. The child who already shows the desired behavior is eager to maintain superior status and is jealous of any progress made by the child who is being urged to improve. The child being urged becomes discouraged, rather than encouraged, by the comparison. Parents have only highlighted areas of inferiority.

Teach your children to overcome physical obstacles, rather than other persons. If they want challenge, let them compete against their own past performance in developing a new skill. Let them master environmental obstacles by learning how to manipulate, build, control, enhance, and beautify things. Steer them away from trying to conquer and control others.

The tenor of your marital interaction also influences the level of contention among your children; the relationship between parents, even after a separation or divorce, sets either a competitive or a cooperative atmosphere (see Chapter 9). An intensely conflicted marital relationship plays into sibling rivalry. Children often choose sides and form alliances. Try to set the best possible example of problem solving and decision making from a perspective of mutual respect and coordination of effort.

Increase your support of each child's individuality and uniqueness as expressed in tastes and preferences. Stay aware of evolving talents, social activities, and accomplishments. To the extent that each child feels affirmed as a unique individual, there is less need to be treated the same as siblings. To the extent they think there has to be a winner and a loser, your children are likely to become hostile and jealous toward each other. Teach them that compromise and cooperation are much better ways of dealing with others and getting rewards in life.

Encourage actions and statements reflecting courtesy, negotiation, sensitivity, sharing, and cooperation. Give them attention, encouragement, and appreciative comments when they share or compliment each other. Encourage your children to show flexibility rather than demanding their own way when playing with each other. Let them experience the direct benefits of being kind and thoughtful. Assist smaller or less communicative children by expressing gratitude for kindness shown to them: "I'm sure Jeff appreciates your helping him pick up his toys." . . . "It feels good to help Jeff now and then, doesn't it?" "When you did that, it allowed Anne to rest for a few minutes. You really helped Anne that way!"

Counter all egotism and selfishness about time, ideas, or material objects. Encourage the sharing of skills and knowledge among your children: "Now you can play pretty music for all of us." "Can you help teach Jamie how to do two-place subtraction?"

Encourage sharing and generosity about ideas as well as things. Teach negotiation and assertiveness skills. Train your children to discuss and settle issues by mutual consent after exploring each other's wants, rather than by bullying or competing. Help them have their "day in court" with each other. Guide them to state what their needs and wants are and to develop possible solutions that might lead to the fulfillment of those needs. Show them how to make deals that allow them to help each other attain their goals and wants. Turn emphasis away from giving in to each other and toward developing win-win solutions.

Promoting Assertiveness

Help your children learn to express their feelings in words, as a first step toward problem solving. Teach them to ask directly for what they want, rather than screaming, whining, hitting, or grabbing.

Help annoyed siblings learn how to handle their anger. Their anger is not directed so much at the bothersome child as at the irritating behavior, which acts like a wall that prevents them from enjoying and making contact with their brother or sister. Another important aspect of anger for your children to understand is that by allowing themselves to become angry they give the bothersome child undue power and influence over their lives and their happiness. Encourage them to be flexible in their needs concerning the bothersome behavior. Though it would be pleasant to experience an improvement, it is not crucial to their survival that the child change.

Your child might misbehave simply to gain attention. Give any pestered child some simple ways to defuse the situation so intense conflict doesn't have a chance to develop. If one child starts being a nuisance, the other child has three alternatives: (1) leave the scene, (2) get the hyperactive sibling to stop being a nuisance, or (3) agree to pay attention to the bothersome sibling.

If your child chooses the first option, suggest a private place such as the bedroom, or invite the child to come to you. Telling the child to ignore the antics of a bothersome hyperactive sibling generally is not effective and simply goads the misbehaving sibling to intensify her efforts.

If the child wants to confront the bothersome sibling and stop the annoying actions, show him how. Suppose your child is being bothered by Cassie:

> Stop whatever you are doing and look directly at Cassie. Ask her what she wants. Make a deal with her—you let her have her way to some extent, in exchange for her no longer bugging you about it. End your conversation with a firm statement of exactly what you want from Cassie. For example, you can play with her in twenty minutes after you have finished your school work, and in the meantime she is not to talk to you.

The third option is simply for the bothered sibling to stop whatever was occurring and pay attention to his sister. This choice can sometimes be quite suitable, so don't rule it out.

Giving Siblings an Expanded Role

The best solution for the carousel effect is to give the formerly better-behaved siblings new ways to be angelic that allow them to reclaim the specialness lost when the ADHD child improved. The most beneficial roles for siblings to adopt are as special helpers to you and to the hyperactive child. By emphasizing these important roles, you can turn a potential negative into a giant positive. Special helper roles provide a new importance and circumvent the need to take over the position of best worst in the family. The benefits of treatment don't stop with the hyperactive child but extend throughout the family. Since all partake of the benefits, all need to share in the responsibility of making those benefits work.

The helper role involves several key aspects.

One important aspect is helping the hyperactive child

recognize the improvements occurring as a result of treatment. Strengthen awareness of the before-and-after contrasts that are so vital to ensuring continued cooperation with the treatment program. Another facet of the helper role is to provide a model for more appropriate behavior—to set an example for the child to follow—and to show gratitude for the improvements by giving sincere compliments that include a gratitude component: "Thank you for playing so calmly with me."

Being the sibling of a hyperactive child is the world's best training ground for practicing the art of forgiveness. You can use your parental role to guide siblings toward accepting the imperfections of others, especially the shortcomings of their hyperactive sister or brother. Urge them to build bridges to replace the walls that developed prior to treatment. One way to facilitate forgiveness is to urge the siblings to give the child credit for the improvements and to stay current in their emotional reactions toward the child. If siblings are no longer embarrassed in front of their friends, they can start treating the child less like a nuisance and more like a valued friend. Ask for help in thinking of activities for them to do together.

Another aspect of the helper role is to assist in interpreting for others the fact that the child has changed and standing up for the child in stressful situations. It also involves assisting in their sister's or brother's self-control, such as by reminding to use the six A's of apology (explained later in this chapter) when the opportunity arises.

In their expanded roles, siblings can help you monitor the effectiveness of the treatment program, including the occurrence or absence of ADHD symptoms, side effects if medications are being used, and day-by-day fluctuations in the effectiveness of the treatment. They can provide additional pairs of eyes and ears to assist you in engineering the project. If siblings still find it difficult to turn their relationship in a positive direction to coincide with the improvements in their sister or brother, seek professional counseling for the family.

PEER GROUP TENSION

Whether it be the neighborhood, the classroom, or the family, other children are often concerned about the hyperactive child's effect on the group. Playmates fear they will lose permission to play in certain locations or with certain children because of the hyperactive child's actions, and classmates fear the entire class will be penalized because of the child's antics. Peers are often embarrassed by the child's behavior.

In their attempts to lessen the effects of an ADHD child's behavior on their groups, children start to reject the child and take advantage. In games such as tag, the hyperactive child may be "it" most of the time. If children are taking turns riding a wagon, he may do most of the pushing. Although this strategy provides the other children some temporary relief, it serves to further the distrust and enmity that plagues the child's relationships with other children.

One helpful maneuver is to arrange a temporary separation of the ADHD child. A better long-term approach is to teach the other children that they are creating their own discomforts. Only the misbehaving child should experience whatever reaction the behavior receives from other people. Remind children that whenever they react to inappropriate behavior, they are allowing the offending child to control the situation and to prevent them from enjoying the event. Children must learn to stand aside psychologically and avoid being in the middle between the hyperactive child and others who are upset by the misbehavior.

Teaching other children how to deal with their anger is an important and difficult responsibility for you as a parent or teacher. Use the same strategies given in Chapter 6, but teach them from the point of view of the other child who is becoming angry at what the ADHD child does.

TEACHING SOCIAL SKILLS

Hyperactive children suffer peer difficulties because their intrusive, obnoxious behavior and poorly developed social skills make them unattractive. Impulsivity is another socially devastating trait closely associated with the amount of rejection these children typically receive from their peers, which can lead to mental health problems.

Among the most common difficulties for ADHD children and adolescents are the following:

- *Reciprocity:* entering an ongoing conversation, interrupting courteously when interruption is necessary, joining group activities, waiting for one's turn in line or in a game, being a participant without dominating
- *Handling negatives:* accepting criticism, accepting a no to a request, responding to teasing, losing gracefully in a game—being a "good sport," disagreeing without criticizing
- *Self-control:* handling peer pressure, making decisions without assistance, resisting temptations
- *Communication:* understanding and following instructions, answering questions, conversing well, being an alert listener, using eye contact, showing empathy
- *Winning people over:* giving compliments, showing gratitude, encouraging others, hello and goodbye skills, apologizing, being a friend, smiling correctly, honoring others' "boundaries," being courteous, using proper language, inviting others to play, noticing and commenting on the good news in others' lives, doing favors, giving thoughtful gifts, lending, sharing, being hospitable, showing interest in others, self-disclosing without bragging

Research has verified that ADHD individuals who are weak in these skills have more adjustment difficulties, including juvenile delinquency, dropping out of school, troubled relationships with peers and authority figures, bad conduct military discharges, and mental health problems. Their academic progress is also impaired throughout childhood because of difficulty following directions and conforming to the requirements of behavior and productivity in the classroom.

Social skills are the specific behaviors during interpersonal contacts that gain positive responses and encourage ongoing transactions. They can be learned through observation and imitation as well as rehearsal of specific aspects that seem to require adjustment. For social competence, children must be able to discriminate situations in which social behavior is needed, choose the best skills to use in that particular situation, perform those skills, notice how the other person reacts, and adjust to the other person's response.

There are three basic social skills training methods. The *mentor method* involves learning from an older child who has refined social skills and would be a suitable model. Arrange for this child to give your child feedback and suggestions for improvement after observing some moments of play or other interaction. This method is convenient if your child trusts the judgment of the older child and is willing to listen to the feedback and advice given, and if the mentor is available often enough to provide helpful instruction and corrective information to your hyperactive child.

The second is the *counseling method*, which involves enrolling your child in group or individual counseling that includes discussion and practice of social skills. In a group setting, social skills training can be a powerful technique. The children can role play their skills while gaining feedback and encouragement from the group and the therapist.

The third is the *parental instruction method*, which allows you to give your child experience at refining social skills within the protective and encouraging confines of your home. Select a day, time, and location that afford privacy and allow you and your child to devote full attention to improving social skills. Confine the training sessions to a maximum length of fifteen minutes. This method consists of six steps, the first letters of which spell *scored*.

1. Show. Demonstrate how to perform the skill by acting it out.
2. Coach. Describe the skill step-by-step; instruct how and when to use it; explain how the skill is helpful, pointing out its short- and long-term benefits. State briefly why it is important, specifically illustrate its benefits in a social situation, and point out the negative results of not performing it adequately. Convey excitement and optimism that the skill you are about to teach will help your child avoid in the future difficulties that have occurred in the past.
3. Offer self-reminders. Provide self-reminding statements to decrease interfering tendencies and to remind how and when to use the newly learned skill.
4. Rehearse. Let your child perform the skill by role playing in a realistic simulated situation. Give feedback as to how your child is looking and behaving. Practice a situation until your child develops poise and quick, accurate judgment about how to respond. Use scripts, reminder cards, tape recordings, mirrors, or any other helpful training device.
5. Encourage. Comment favorably on your child's attempts and correct any aspects needing refinement. Give plenty of encouragement, express confidence, and share your child's joy about progress.
6. Debrief. Encourage your child to gradually apply the skill to real-life situations. To provide a quick victory and build confidence, start with an easy situation. Have a goal of one instance per day in which your child applies the currently emphasized skill.

Consider reviewing progress at each day's bedtime tuck-in or at the next PPI meeting (see Chapter 13).

Suppose, for example, you want to teach effective greetings and goodbyes. Tell your child the exact words to say and illustrate the proper voice inflections to convey friendliness and interest. Have your child role play word choice and voice inflection until he has mastered the art of opening and closing social contacts. Then as these methods are applied in the days and weeks following the initial training and practice, review the results and give further encouragement and corrective instruction if needed.

ADHD children tend to be weak in their ability to decipher others' feelings as well as their own. A useful starting point is to practice labeling emotions correctly. At the end of the day, discuss the feelings your child has had during the day and help find correct labels for those feelings. Provide examples of those emotions occurring in others. Discuss the situations that provoke those emotions as well as alternative ways of handling those situations in the future.

Consider having your child cut out magazine pictures of people in emotional situations and define or label the emotion being pictured. A variation is to have your child make up a brief story of events leading up to the emotion being shown, then possible solutions to unpleasant emotions or aftermaths of positive emotions. You can magnify the impact of this exercise by role playing a similar emotion.

Overcoming a Bad Reputation

Peers are generally rather slow to accept the idea that a hyperactive child can change so dramatically after the start of biochemical treatment. Prior to treatment, the peers might have excluded the child from their alliances.

Therefore, even more time is needed for breaking into the preexisting friendship networks and winning new friends. Some differences remain after treatment that can interfere with a smooth reentry into the accepted social network among classmates and neighborhood friends. The disappearance of disruptive behavior doesn't necessarily bring with it the degree of social polish that makes your child an enjoyable partner in peer activities or attractive as a potential friend.

Your child may have developed a reputation in the neighborhood or at school that follows him or her around and keeps the waters of social relationships churning—referred to as the wake effect because it is analagous to the wake behind a boat that moves across the water.

Think of the child as a speedboat, the hyperactivity as the motor, and the water as the child's relations with others. The motor propels the boat rapidly through the water, splitting and dividing the water. When the motor stops, the boat no longer moves across the water, so it stops splitting the water. However, the wake will catch up with the boat and rock it. In the same way, a hyperactive child builds up a reputation among others that will keep him in a disruptive role long after he stops being hyperactive. The reputation will continue to plague the child long after the behavior has stopped.

A startling example of how pervasive a neighborhood-based wake effect can become involved the family of a 9-year-old ADHD boy, whose mother reported:

> I take each day as it comes, not knowing what the day will hold. I have even received an anonymous clipping in the mail with no return address: "Pointers on How to Raise Juvenile Delinquents." Josh can't even breathe without everyone jumping on him. Our lawyer sent a private investigator into the neighborhood and I couldn't believe it. Everything that happens is all Josh's fault and he has everything coming to him and then some.

Your child needs to undo the wake effect directly after the ADHD symptoms are successfully treated. The moment the symptoms are controlled, the burden is on your child to demonstrate to all that things are going to be different. Others might not believe the claims of differentness at first. They are likely to react to your child as if the Old Wild Self is still in charge. My experience is that it can take a year or longer for most hyperactive children to undo their reputations, replace friendships, and revise expectations about their behavior. Your child must prove to others the hyperactivity will no longer occur by showing and telling them at the same time. Those claims must be matched with changed actions. Your child must *show* others the hyperactive behavior has stopped, not just *promise* it has stopped.

The direct undoing of the wake effect is very effective. If your child has difficulty with the method, talk individually with adults who regularly see your child. Explain the wake effect to them and tell them of the improvements that are occurring. Ask them to help undo the wake among your child's classmates and playmates.

One of the most useful general-purpose statements for your child to use to accomplish this goal is "I don't do that anymore." Instruct your child to say it whenever others are assuming that no changes have occurred. It is also useful when invited by peers to misbehave.

You can explain the wake effect and how to undo it to your child:

> Other people expect you to still act like the Old Wild Matt instead of the New Calm Matt. Even your teacher expects you to still be like Old Wild Matt. You need to convince them you are now the New Calm Matt. Tell them "I don't do that anymore" whenever they act as if they expect you to still be Old Wild Matt. You might want to say something else along with it, like "I would like to be your friend, and I don't do that anymore."

Getting realistic feedback from others, such as during a group counseling experience, can aid greatly in undoing the wake effect and giving your child the needed suggestions for refining social skills. Switching to a different classroom or school is also an option that opens new friendship possibilities if all else fails.

Learning the Six A's of Apology

A crucial part of your child's overcoming the wake effect is learning to backtrack successfully after an error or misbehavior has offended or hurt someone. Here is a simple-to-learn formula I have developed to guide ADHD children and adolescents to successfully undo their mistakes. It consists of six steps, each beginning with the letter *A*. The suggested wordings given here should be revised if necessary to fit your child's level of understanding.

1. ADMIT. Admit you did the act, and do so without telling lies about it first and without having to be asked. In other words, volunteer the information to the offended person.
2. ACCOUNT. Explain what you were trying to accomplish or what you were thinking at the time, even if you were just being careless and not thinking about it.
3. ACKNOWLEDGE. Indicate you are aware of the pain, hurt, or inconvenience the other person is feeling. Express the wish that you had not caused these hurtful things to happen, and that you are feeling bad because of the hurt you caused.
4. AFFIRM. Indicate you still want the person to be your friend, to like you, and to forgive you. Ask for the person's forgiveness. Affirm your desire to maintain or improve your relationship with the person.
5. AMENDS. Make amends by doing something to show

your desire to make up for the pain you have caused. Do a favor, bring a gift, do chores for the person, or invite the person to do something fun with you. Explain that you want to repay the person for the hurt you have caused.

6. ADJUST. Think about what you can do differently next time so that you won't repeat the mistake. Change something to prevent it from happening again.

Rehearse with your child and consider collapsing some of the points if giving all six steps is too cumbersome. Suggest a specific wording during the rehearsal, such as: "I'm sorry I did that. I still want to be your friend. Let me make it up to you. I would like to do this favor for you to show you I'm really sorry."

A begrudging, mumbled "I'm sorry" is not sufficient, nor is the false apology "*If* I lost your toy, I'm sorry."

Cultivating Friendship Skills

Your child does not learn social skills by pretending to be a hermit. Don't support attempts to reject other children. Instead, assist your child in rebuilding stressed relationships or developing new ones. The best way to accomplish these goals is to invite individual children as guests in your home for brief periods. Observe how they interact with you, your family, and your child. At the same time, notice your child's style of dealing with them. Guide her and her peers in selecting attractive activities such as a trip to a theater, amusement park, or zoo; dinner at a restaurant; table or video games; video movies; and snacks.

This method also encourages everyone to regard your home as the center for fun activities and opens the door for your continued monitoring of your child's relationships. Preparing light snacks is an additional form of involvement for your child in the exciting project of developing new friendships, gaining a sense of accomplishment, and becoming a special opportunity for companionship for you and your child. Remain nearby as your child plays with potential new friends and notice the general trends in the conversation and cooperation between the youngsters. Determine what your child does that creates problems in relating to other children.

Your child needs basic guidelines to cling to in various circumstances. Rely on simple rhyming or sequential self-reminders. Overstate and simplify principles rather than drawing fine distinctions or being too technical. I have developed the following list of friendship principles for those who have difficulty making friends:

- Talk to potential friends rather than remaining silent.
- Talk about what they want to talk about.
- Ask questions so they will talk to you.
- Do what they want to do.
- Smile.
- Exchange small gifts and favors.
- Show you understand how happy they are.
- Talk about the potential friend rather than yourself.
- Get them to talk about themselves.
- Invite them over and be a friendly host.
- Let guests have first choice of what topic to talk about, game to play, movie to watch, or food to eat.

Have your child write this list and then make a project of memorizing it. Post a typed version in her bedroom or near her study desk. Invite your child to carry a copy and look at it occasionally.

Emphasize honest ways of relating, being a true friend, and showing sincere interest in other children. You are not trying to train your child to be phony or political. Instead, you are training your child how to be genuinely kind—the essence of increasing your child's attractiveness as a candidate for friendship.

To win people over, the goal is to encourage people by interacting with them. Their lives should be enriched by coming in contact with your child. Teach your child to self-reveal at the same level that others are revealing, aiming for a mix between chitchat and intimacy.

Often relationship difficulties are a result of mistaken beliefs about people and feelings. If your child has an attitude that interferes with friendship building, describe a more constructive belief and demonstrate the logic behind it. For example, your child might purposely be brash and unkind out of a belief that other children would interpret kindness as weakness. Explain that being kind doesn't automatically lead to being victimized and then correct any mistaken understanding of strength as it relates to being a cooperative and helpful person: "If you are going to get along well with other people, you need to act in a way that makes them feel grateful and happy to be around you."

Two self-reminders are especially useful in helping the ADHD child who has an irritating tone of voice or who calls out inappropriately: "Zip my lip and I won't get into trouble" and "Tell them calmly what my problem is."

To increase harmonious play, teach two rules. The first is the 50/50 rule, which indicates that choices are to be distributed evenly. Suppose your child and another child are playing with a set of toy soldiers. To start the play session smoothly, both children obey the 50/50 rule: "You name your soldiers and I'll name my soldiers." Your child can also use this rule for determining what to play: "First let's play what you want, then we can play what I want."

The second is the freedom to stop rule. Neither child is to become angry or insist that the playmate remain, and is to cooperate in moving on to another activity. There are no attempts to control or coerce. Either child is free to depart at any time, and all participation is voluntary.

Point out noncritically anything your child is doing that leads to dissatisfaction among other children. Whenever you bring up a negative, offer a positive, such as a suggestion to help make things better next time.

Don't let your child become a couch potato. Look for activities and new skills to develop. Take advantage of common interests your child shares with other children. Lean toward activities in which your child wants to excel and the arena for accomplishment includes opportunities to expand friendships. Your child has much to offer. Many ADHD symptoms can be positively channeled. Your child's intensity, for example, can be focused on providing the zeal and determination to motivate others toward achieving goals.

Children sometimes engage in activities in which they must struggle too hard to keep pace with the others. Carefully select activities your child already does well and ones reasonably easy to master, especially if they are competitive. The local YWCA or YMCA, clubs, civic organizations, church youth groups, sports activities sponsored by community park and recreation departments, scouting, extracurricular school clubs and groups, exercise and dance classes, children's bowling leagues, and gymnastics and martial arts classes often offer activities geared to varying age and skill levels.

Help your child improve knowledge of the rules and strategies of the activities. Also consider helping your child improve any physical skills needed to participate successfully in the activities.

Show your child how to ask questions to discover areas of overlapping interest and experience with prospective new friends—how they spend time, where they have lived, interesting places they have visited, and hopes for the future. Teach your child to talk about what the other child wants to talk about. If a friend wants to talk about something unfamiliar, the conversation can become an interesting learning experience.

Teach your child how to strengthen friendships with genuine gratitude. Suggest specific wordings for giving sincere compliments without sounding phony or patronizing. Teach how to return favors and how to show appreciation by acts of kindness, gifts, and favors in addition to verbal thank you's. Sincerely expressed gratitude also prevents others from feeling they are being taken advantage of.

To improve listening skills, the simple technique of eye contact will help refine concentration and listening skills. Tell your child to look directly into the eyes of whoever is speaking.

Handling Conflicts

If a disagreement with another child occurs, ask how each combatant could have prevented the fight or could have reduced the amount of anger involved. Help your child anticipate some possible results of taking different approaches next time (always safe to talk about because it hasn't happened yet). Use the "what would happen next time if . . ." approach.

> Next time, what would happen if you stopped and thought about what else you could do? . . . Could you invite your friend over to our home? . . . Would you be willing to go with her to that place? . . . Would you say to him very clearly that you didn't want to play that game but would be willing to play some other game?

To deal with teasers, take the teaser and your child aside and treat the incident as an opportunity to teach some important facts to both children. If the teaser wants nothing to do with your child, then the teaser should be asked to leave. If the teaser is actually fishing for more contact, suggest better ways than harassment.

If a friend disagrees with your child, try to get your child to understand the other person's point of view. Using a standard phrase such as "You might have a point there" can often sidestep an argument. Point out that nobody wins an argument. A damaged friendship is much worse than an agreement to disagree peaceably.

Teach your child how to handle feedback or criticism from others in a way that allows the experience to result in personal improvement. Emphasize taking feedback seriously as a basis for making self-changes. If the feedback correctly identifies a negative trait, help your child overcome it so he can do better next time.

Handling Undesirable Friendships

If you have concerns about peer influence, study your child's friends, their interests, and their influence. Involve your child in other, new activities that exclude the less desirable peers or forbid any nonobligatory association with them.

If the choice of friends reflects poor judgment, encourage more wholesome relationships by offering potential new friends. Ask the teacher to plan activities that pair your child with children who are likely prospects for wholesome friendships. The school counselor might conduct group therapy or group discussion sessions that could include friendship skills and companion selection as topics.

Once you have established more wholesome peers as possible new friends, contrast the desirability of the two groups. Discuss the qualities of a good friend and compare both groups of peers against those standards. Don't force the issue, but plant the seeds so your child will consider standards for whom to befriend. State your intention not to try to stop any friendships, unless absolutely necessary, but that you want your child to consider these matters very carefully. The weekly PPI meeting discussed in Chapter 13 is an excellent time for this conversation.

Often children who have the least desirable influence on ADHD children come from poorly functioning families and need help themselves. Your child might be trying to rescue or be the only friend of an undesirable peer. In your discussion of the qualities of a good friend, your child might try to defend this friendship as a project. Gently set limits on the relationship. Insert yourself as a sieve between the two children, filtering and supervising the amount and type of contact they have with each other. You might want, for example, to confine contact to infrequent visits to your home, and only when you are present. Explain it is not your child's responsibility to solve any of his friend's family problems. Explain clearly your concerns about the undesirable influence the child might represent, but indicate your concerns do not mean you doubt your child's judgment or ability to resist temptation.

Several key steps can help you train your child in the skills needed to refuse invitations to mischief.

Lower the Attractiveness of Temptations. Start by making thoughts appear drab and senseless. By approaching them from a purely scientific, unemotional viewpoint, you deprive them of their validity and their impact on your child by first listing, then analyzing them.

Introduce the process as a special game you want to play.

> Let's play a special game of listing all of the ways those children have of trying to convince you to get into mischief. I know a couple of them to start our list. Then you help me add some more. "Everybody does it . . . you are chicken if you don't . . . we won't get caught . . . just this once would be okay . . . I did it so you have to do it too . . . if you were really my friend you'd do it . . . it will be fun . . . I won't do what you want me to do unless you do this for me . . . I dare you."

Continue helping your child list others; then explain each one of those approaches as a distortion intended to manipulate and to rob her of power and control over herself.

Provide Self-Reminding Statements. Point out statements to strengthen self-determination, such as:

> I will control me and not let others control me. . . . They are trying to control me—I won't let them. . . . Stop and think, what should I do now?. . . What would [Mom, Dad, Grandma, Grandpa, Mrs. Jones, Jesus] want me to do now? . . . If I do that, what will happen? [undesirable consequences]. . . If I refuse, what will happen?" [desirable consequences].

Practice Refusal Statements. Teach your child to say no, suggest a better idea, and quickly change the subject rather than debate the issue. Have your child practice saying no and stating refusals, such as:

> No thanks . . . not me . . . absolutely not . . . You can get into trouble if you want to, but not me . . . I don't want to . . . that's dumb . . . That's wrong and I won't do it . . . forget it . . . no way.

Magnify their impact by getting your child to use body language—head shaking and hand gestures—at the same time.

Emphasize the "Broken Record" Method. This assertion technique involves purposely not justifying or explaining the refusal to go along with a temptation. Your child simply repeats the refusal statement without elaborating. The entire conversation goes like this:

Peer: "Let's push over Mr. Brown's garbage can!"
Your child: "Nope; no way!"
Peer: "Aw, c'mon, what's the matter with you?"
Your child: "No way!"
Peer: "Why? Don't you want to have fun?"
Your child: "Not that way!"
Peer: "Then what would you like to do, chicken?"

Your child: "I'd rather play catch in our backyard. Let's go do that."
Peer: "Well, okay."

Invite a Once-and-for-All Decision. Your child has already made several once-and-for-all decisions—to eat rather than starve, to sleep at night, to perform routine acts without stopping to redecide each one. Simply invite some additional similar decisions. Ask your child to make a decision never to get into particular types of trouble and not to follow the lead of a certain troublesome peer. Don't push too hard with this technique, because you don't want to generate false promises.

Teach Your Child to Give Two No's, Then Leave. Your child needs to settle the matter by giving two refusal statements, then leaving the scene, which comes after the refusal, not before it. Staying and arguing with the peer leads to weakening and becoming persuaded or bullied into false promises.

By allowing experience uniquely suited to each of your children, you can reduce sibling rivalry. Giving brothers and sisters meaningful new roles to fulfill and minimizing competition in the family also help. By strengthening your child's social skills, teaching the six A's of apology, cultivating friendships, and guarding against undesirable peer influence, you can assure your child of new, more successful interpersonal relationships. Chapters 8 and 9 focus on the stresses the ADHD syndrome imposes on you and your marital relationship.

8

Understanding Your Own Feelings

As the parent of an ADHD child, you have the distinction of being a member of the most misunderstood, overburdened, and underhelped group in the world. The emotional stresses you face are beyond what most people can comprehend. They represent strange contortions and twistings of your psyche and clashes of basic sensibilities such as wanting to love and protect your child, yet feeling incredible rage against your child's behavior. This chapter details the typical reactions to the emotional stresses of having an ADHD child, particularly those experienced in the period prior to starting biochemical treatment.

THE EARLIEST EMOTIONAL STRESSES

Even before birth, the ADHD child can manage to stir up negative reactions in parents. The list of indicators during pregnancy and childbirth is enough to cause resentment, fatigue, and worry in the expectant parents. Hyperactivity in the womb keeps the mother-to-be awake at night, which makes the birth process all that much more taxing on her body. The numerous signs of disrupted body chemistry during infancy bring with them urgent demands for continual parental attention, which further drains both parents. The colicky, unsoothable baby creates physical and emotional stresses that often take months to unravel.

The key to emotional survival during the infancy of a severely symptomatic ADHD child is to arrange rest breaks and times away from the burdens of caring for the infant. Try rotating baby-care duties or get help from a relative, friend, or paid caregiver.

LATER EMOTIONAL STRESSES

The feelings many parents of ADHD children experience represent an emotional roller coaster. Typically, they appear in this approximate order, each step leading to the next:

1. Feeling misunderstood and criticized
2. Feeling guilty and inadequate
3. Feeling the need to serve and protect
4. Feeling angry
5. Feeling emotionally bankrupt

Feeling Misunderstood and Criticized

Prior to identifying the source of the child's difficulties, the parents are confronted by an army of outsiders who have advice about how to solve the many problems that are occurring. Teachers, in-laws, neighbors, friends, strangers, clergy, physicians, mental health professionals, and others offer suggestions that, when added together, are confusing as well as insulting. The two most prominent criticisms are that the child is not receiving enough love and that the child is not receiving enough discipline. If the parents would just shape up and give more love by not using such a harsh tone of voice and by being more patient, everything would be solved. Or if the parents would just stop letting the child get away with so much, stop being so inconsistent, and use firmer discipline, everything would be solved.

The parents understandably feel very alone and misunderstood, undersupported, and overcriticized. They soon become aware that others really don't understand what it is like to raise this child. One parent expressed this feeling to me in this way:

> If they could have my child at their home just one evening—even just one hour—they wouldn't say the things they've said to me about how I should be calmer and boys will be boys. I'd like to see how calm they'd be when he attacks their children, has tantrums when you make a reasonable request, turns off the TV when everyone is watching, and can't remember anything you tell him for longer than thirty seconds.

After diagnosis of ADHD, a new volley of criticisms can occur. Many people simply deny such a disorder exists. Others deny your child has it. Your uncovering of the correct diagnosis may be condemned and regarded as prejudicial labeling and scapegoating. You might be criticized for trying to explain away your own ineptness at showing proper love and discipline by blaming everything on a disorder in your child.

As if all of these attacks aren't enough, once you start biochemical treatment you open yet another source of complaints from outsiders. Some automatically equate the notion of prescribed medication with addicting your child to drugs, turning your child into a zombie, or training your child to become a future drug abuser. Others regard any interest in the Feingold Program as equivalent to a fad diet for health food fanatics.

It is important to have the facts straight and use correct terminology when talking with, as well as about, your child. Doing so will enable you better to fend off criticism, accurately inform others how they can help, and reassure your child.

React to these people as if they need more information —which indeed they do. If they genuinely want to help, give them more information, such as by referring them to relevant sections of this book. You are aware of the controversies surrounding diagnosis and treatment, have taken all of these considerations into account, and have decided on a treatment program for your child. Illustrate your awareness of the concern shown by the other person: "Thank you for your interest in my child's welfare. I know you mean well and have my child's best interest at heart. People have many different opinions. I am very aware of these issues and have thought them out already. The bottom line is that the best help for my child right now is to use this treatment."

Ask them to respect your stewardship over your child; then ask for whatever specific help you desire from them. Refuse to lose your self-respect over these comments. Observe the principle of pleasing yourself first rather than worrying about what others think. You know what you are doing. Accept comments based on knowledge, understanding, and empathy, but reject comments based on ignorance.

If others' objections seem compulsive, out-of-balance, and vindictive, their need is probably to attack you rather than learn more about how to help. You must be self-caring enough to insulate yourself against the sting of this criticism. Regard such criticism as coming from weakness, ignorance, or emotional need, but not from a reality-based exploration of the facts. Do not give any validity to what they are saying. Refuse to be surprised by these uninformed comments. Remember that they are not new, you have heard them before, and you will hear them dozens of times in the future. In this way you can drain the comments of some of their power. Calmly and quickly end the conversation.

In some cases a letter can convey your feelings more effectively than a conversation. Write a detailed letter to the critic, asking for understanding and for an end to his or her suggestions. To keep a friendly tone in the letter, you might also want to express appreciation for the person's concern. I have found this written confrontation usually does the trick for hard-to-convince critics.

Feeling Guilty and Inadequate

If the barrage of criticism takes hold, parents of ADHD children quickly sink into believing what their criticizers are saying. Sometimes this process is helped along by such circumstances as a poorly timed pregnancy, marital conflict or divorce, job stresses, frequent moves, or other disruptions in parenting functions. Feelings of failure, helplessness, and self-pity can evolve into a defensive anger against the child, for which the parents then feel guilty. The result is conflicting feelings of (1) intense resentment of the child; (2) guilt over that resentment; (3) an urge to protect, love, and help the child; and (4) guilt about not having been a caring parent. Though parents may not realize it, resentment and protectiveness are natural results of raising an ADHD child, and there is no need for guilt feelings.

The gripping tentacles of guilt are illustrated in one parent's confession in dealing with her 4-year-old prior to starting biochemical treatment.

> Each day is a giant struggle, and I pray for patience all the time. Every morning when I wake up I tell myself: "Today

> I will be calm and loving." And before I am through the morning, I've already failed.

It has been my privilege to provide many parents with the first mention of the ADHD diagnosis after a review of the child's and family's history, checklist results from home and school, and observation and interview of the child. There is a great lifting of the burden of guilt when a cause is finally recognized as the mechanism behind the child's troubles. The joy of a similar moment was captured by a mother who heard me discuss ADHD on a nationally broadcast interview.

> I had never imagined that hyperactivity might be our problem. I listened to the list of twenty-one behavioral characteristics of the hyperactive child and by the end of the list my mouth was open in shock. . . . Our son manifests *each* of the twenty-one. At last, to know what it is that we're dealing with, it's such a relief! It has helped to ease the guilt that I'd heaped on myself and has given me determination to deal with the behavior in a constructive way.

Of course, every parent who suspects ADHD should seek an appropriate professional diagnosis rather than relying on media shows and a checklist. The feeling of relief this mother expressed, however, is typical of that experienced by parents of ADHD children when the diagnosis is finally established.

It is natural to feel overwhelmed by such a potent force as ADHD. The fact that you may at times feel inadequate to the task says nothing about your abilities as a parent, except that you are not superhuman.

The failure to receive affirmation of your parenting skills can make things worse. Hyperactive children are poor at showing appreciation. It is easy to perceive any child who is disobedient or inconsiderate as a reflection of poor parenting. If you have at least one non-ADHD child, notice that child's strengths, cooperativeness, and ability to give and receive love. Such qualities are proof of your effectiveness as a parent. Reassure yourself by your success with that child and put the cause of the hyperactivity where it belongs.

A common difficulty in any intense emotional relationship between two persons is a tendency to be blinded by negative feelings of anger and resentment. The positive feelings of love and caring then seem to disappear. Once a solid love bond with your child is formed, it is permanent and indestructible, despite the development of some negative feelings. This ambivalence is perfectly normal, especially in such an intense and potentially conflict-laden relationship. Accept that fact and free yourself to feel occasional resentment, without guilt, toward the disruptions caused by your child's disorder.

Feeling the Need to Serve and Protect

Partly in an attempt to compensate for guilt feelings and partly out of a realistic concern for the child's difficulties, parents of ADHD children often attempt to run interference. They become overinvolved in the child's life and physically and emotionally drained. This overinvolvement reflects too tight a meshing of the parents' efforts with the child's life. Brothers and sisters witness this seemingly excessive service, devotion, love, time, energy, and concern, and they feel a need to counterbalance. The result can be disastrous for all concerned.

Five types of overinvolvement often develop between parents and their ADHD children.

Overprotecting. The child's lack of caution spurs parents to become overly watchful for potential dangers. Fearing that bad or overwhelming things might happen to the child, they overprotect the child from potential danger or unkind remarks. The parents feel a need to intervene so that no misfortunes occur, and they develop the habit of automatically defending the child. This tendency is reflected clearly in the comments of one mother of an ADHD boy.

> I know I am way overprotective and I do take up for Kevin. But if I don't stand up for him, who will? When he was younger, before being diagnosed hyperactive, I was afraid to answer the phone or door for fear of what Kevin has done now.

When parents place restrictions such as "Don't climb the ladder; you might fall off"; or "Don't go outside without a jacket, you might catch a cold," they rob their child of the opportunity to learn how to cope with difficulty or responsibility. They also reinforce their own doubts about the child's ability to cope. The child, furthermore, becomes discouraged and convinced that life is overly difficult. Certain every situation is full of danger or defeat, the child becomes able to cope with only the mildest challenges. Eventually the child shrinks from almost any circumstances that involve unknowns or risks and becomes a prisoner of fears.

NAGGING. Research has indicated that, in contrast to mothers of non-ADHD children, mothers of hyperactive children are more likely, particularly on difficult tasks, to provide direction, supervision, and structure. They have learned well that ADHD children require such assistance, but the tendency may be to overdo it somewhat. Research has shown (thankfully for mothers' self-esteem) that these maternal controlling behaviors are clearly the result of a need for them and are the reaction to their children's noncompliant behavior.

Nagging is probably the most common error made by parents of children in general and of ADHD children in particular. The child's lack of diligence—combined with a short memory for verbal messages—leads parents into issuing an endless string of directives, reminders, commands, and suggestions. They gradually lose trust in the child's ability to do anything without being nagged about it. As the nagging increases, the child becomes sloppier, slower, and more forgetful, thereby giving parents further reasons to nag. This cycle continues until parents are constantly giving the same message to obtain cooperation on just about everything. My worst case of this nag cycle involved the mother of a 7-year-old hyperactive boy who claimed that, on the average, she repeated each request or command seventeen times before her child would respond!

Spoiling. Overindulging the child means trying to shield the child from every frustration. The parents give excessive service and attention to the child and end up doing many things the child ought to be able to accomplish independently. One father indicated this tendency to spoil with this motto: "You just breathe; I'll do all the rest for you!" If patronized and overindulged, children become increasingly demanding.

Pitying. The misfortunes of the hyperactive child can remind guilt-ridden parents of their own self-assumed responsibility for having created or worsened the child's problems. A common mistake is to pity the child by overly sympathizing rather than showing strong caring and concern. An example is allowing little violations of medication treatment or the Feingold Program, which end up only harming the child in the long run.

Babying. Running interference is sometimes necessary in raising a hyperactive child, but when it is carried too far, the child remains ignorant, relatively helpless, and poor at social and academic skills. The net result, for example, of parents' doing the child's homework for him is that he doesn't learn good study habits or gain needed academic knowledge. In response to their need to overprotect and serve the child, the parents perform so diligently that the child can also fail to develop ordinary social skills. If the child has a tantrum, his demand is fulfilled by the exhausted, guilt-ridden parents. Robbed of the opportunity to develop coping skills by struggling with age-appropriate challenges, the child remains socially and emotionally immature. Overprotected, overindulged, nagged, spoiled, and pitied, the child has little choice but to think of the world as a totally overwhelming place that requires the constant service of adults to insulate her from its demands.

Feeling Angry

Anger can be one of the most difficult and potentially destructive emotions within a family. It can be understood as an emotional defense against stress from outside sources, including the unfairness of others. It can be used in a controlled, manipulative fashion; people are not at the mercy of anger but are, instead, the creators of their own anger. Seething anger and resentment, which in some cases build up to tremendous proportions, are quite common among parents of hyperactive children, because of the emotional and physical stress they experience.

One source of emotional stress is coping with conflict among the children in the family. Parents may find themselves faced with the almost impossible choice of defending the hyperactive child against an angry sibling. The sibling may assert that the parents are unjust and unfair and become angry with them and the hyperactive brother or sister (see Chapter 7).

Parents may discover they cannot be alone as a couple without interruption and pressure from their hyperactive child. They may have their periods of renewal and relaxation hampered or even ruined. They may feel like his prisoners, obliged to supervise him constantly, and unable to leave him alone for fear of what might happen. Over the years they may grow to resent their lack of personal space, a condition caused by the child's hyperactive behavior.

They may need to walk on eggs because the child's emotions are extreme and unpredictable. They may be embarrassed in public, hesitant to entertain visitors when the child is home, and angered because she prevents them from presenting a good appearance to the world.

They might feel manipulated and used by the child. They may defend the child in public in a certain situation, only to discover that he suddenly acts calm and orderly, making their concern appear foolish and excessive.

Most parents of a hyperactive child sense an invisible psychological wall or barrier between the child and others, including themselves. They are aware of never having truly made contact with the child in the sense of closeness of spirit or emotional intimacy. Parents can become angry about this barrier.

Parents' anger is perhaps most easily aroused when the hyperactive child flagrantly and defiantly refuses to cooperate with their requests and rejects their leadership. They may feel a strong need to bolster their position and defend themselves against the child's rebelliousness by angrily forcing the issue.

Parental anger can be handled in many different ways. Much of it may never be directly expressed. That which is expressed may be aimed at the physician or counselor or teacher, at the child, or even at God with the question Why me? Anger directed inward can turn into self-pity, self-criticism, or depression or trigger various emotional and physical ailments.

Don't pin the responsibility for your anger on any external source, including your hyperactive child. Your child does not make you angry, any more than someone whom you love makes you be in love with him. Instead, realize that you create your own anger. "I'm getting angry as I listen to you talk" is a much more accurate statement than "You are making me angry by what you are saying." Accepting that the source of your anger is within you brings it within your grasp and potentially under your control.

Understand that anger is a secondary reaction to an earlier, primary emotion that involves some perceived hurt or stress. Although it is possible to focus on trying to decrease your anger, it is generally more efficient to focus on decreasing the primary hurt. It is basically much easier to deal with primary hurts than with their secondary offshoots.

Embarrassment, like anger, is reflexive; we make ourselves feel embarrassed. If you become embarrassed when your hyperactive child misbehaves in public, realize that your primary emotion is embarrassment, not anger. Then focus on taking action to prevent the embarrassment rather than trying to prevent the anger. You might, for example, remind yourself that your embarrassment is needless and perhaps excessive. Remember that it is the child and not you who is creating the scene, and that not getting upset is more important than what a handful of strangers may think about you as a parent.

Differentiate between the child and the child's behavior: the hyperactivity, not your child, is the culprit. If your child had the measles, you would be loving toward him or her and would hate to see the red spots and the other signs of the disease. You would be able to say, "I love you, and I hate your illness." In the same way, the hyperactivity can be considered the equivalent of ugly red spots that you as a parent don't like and, in fact, may learn to hate. Understand that the source of your primary hurt is the hyperactivity, not your child.

Your anger may sometimes be directed at yourself for not being able to deal more effectively with your child, as much as it is toward the child. Try to become more aware of the times in which you sound as if you are angry only at your child but actually are also angry at yourself. Once you have separated the two types of anger, you can dispose of them in separate maneuvers, starting with the inward-directed anger. "I'm frustrated because I don't know what to do" is more accurate than "You are frustrating me."

Remind yourself that everyone has problems in life. There is no particular injustice in the fact that you are facing the problem of hyperactivity. Don't stop to ask fruitless questions about the justice of it all. The answer to "How could this happen to me?" is "Very easily, because it *is* happening!"

Lessen stresses by stopping them early. Set limits calmly and firmly. Make a clear, simple statement that the child is crossing your boundaries and that you want her to stop immediately. Back up your brief statement with a dramatic, firm, silent action that indicates your intention not to allow her aggravating behavior to continue. The limit-setting action should be a logical consequence or restructuring technique as described in Chapter 13.

Feeling Emotionally Bankrupt

The parents of a hyperactive child often end up feeling completely defeated, drained, and at the end of their rope. They may have been faced with the medical stresses, feelings of guilt and inadequacy, and the emotional exhaustion of overinvolvement in efforts to save the child from impossible situations. They may have had endless worries, a flood of unanswerable questions about the child's future adjustment, and a welling up of deep-seated anger and resentment toward the child. There may have been disruption in the family, bombardment with destructive criticisms from outsiders, and a barrier between themselves and the child.

The parents may feel as if they are trying to put sixty jigsaw puzzle pieces together to make a picture that requires only fifty. Every time they make a move in one direction to get something to fit, some other situation needing their attention pops up. Needs become stacked up against needs, so that meeting one results in others' going unmet. Their daily lives may become an endless struggle for peace, quiet, and calmness for themselves and their family.

Emotional bankruptcy occurs when the parents realize no ordinary change in parenting technique will prevent the problems the hyperactivity creates. Treating the hyperactive child just like other children does not solve matters. Using ordinary techniques for showing love, techniques that the parents had learned to rely on with their other children, proves ineffectual. Relying on ordinary sources and standards for child rearing, such as how their friends handle their children, or what their parents did in raising them, does not work. Punishments that are dramatic and even overwhelming for other children often have no effect when applied to a hyperactive child. Spanking may bring out more intense defiance or send the child into a frenzy. There may seem to be nothing left but to yell and scream, but yelling and screaming do not solve anything. The parents try everything and find that nothing works. They then feel guilty because they know that yelling and constant punishment serve only to make everything worse. There may be "How many times do I have to tell you?" lectures, coupled with endless nagging. They then become as angry with themselves as with the child.

A sure sign emotional bankruptcy has been declared is the parents' sense of defeat and the almost complete lack of any positive or loving communication between the parents and the hyperactive child. The result is that the parents run out of options, give up, and start to feel defeated and depressed.

Feeling robbed of tools, techniques, options, and energy, parents may conclude there is no way out of the situation. One parent may then react by trying to dump parental responsibility onto the other parent or to legally remove the child from the home.

There may be a great sense of personal relief whenever the parent is separated from the child. Neglect and abandonment of the child can sometimes occur. The parents may stop trying to exert any influence on the child, expressing their sense of helplessness with a "What's the use" attitude.

A tragic reaction at this stage is child abuse. Hyperactive children are overrepresented among the victims of all types of child abuse: verbal, emotional, physical, and sexual. The likelihood that a hyperactive child will be abused increases if one or both parents is hyperactive, has a character disorder, or abuses drugs or alcohol.

Verbal abuse includes excessive bossing, criticizing, swearing at the child, name-calling, use of sarcasm, threatening, insulting, belittling, yelling, dwelling on weaknesses and failures, unfavorable comparisons to other children, and undermining his sense of worth and humanness.

Emotional abuse includes withholding love. Many parents relay nonloving messages verbally. When these nonloving messages are also reinforced by acts of rejection, they constitute emotional abuse. The parent who will not do favors for the child, who avoids affectionate touching of the child, who is spiteful toward the child, who does not provide gifts for the child when gift-giving is expected within the family, who overreacts to the child's actions on some occasions and underreacts to identical actions on other occasions, or who gives the child "I hate you" messages is committing emotional abuse.

Physical abuse includes hitting, slapping, strapping, kicking, hair pulling, throwing, biting, shoving, burning, spraying, shaking, excessive twirling, excessive tickling, or excessive spanking. More extreme and bizarre forms of physical abuse include forcing the child to eat or drink foreign substances, stabbing the child with pins, putting the child in bath water that is too hot, and similar acts of brutality.

Sexual abuse includes forcing, tricking, or persuading the child to witness or participate in sexual activity. Hyperactive children are also overrepresented among sexual offenders to other children. Not only are they more likely to be molested, but they are also more likely to molest than non-ADHD children.

All the actions listed here are not always abusive. They become abusive when they are nonaccidental, excessively frequent or severe, or have a destructive effect on the child. For example, almost every parent feels the urge at times to spank or slap the child. When these impulses become excessive and sadistic, they constitute child abuse.

If you are at the end of your rope, you need to separate yourself not only from the child but also from the routine surroundings in which you relate to the child. Take a vacation; relax for a couple of days, either alone or with a friend, relative, or your spouse. You need to regain your sense of emotional balance and self-respect as well as your inner calmness and sense of personal strength.

It is much easier to *prevent* emotional bankruptcy than to get rid of it once it has started. Try to learn to surrender your need to control the child's behavior. When you have less investment in making the child act differently, the child will have less need to prove to you that you can't do it. There is only one person in the world whom you can control, and that person is yourself. Emphasize controlling yourself and your own emotional reactions to the child's behavior, rather than controlling the child.

Eliminating the feeling of desperation and returning to a calm and productive way of dealing with your hyperactive child is next to impossible to do by yourself. Seek professional counseling if emotional bankruptcy is occurring.

REDUCING OVERINVOLVEMENT

To reduce overinvolvement, encourage your child's efforts. Strength comes from practice and from accepting life's challenges. Be grateful for each step taken toward mastery and competence. Be concerned and involved, but don't overdo it. Avoid the extremes of little concern and involvement on the one hand, and overconcern and over-involvement on the other. Give help without excessive service. Reduce stresses without taking away your child's opportunities to learn to face challenging situations.

Refuse to be tricked into guilt-motivated servitude to your child. If you are already overinvolved, your child may want to perpetuate the situation with invitations designed to remind you of your own guilt feelings: "If you were nicer, you would do this for me. . . ." Be alert to manipulation and do the opposite.

Avoid the "I can do it faster and easier" trap. Your child can learn far more by being unsuccessful at completely mastering a difficult situation than by simply watching you master it. Your child cannot learn to swim by sitting on the shore and watching you swim.

Concentrate on reducing the number of verbal directives you give, putting the emphasis instead on setting up the structure and routines to support what you want your child to do. This procedure is given in detail in Chapter 13.

The key to regaining your emotional composure about your child's behavior is to keep the condition's effects as minimal as possible. Follow through with biochemical treatment, if it is indicated, and practice the additional psychosocial helps outlined in this book. Don't be afraid to obtain the services of a skilled therapist or counselor for your own sake and that of your family. Professional assistance in unblocking your built-up feelings through counseling or psychotherapy will be a beneficial and wise investment of your time and energy. Be determined not to let negative emotional responses sabotage your efforts to make life work for your child, for you, and for your family.

9

Coping During Marital Stress

Your marriage is the foundation of all other relationships in your family. It sets the tone for the ways in which your children will relate to each other, and your behavior helps determine how your children relate to the two of you. Much of your impact is created by the example you set. The ways you settle conflicts with each other, express affection toward each other, handle difficulties together, and talk with each other teach your children important lessons. Therefore, the state of your marriage must be given the highest priority. One of the greatest gifts a child can ever receive is happily married parents.

Hyperactivity can be a dangerous threat to any marriage. It usually exerts a heavy stress in many ways. Each parent undergoes various emotional stresses in trying to deal with the child's hyperactivity. Meanwhile, the two parents must continue to deal with each other. The constant change in both persons, caused in part by reactions to the child's hyperactivity, puts additional strain on the marital relationship. You and your spouse may have very different reactions to the same stressful situation. You will have to adjust to your spouse's reactions in addition to adjusting to your child.

As a couple, you have all of the responsibility for the usual tasks of parenting: family nest-building, homemaking, and maintaining a calm, affectionate marital relationship. In addition, you must deal with your child's hyperactivity, resolve the differences between your reactions to your child, and deal with the various stresses on any siblings.

RECOGNIZING DESTRUCTIVE MARITAL PATTERNS

Twelve common marital destructive patterns often result from hyperactivity. Not all of these patterns will occur in any one marriage, and additional patterns may occur in some marriages.

Though reading this section may be discouraging or even frightening at first, it is important to be aware of the potential pitfalls that can and do happen. Many situations evolve so slowly the husband and wife do not realize the patterns are developing. Few parents would intentionally create these situations to disrupt their marriages, but they occur in a strikingly high proportion among parents of hyperactive children.

Partial Denial

In the partial denial pattern, one spouse denies the hyperactivity while the other recognizes and correctly labels it as hyperactivity. The spouse who recognizes the hyperactivity may be criticized by the denying spouse as being too emotional or overprotective of the child. The denying spouse clings blindly to the belief that nothing is wrong with the child.

Joint Denial

The second parent joins the first in denying the existence of hyperactivity and both parents are left with inadequate and self-defeating explanations for the child's bizarre behavior. Their methods of dealing with the child are likely to be equally inappropriate and destructive. Never recognizing what they are dealing with, they remain ill-equipped to help the child, whose behavior becomes increasingly out of control as time goes on.

Partial Abuse

This pattern occurs when one parent becomes abusive. The abusing parent may blackmail the other parent by threatening to cease all parental functions if the nonabusive parent complains about the abuse. Not wanting to assume the entire burden of raising the child, the nonabusive parent stops criticizing the abusive parent, who continues to abuse the child. Sometimes the nonabusive parent will not reveal the child's misbehavior to the abusive parent to protect the child from the abusive parent's temper. Other reactions of the nonabusive parent include assuming most or all of the parental duties, becoming overinvolved with the child, and reminding the abusive parent in holier-than-thou fashion: "*I* don't abuse the child the way *you* do."

Joint Abuse

Both parents abuse the child verbally, emotionally, or physically. The second parent's response to the first parent's abusiveness is to join in the abuse, thus both justifying and denying the abuse. Couples who indulge in child abuse usually manage to find reasons for continuing their actions. When the abuse comes to the attention of social agencies, such couples often move out of the area rather than face the risk of losing their children. A large number of abused children are, in fact, hyperactive.

Partial Overinvolvement

One parent becomes overinvolved with the hyperactive child. This parent develops a habit of running interference to the point of overprotecting, nagging, spoiling, pitying, or babying the child. The other parent often wants to correct the situation, and the resulting conflict puts additional strain on the marriage. The second parent might react by overcompensating in the opposite direction and therefore becoming somewhat abusive toward the child, or playing one-upmanship.

Joint Overinvolvement

Both parents become overinvolved and overprotect, spoil, nag, pity, or baby the hyperactive child. The result is a demanding child who is unprepared to meet the challenges of life and who is catered to continually by two exhausted and guilt-ridden parents.

Partial Emotional Bankruptcy

In this pattern, one parent declares emotional bankruptcy, forcing the other parent to assume the total burden of parental responsibility. In this one-sided situation, the parent with the entire burden may start to feel angry and resentful toward the bankrupt parent and the hyperactive child. The bankrupt parent may feel guilty for creating such a lopsided situation but may also be quick to justify his or her actions by blaming everything on the hyperactive child with an "If it weren't for that child!" attitude.

Joint Emotional Bankruptcy

Sometimes both parents declare emotional bankruptcy. The second parent responds to the first parent's bankruptcy, and they attempt to unload their parental responsibility onto an external source by trying to give the child away, abandon the child, or offer the child to a social agency. If the child remains in the home, there may be gross physical and emotional neglect.

Another aspect of this pattern is that both parents become too dependent on outside help for advice. They gradually stop making their own decisions and thus slowly surrender their leadership function within the family.

Partial One-Upmanship

The second parent criticizes the first parent and eventually feels self-righteous and superior. The first parent feels misunderstood and senses a lack of empathy from the second parent. The second parent seems not to understand the stress that the first parent is experiencing in trying to deal with the hyperactive child.

Both parents allow the primary burden of child rearing to fall on the first parent, who suffers not only from the burden of dealing with the child but also from the critical attacks of the second parent. The second parent typically claims everything would be all right if only the first parent would change.

The second parent gains a sense of superiority by trying to label the first parent inferior, inept, uncaring, ignorant, weak, or sick. The second parent's motive is to avoid focusing on his or her own inadequacy by keeping the spotlight on the alleged shortcomings of the first parent. Meanwhile the first parent is kept weak by the second parent's efforts to undermine any improvement the first parent tries to make.

The first parent is often overburdened. The parent who is in the one-up position is, in fact, more at ease with the child, partly because he or she is also underinvolved in the day-to-day raising of the child. This parent can announce self-righteously that he or she knows how to handle the hyperactive child and does not have so much difficulty as the first parent.

The parent who is in the one-up position can destroy the other parent's efforts by not showing empathy for the spouse's emotional stresses. The one-up parent may criticize the first parent for always wanting to prove that the child is defective. The one-up parent may not support the first parent's attempts to learn about hyperactivity or parenting skills and may scold the first parent for seeking professional counseling. The second parent might disguise these destructive actions by claiming the first parent ought to be able to handle the child without outside help, without taking breaks, and without trying to attach a label to the child.

Mutual One-Upmanship

When the first parent counterattacks after being criticized by the second parent, the two parents are then unable to negotiate mutual decisions about child rearing. They struggle for prestige and status, each attempting to feel superior to the other. Each wants to pin the blame and the responsibility for their child rearing difficulties onto the other. Each considers the other weak, incompetent, abusive, and unfit. Both assert that everything would be all right if only the *other* parent would change. Sometimes they vie for the one-up position. If the first parent goes for professional counseling, for example, he or she may criticize the other parent for not being mature enough to accept counseling, while the other parent criticizes the first parent for being weak.

Sometimes the parents will weaken each other's position when one puts the other into a stress situation that he or she cannot cope with, then scoffs at the resulting incompetence and inefficiency. If this pattern continues and develops, it can easily end in divorce.

Divided and Conquered

Primarily through lack of communication, the parents can be deceived by the child's manipulations. As a result, the situation deteriorates to the point where the child needs to deal with only one parent, rather than both. Thus, the parents are first divided, then conquered, by the child.

The child may have become adept at using deceit to play one parent against the other. The child may find the "softy" and ask him or her for permission to do things he knows the other parent would not allow. Another common manipulation occurs when the child, after being denied permission for something from the first parent, tells the second parent the first parent has granted permission if the second parent agrees; or the child, after rceiving a noncommital answer from the first parent, tells the second parent the first parent has given permission.

The child may keep pestering one parent until the parent gives in to end the harassment. Like a bulldozer, the child keeps driving forward, pushing everything, including the parent's resistance, out of her way to get what she wants. The child does not go from one parent to the other in this case, but bullies either parent into changing no to yes.

Hyperactive children are particularly good at bulldozing. They learn if they nag and yell all day, the parent will be worn out and they will get their way. The result is that the child resorts to bulldozing and badgering for great lengths of time, knowing that eventually the parent will wear down and surrender.

The child may bully by threatening to create an uproar. The child promises he will torment the parents with endless pestering or tantrums. To the parent who likes peace and quiet, it is easier to give in to the child than to face a tantrum.

The child may also bully by threatening the parent with physical assault, by destroying property, or by hurting others. The child may defy the parent and dare him or her to use disciplinary techniques. As a power ploy, the child may goad the parent in a "Go ahead, see if I care!" fashion.

Often the child does not have to announce her blackmail weapon. The parents may already know it exists and may apply it to themselves with little or no provocation from the child. The parents may tell themselves: "If I don't give in, she will (destroy my things, scratch the paint on the car, attack her sister, steal it if I don't buy it for her, and so on)."

Sometimes the child's manipulation involves taking unfair advantage of a conflict that already exists. If the parents cannot agree on a child's allowance, for example, the child will approach the more generous parent for money. A variation of this type of manipulation occurs when the child starts fights and arguments between his parents after he has obtained what he wants.

Overcompensation

The excess of one parental trait in the first parent is responded to by the second parent, who develops too much of the opposite trait. The patronizing parent, for example, feels no license to be firm with the hyperactive child, because the other parent is already too harsh toward the child.

The crucial factor is not that the two parents differ in their preferred amount of softness or hardness toward the child; it is the increase in the severity of their approaches. Instead of being pulled together, the parents drive themselves farther and farther apart. The patronizing parent, for example, becomes increasingly patronizing and avoids all strictness, while the strict parent feels no license to give in because the child is already being excessively given in to by the patronizing parent. Each time the child is treated softly, the firm parent will become more firm; each time the child is treated firmly, the soft parent will become more soft.

At any specific moment, the child is treated either too firmly or too softly, depending on which of the two parents is more in control of the situation at the time. Either parent can become the too-harsh one, depending on whether dad's tools or mom's cosmetics are the targets of the child's antics.

Combinations of Patterns

These twelve destructive marital patterns can often evolve in sequence from, for example, emotional bankruptcy to divided and conquered. In this development, the bankrupt parent becomes the target of the hyperactive child's bulldozing manipulations and the child can then get his way with little or no resistance from the parent.

A particularly dangerous but common sequence is a progression from one-upmanship to mutual one-upmanship to overcompensation. Slight differences in approach toward the hyperactive child become magnified. The parents attack each other for their differing approaches. Finally, they try to outdo each other by becoming more polarized and more extreme in their respective ways of dealing with the child.

Several of these twelve patterns can occur at the same time. For example, an abusive parent and the over-involved spouse can argue about the faults of each other in mutual one-up fashion, while the hyperactive child divides and conquers them by bulldozing the overinvolved parent.

OVERCOMING DESTRUCTIVE PATTERNS

The first step in dealing with these stresses and the destructive marital patterns that can result from them is to recognize them. Spot the patterns that seem most likely to develop in your own marriage. Awareness opens the door to reversing these trends. Without awareness, there is no chance for an effective solution.

The greater the amount of stress in your marriage, and the more these patterns have developed, the greater the need for activities that strengthen your marriage. Regardless of how pressured or discouraging the situation is, there is always hope for improvement as long as you are aware of what is occurring.

Hunt for the Good

Don't allow the hyperactivity to dominate your family. Identify and emphasize all the positive aspects of your family. Help your spouse appreciate all family members. Although your glass may seem half empty, remember that it is also half full.

Don't Expect a Perfect Solution

Realize and accept that there is no perfect answer to the many difficulties your family experiences. Part of the risk and responsibility of life is finding the best available method to adopt in any specific situation. None of the available methods will be perfect.

Seek Constant Improvement

The more confident you are as parents, the more easily you will respond to the stresses of your child's hyperactivity. Everything you can do to increase your parental skills and knowledge will help.

In addition to improving your parental skills, improve your marital skills. Study and learn as much as possible about your relationship. Attend workshops, seminars, classes, retreats, and similar programs that focus on marriage enrichment, and read instructive materials.

Sometimes it is best to seek assistance from a mental health professional who is knowledgeable in family relationships and hyperactivity.

Defend Against Outside Criticism

One mother of a hyperactive child expressed her thoughts this way: "Negative responses are like negative fields of energy—they can't do any harm if they remain grounded. I try to latch on to all the positives—friends who are understanding, a success for my child, realizing nobody is to blame when I know I have tried my hardest. If people criticize my parenting, I have begun to realize that this is *their* problem; it has nothing to do with me."

Acknowledge Your Anger

Discuss your anger and criticisms with your spouse and urge your spouse to do the same with you. The use of anger as a weapon will decrease when you both can frankly acknowledge it is self-generated.

Recognize Your Child's Manipulations

Notice your child's attempt to play one parent against the other. Does she bulldoze one parent? Does she find the weak spots because the two parents differ about whether or not she should be allowed to do certain things? Does she hide behind the softy and push for all she can get? Bring your child's manipulations to the forefront and deal with them as misbehavior.

Consider the events that occurred just before you entered the situation. Before criticizing your spouse, be willing to consider an instant replay of the preceding moments. Find out what happened with the child and with your spouse during these moments.

Avoid Overinvolvement

Avoid running interference between your child and others. Let others deal directly with your child. Stand united as a couple *behind* your child, not protectively in front of your child.

Accept Differences in Approach

Accept the fact that you are both trying to do what is best for the child. Even if your approach to a particular situation is different from your spouse's, support the spouse's effort. There are usually a number of ways to handle a conflict situation, and your method may not be the only effective one.

Rise above mutual criticism. Don't try to pin blame on each other. Deal with the specifics of the situation in a spirit of mutual respect and acceptance. There is nothing wrong in your spouse's being different from you, so don't attack or blame your spouse for being different.

The important question in each situation is "What is the best type of parenting for the child now?" rather than "Who is the better parent?"

Switch Parental Duties

To aid your understanding of how your spouse feels, exchange roles for at least one full day. This measure is especially useful when one parent is near the point of having to declare emotional bankruptcy. The spouse can take over while the overstressed parent receives much-needed relief from the constant pressures of dealing with the hyperactive child. Switching duties is a cooperative adventure; it must never be done with resentment or as part of one-upmanship.

Be Willing to Negotiate

Be flexible. Be willing to listen to new ideas and to the wisdom of your spouse. Remaining blindly rigid is the beginning of many destructive marital patterns. When one parent loses flexibility, the other parent may overcompensate in the opposite direction, or fall into a one-up pattern of bitter argument toward the inflexible parent. Adhering to inefficient techniques forces the other parent to go to extremes to start good disciplinary methods again. Sometimes these extremes are worse than the original techniques, because they create resentment between the parents. Try to come to a mutually negotiated agreement, especially in a disciplinary situation.

Use the Co-Parenting Technique

The principle of co-parenting is one of the most useful tools for preventing destructive marital patterns. Co-parenting means simply checking with each other before giving an answer to the child's request. The answer is a mutually agreed-upon solution, developed by quick negotiation between both parents.

The negotiation should take place immediately, and it should be in private, away from the child. If you cannot arrange to discuss the matter immediately, arrange a time of day as a deadline for giving the child an answer.

Co-parenting allows both parents to naturally and constructively balance each other. It welds the two parental styles: parents become less extreme, less one-sided, and more flexible in coping with the total needs of the situation. The softy, for example, can help the firmer parent's point of view and can learn some reasons for being less soft and more firm. The firm parent, at the same time, can hear reasons for being less firm and more flexible.

Co-parenting protects each parent from being canceled out by the child's manipulations. The child faces two parents, not one. The parents have arrived at a unified decision through cooperation and negotiation. Playing one parent against the other is now impossible for the child.

Not all decisions need to be co-parented. Discuss with each other ahead of time those areas that can be decided individually. Save for co-parenting only the situations in which the child is likely to try to manipulate.

Arrange for Time Away

Being a twenty-four-hour-a-day, seven-day-a-week parent of a hyperactive child is an emotional impossibility. Allow various breaks—rest breaks, vacations, nights out, and similar opportunities to relieve the intensity of the relationship between the hyperactive child and the parents. Parents who are homebound with a hyperactive child day in and day out run a risk of becoming depressed and emotionally bankrupt.

Take time for individual pursuits. Visit friends, develop a hobby, or become active in church or community work. Every person needs time alone in which to think peacefully and to enjoy a pleasant, restful activity.

A crucial type of time away is time away together. At least once each week, spend a few hours with your spouse in an enjoyable activity. Time together helps uphold and sustain the romantic, nurturing part of your marital relationship. Unless you make sure this special time is reserved during your weekly schedule, it can easily slip away. Nurturing activities will then be doubly needed, and your efforts will be toward making up for lost time rather than toward moving your relationship forward. Do not worry about leaving the children at home for these few hours. It is far better to have your children under the care of a sitter for a few hours each week than to have them in the hands of overstressed, overcompensating, emotionally exhausted parents who have no opportunity to strengthen their love for each other.

The importance of time away cannot be overemphasized. If you do not build in enough of it, the times when you and your spouse are together might be usurped by the practical but non-nurturing decisions that are always a part of the responsibility of leading a family.

The quality of time spent together is very important. Try to have a relaxing and intimate talk, along with periods of recreational activity. If you go to a theater, talk about the program at intermission or afterward. The most crucial part of time together is the sharing of feelings in a romantic, mutually affectionate, and accepting spirit. Time spent together without talking with each other is not as productive as time spent in open communication. The choice of a restaurant, for example, is not as important as the quality of the conversation while dining.

Have Regular Business Meetings

Your family pivots on your marital relationship, and your marital relationship pivots on your love for each other, which must be nurtured by romance and companionship. Having regular business meetings allows you to reserve your weekly private time together for its intended purpose—romance, not problem solving.

At regular intervals discuss with your spouse the routine problems and make the routine decisions that are a necessary part of family leadership. Decisions about time schedules, meals, shopping, home improvements, and dozens of other matters have to be made almost daily. Keep such matters in the regular business meeting, where they belong.

REBUILDING HARMONY IN YOUR FAMILY

As you become more proficient at overcoming destructive patterns and strengthening your marriage, family harmony improves. Love and discipline are the twin bases for effective leadership and harmony. If there is too much or too little for each child, the family relationships become strained and children's misbehavior increases.

Of the two, love is the primary need. It is the rock on which sound discipline must rest. Without love, discipline can be unauthentic and uncontrolled to the point of child abuse. The most successful method of restoring harmony in your family is to provide judicious, balanced discipline as well as genuine love to all of the children. Effective parents are very firm *and* very loving.

Rebuilding Family Harmony Through Increased Love

As your child's behavior changes and improves, your approach, and that of relatives, teachers, and friends, must also change. Improvements must be acknowledged and appreciated. Discontinuing your old habits and responses are important aspects of adjusting the love and the discipline you give your family. As your child responds to your increasingly effective disciplinary approaches, harshness or anger that formerly may have seemed necessary will become excessive. There will be fewer moments in which a raised voice or an angry look will be appropriate. When you receive a negative report about your child, give yourself time to analyze the complaint. Control your reaction, and avoid taking sides if possible.

The expectation that the hyperactive child will be the main source of irritation in most conflict situations is a difficult habit to break. As the child's behavior becomes less frequently the true cause of difficulty, you will be able to see more clearly the roles of others, particularly brothers and sisters, in leading to adults' anger. The habit of expecting the child to oppose you whenever you ask him to do something may also be difficult to stop.

The temptation to rely on punishments as solutions to conflict, the tendency to nag and scold repeatedly, the desire to ignore the child's behavior, and parental tantrums are all responses that must be toned down and eventually eliminated. These inefficient disciplinary methods will slow the progress of your child's improvement.

Introducing more love into the family will be much easier if both parents share this goal. Any improvement in the marital relationship will, of course, promote an increased feeling of love and harmony throughout the entire family.

Find occasions to thank your children for doing things.

Too often, children hear about the things that they *don't* do, or don't do correctly. Even little acts like bringing in the newspaper or the milk can be noticed and appreciated. Doing small favors provides ways for everyone in the family to show their love for each other on a daily basis.

Make every holiday a chance for the entire family to join in the fun and enjoy each other. Show family movies and slides often, and assemble picture albums and family scrapbooks. Have pictures of family members on the walls of your home. Be alert for opportunities to give all family members a greater sense of unity and togetherness.

The following activities will also help promote harmony in your family by increasing everyone's sense of being loved.

Cooperative Ventures. Work and play together as a family unit with the common goal of cooperation and companionship. Anything from cleaning house to building a sand castle together can sustain and enhance the family's love for each other. Focus on the positive aspects and not on the shortcomings of the activity. The project should involve something for the entire family: planting a family garden, pitching a tent, painting a trailer or a boat, setting up a model train layout, or doing home remodeling, for example.

Talks About Feelings. Have family conversations in which members take turns talking about gaining new insights, avoiding self-defeating behavior, being fulfilled and excited, having a success experience, or similar good feelings.

Thanking Each Other. Expressions of gratitude sustain love. The family can sit together, with each member expressing thanks for something another family member has done recently. The gratitude can be on behalf of someone else, so that the person expressing thanks need not be the person who was directly benefitted by the person being thanked. Each person can be asked to tell at least one other family member the circumstances in which he or she appreciates the other family member the most. Another idea is to have a thanks-sharing circle, in which the family sits in a circle and each person gives a sincere message of gratitude to the person next to him. Variations on this theme are endless. One family has a love message center consisting of large envelopes with pockets. Family members write notes of appreciation to each other and deposit them in the envelopes; the messages can then be read privately or shared with the family once a week.

Gift Exchanges. Some parents have not learned to be comfortable about accepting gifts from their children. Too often parents reject offerings from their children or dismiss the gifts as unimportant. Gift exchanges usually work best if family members exchange gifts with each other. Gifts can be tangible or can involve a service or activity such as playing a game, giving a back rub, or doing a favor. The custom of giving gifts on holidays is a form of love-gift exchange.

Special Days. Give each family member a day to be "king" or "queen" and to do just about anything, including being free of the usual responsibilities and obligations. On the child's Special Day, he or she can have a special table setting to eat from, wear a special hat, have favorite meals, and choose family fun activities for that evening. Special days can be given whenever something out of the ordinary is happening for the child, such as a birthday, a job particularly well done, or the first or last day of school. They can also be arranged for fun reasons, such as an unbirthday, half-birthday (six months from birthday), kindness shown to others, or just because.

Togetherness Times. Arrange regular times during which the entire family gets together for work, discussion, or play. Put all other matters aside so that every family member can give full attention and involvement to the family activity.

Parent-Child Pairing Times. Each parent should spend some time alone with each child, devoting his or her full attention to that child in an activity the child enjoys. The child basks in the full and undiluted love and attention of the parent. These times provide good opportunities for closeness to develop between parent and child, especially for the parent who is uncomfortable at showing affection in front of other family members.

Family times and parent-child pairing times need not always involve games. Simple companionship activities that are enjoyed by all participants can enrich the family's love for each other. Reading stories, playing with toys, exercising, taking a walk together, and similar activities will all prove useful for this purpose. Whatever the activity, it is important that parents and children come away from it enriched and renewed in their love for each other.

Surprise Times. Weekly notes describing pleasant surprises can be included in each child's lunch box or given in some other way. The surprises can include favors and privileges, such as lunch in a restaurant of the child's choice. Surprises should not be coordinated strictly with the children's behavior; they are more effective if given for no particular reason as an indication of constant love.

Rebuilding Family Harmony Through Cooperative Play

One of the principal ways to increase love in the family is to have a regular playtime, which can involve parent-child pairs or the entire family. A regular playtime has several advantages for the parents as well as for the children, as discussed in Chapter 14.

Play is an activity through which learning takes place, and among the things learned in play are attitudes toward interpersonal relationships. Cooperative family activities are important aspects of your family's relationships, and cooperative games can be a great help in rebuilding harmony in your family. Self-love and love of others cannot blossom in a competitive atmosphere but can flourish in an atmosphere of cooperation and mutual respect.

Cooperative games differ from competitive games in that the factor of persons being pitted against each other is minimized or absent. If the play activity is bitterly competitive, some unfortunate attitudes may be learned by the winners as well as by the losers. Instead of a winner who defeats a loser, all players work toward a common goal. All players win if the goal is reached and all lose if the goal is not reached. The other uncertainties and obstacles of games, such as skill and chance, remain.

The goal might be that all players finish their parts of the game at the same time. In cooperative Chinese Checkers, for example, all players try to place their last marbles into home place on the same round. In cooperative regular checkers, the players try to change the black and red checkers to opposite sides of the board at the same time with no jumping or moving backward. Players can take turns, one after another, in reaching the final goal.

All players can try to coordinate their timing and actions with other players so that a smooth pattern develops. In cooperative ring toss, for example, one player holds a stick and tries to catch rings that are thrown toward the stick by the other player. In cooperative jacks the first player picks up one jack, the second picks up two, and so forth, until the goal of a certain number of jacks is reached.

In cooperative sentence writing, the players take turns adding a new word to the sentence. Players do not communicate with each other about what the sentences will say. Any player can add punctuation in addition to a word during his turn. The sentences that result can be read aloud for everyone's enjoyment. In cooperative picture drawing, each person makes a pencil or crayon stroke (or chalk on a chalkboard) during his turn. Each player adds a little bit to the drawing during each turn, with no communication between players. The picture evolves naturally from the cooperative spirit and creativity of the players.

Sometimes a total score for the entire group can be agreed upon before the game starts. In four-player card games there are thirteen possible tricks. Before any player sees his own hand, the number of tricks he must take should be agreed upon. Players can then cooperate in trying to help each other take the correct number of tricks.

With no other teams or players to compete against, players can agree on modifications of the game as it progresses. This flexibility provides more creativity and more variations; new games result. More planning takes place while the game goes on, and the entire experience becomes a more fulfilling activity than an ordinary competitive game.

There is less resentment toward any one player's errors or inefficient performance. For children who have coordination problems, this aspect of cooperative games makes them especially helpful. The group as a whole often attempts to compensate for errors made by any one player. Fewer quarrels break out; children seldom accuse each other of cheating, lying, not knowing how to play, being afraid, being weak, being poor losers, or being show-offs. Any one person's outstanding abilities become assets to the entire group rather than becoming obstacles to opponents.

Storytelling can also be a delightful family activity.

The children can take turns acting out the story being told, or they can take turns adding segments to the story.

Those times in which the entire family is together in a car are also an opportunity for cooperative family fun. Many varieties of word games and guessing games can be used, in addition to such cooperative activities as singing and telling jokes.

In many cooperative activities, coordination, timing, and rhythmic movement are involved, so that a pattern of motion and momentum develops. Cooperative games are generally enjoyable from a physical standpoint as well as from a psychological one.

Rebuilding Family Harmony Through the Family Council

The family council is one of the most powerful tools for rebuilding and maintaining a new level of harmony in your family. The basic idea is simple: regular meetings of the entire family to discuss issues, make plans, voice concerns, solve problems, agree on solutions, and celebrate your love for one another. The family council is essentially a method of allowing your children a voice in family affairs while providing you with an avenue for exercising your leadership in a benevolent way.

A typical family council meeting might have a schedule similar to the following:

Review of Last Week's Activities. The pleasant activities of individuals and of the whole family during the preceding week are discussed to refresh memories and to bring everyone up to date.

Notes From the Last Meeting. Notes from the preceding meeting are read aloud. They include the issues discussed as well as the agreements, decisions, and plans that were made.

Personal Schedules for the Upcoming Week. Transportation, child care, meals, and similar routines may need to be modified for one or more family members during the upcoming week. Any deviation from routine schedules is announced, so all members know where everyone is going and, in general, what everyone is doing.

Family Projects for the Upcoming Week. The group discusses recreational and family fun activities as well as family work projects. Decisions are made about how the family will spend the upcoming weekend.

Chores and Routines. Any family member can make suggestions for changing the routines necessary to keep the family functioning. Discussion includes such items as clothing, meals, housework, lawn care, pet care, car care, and room cleaning, whether previous decisions have been carried out, and if not, why not.

Concerns and Negotiations. Items dealing with long-range family plans, such as vacation planning, job changes, moving, or household remodeling are discussed. Any difficulties or conflicts that any family member is experiencing can be discussed. Various solutions are proposed, and agreement is reached on which solution to try, usually for an experimental period of one week until the next family council meeting. Because the hyperactive child may have difficulty with self-control for long periods of time, he has a greater chance for success if he has an entire week for trying a new routine.

Recording of Agreements. One person takes on the secretarial duty of reviewing and recording the agreements and the plans made during the meeting. This record helps to prevent future misunderstandings among family members. It can be written or tape-recorded.

Lesson. A lesson is taught by one or two family members. The lesson can involve religious, moral, or social values and may include visual aids or other entertaining features. Usually the lesson consists of a presentation followed by discussion that involves all family members.

Allowances. Financial matters are discussed, and allowances are distributed to the children.

Celebration. The council meeting closes with games, singing, storytelling, refreshments, or some similar celebration of family life. Celebrations can be rotated, so that each week a different child is responsible for providing the fun activity or the refreshment. With a little advance planning, the celebration can become a basis for regular parent-child togetherness for the purpose of preparing and cooking the refreshments.

Among the important parental leadership functions during the family council meeting is the guarding of each person's right to express genuine concerns and opinions. In this way the children learn they can have an impact on the family's decisions. As the children learn that their opinions are valued and listened to, they will gradually put more thought into them and will offer more useful suggestions as time goes on.

As each issue is discussed during the family council meeting, each family member needs to examine it from the viewpoint of the needs of the entire family.

The decisions in the family council meetings are agreements; they are made unanimously or by consensus, with each family member participating. Consensus differs from majority rule, in which those who disagree are outvoted. Agreement is reached only when all family members, not just the majority, can endorse and be comfortable with the proposed solution or plan of action.

To attain consensus, a thorough search of all the facts must be conducted. Everyone's opinion must be considered, and the ideas that meet the needs of most family members should be offered as temporary solutions, at least until the next family council meeting. If no agreement can be reached, decisions are postponed until the next family council meeting.

The most important attitude is a spirit of inquiry: What is the situation? How does it look to each family member? What ideas can be proposed to improve it? Which one holds the most promise? What shall we do to make sure that it is tried? Inquiry and discussion are done in the spirit of mutual respect for everyone's viewpoint and everyone's right to make choices.

The most common abuse of the family council meeting is to treat it as an opportunity to lecture to a captive audience. If you use these meetings to preach, scold, or impose your will on your children, their purpose will fail. One way to help ensure a high level of openness of communication is to rotate the positions of chairperson, secretary, and lesson giver so the children gain a sense of participation and responsibility.

The family council meeting must not be allowed to deteriorate into a gripe session. Each person expressing a complaint is also expected, if possible, to present one or more suggested solutions at the same time. The emphasis is not on how any one member should change, but on what the family can do to prevent a certain difficulty from arising in the future.

An additional function of parental leadership at the family council meeting is to make those decisions that are parent-level decisions. Deciding whether the family needs to relocate and if so, where, for example, is essentially a parental decision. The family council meeting is an excellent arena, however, in which to hear the children's feelings about the upcoming move, and to receive their suggestions for making the move more pleasant for the family.

The first few family council meetings should be oriented toward making plans for pleasant activities, such as deciding about weekend projects or vacations. In this way, the family can become accustomed to the concept of regular meetings without having to face difficult or touchy negotiations. Other parts of the typical family council meeting can be included later, as the members gain increased practice, confidence, and trust in each other.

It is helpful to provide a notebook or bulletin board on which family members can write the concerns and issues they wish to discuss at the upcoming family council meeting. In this manner, all conflicts can be brought before the family, analyzed, and used as teaching examples. All members can then learn how to prevent or reduce such conflicts and how to build and maintain harmony. Gradually the family council meetings will reduce contention among family members.

Sometimes a child may feel so out of place and unwelcome that she shuns participation. Also, some children boycott the family council as a way of displaying their power or as an attempt to hurt the rest of the family. All members are invited to participate, but attendance should be voluntary. The best way to lure an uncooperative family member into participation is to conduct effective and interesting meetings. Eventually the member will participate, out of curiosity if for no other reason.

Even preschoolers can participate to some degree in family council meetings. Certainly the younger children can help prepare or serve the refreshments. With the aid of a tape recorder, a nonreader can serve as secretary for the meeting. Whatever their role or contribution, young children can be encouraged and helped by parents to express themselves during the meeting.

By being vigilant for opportunities to encourage acts of love and caring among your children and by minimizing competition, you can strengthen the fiber that binds your family together. By maintaining an open forum where each child feels free and safe to communicate needs and desires, you can prevent misbehavior and further rebuild the relationships that make for harmonious family life.

MEETING THE CHALLENGES OF BEING THE CUSTODIAL PARENT

The struggles of the single parent of an ADHD child are basically the same as those of other single parents, though some of the difficulties are magnified. Single parents with primary responsibility for a hyperactive child may confront problems not encountered in the two-parent family.

Overinvolvement. Because of the forced intensity of your relationship, one of the most likely pitfalls is too much mutual emotional dependency, by you on your child and by your child on you. This overinvestment of energy into the parent-child bond magnifies most of the problems involved with raising the child. Having no partner with whom to share the responsibilities and the frustrations makes parenting even more difficult.

Noncustodial Visitation. During visitations, the child is no longer under your direct supervision, and maintenance of the treatment program, whether medication or the Feingold Program, is left to the child, the noncustodial parent, and others with whom your child temporarily visits.

The Child as a Weapon. During the last part of a visit, the noncustodial parent might allow an off-limits chemical exposure or skip medication, causing symptoms to flare up. Your child then returns in a completely hyperactive state. The noncustodial parent uses purposeful violations of your child's treatment program as a way to cause you additional, unnecessary burdens and suffering.

UNDERCUTTING TREATMENT. The noncustodial parent may wish to impress the child with his or her flexibility and how much fun can occur during visits. Or the noncustodial parent may simply challenge the diagnosis, the need for any treatment, or the specific treatment program you have chosen. Then that parent refuses to maintain the program to prove the point.

LIMITED TIME AND ENERGY. Especially if you are an employed single parent, you may have little time and energy left after earning an income, doing housework, providing meals, and spending a few moments with your child each day. The extra services your child needs to improve social relationships, self-esteem, or school adjustment may simply be more than you can deliver.

FEARS. A major discouragement of a single custodial parent is the belief that you must have a spouse in order to be happy. A common fear is that you can't live on your own and that your children can't possibly be normal in a one-parent household. You may also wonder whether you can ever make realistic arrangements for coping with a child who requires so much extra supervision.

One of the most important sources of help is the passage of time. Time is needed to discover your whole personhood beyond your role as parent. You also need sufficient time to develop confidence in your ability to cope with all that life hands you. Good backup child care is very important, partly because it allows you much-needed breaks for personal renewal.

Make time-saving arrangements and plan how to minimize and streamline your housekeeping chores, including meal preparation. Perhaps a friend or relative would agree to assist.

Avoid being distracted by trivial problems. There are so many battles to fight that it makes no sense to become distraught over little problems, imaginary ones, or future difficulties that you don't need to plan for now.

Perhaps the most important step is to make sure your needs are met in arenas other than child rearing. The best solution for limited time and energy is arranging as balanced and well-rounded a life as possible. Make sure you get adequate sleep, nutrition, exercise, and mental relief from pressures at work. Perform a sieve role for your child—filter and screen your child's difficulties but avoid unnecessary rescues from challenges. Stand by with help from the sidelines but let your child deal as directly as possible with the events in his life.

If the noncustodial parent is allowing your child to deviate from the treatment program, find out why. If the matter is open to negotiation and if the noncustodial parent will listen to your reasons, explain the need for maintaining the program in terms of the pre-post contrasts that have occurred. If there are hard feelings from the marriage and you are the target of criticism or other retaliatory antics, consider reducing your communication to the barest minimum. Converse in a businesslike and courteous manner. Harsh confrontation won't work and reinforces that person's attempts to hurt you and cause more upset in your life.

Let the natural consequences of treatment deviations persuade the noncustodial parent. Though you and your child will suffer from the experience, some undeniable evidence of ADHD symptoms will flare up during the visits. Refer to that fact in your attempts to regain at least a minimal level of cooperation for supporting the treatment during visits. If that arrangement seems unattainable, drop the issue and resume the treatment only during the times when your child is under your supervision and care.

Develop the attitude that no spouse is better than any spouse. Make it clear to anyone you date seriously that you and your children are a package deal. Any potential future spouse should enjoy the children as much as you do and should be supportive of whatever steps are needed to give your ADHD child a successful life.

Left unattended, the stress in a family with an ADHD child can harm the emotional stability of a marital relationship or a custodial parent. By recognizing potential trouble spots early and trying to maintain open, complete emotional communication, you can gain strength against the stresses brought about by the effects of your child's disorder on your family.

The next chapter details how to get help for your hyperactive child from the school.

10

Obtaining the Best Schooling

When asked where the greatest assistance is needed, parents of ADHD children consistently reply "School!" Teachers' expectations are often not consistent with hyperactive children's abilities and readiness. Homework is a major area of concern and conflict among parents, teachers, and ADHD children. An additional concern is whether the school can provide special services to accommodate a child's academic, social, and emotional difficulties.

Prior to the late 1940s, ADHD children were regarded as equivalent to the mentally retarded: unteachable and suitable only for custodial educational services. In the 1950s and 1960s, ADHD children were considered learning disabled and developmentally delayed in the physiological systems necessary for learning. In 1975, Public Law 94-142 (discussed later in this chapter) was passed to guarantee equal education for all children.

School programs for ADHD children range, however, from elaborate special classes to no special help. The extent of awareness and cooperation among teachers and administrators is wide, with flexible individualized approaches at one extreme and outright denial of the disorder at the other.

This chapter examines learning disabilities and how to identify them, how to obtain help through special educational and legal processes, and how to enlist teacher cooperation as you work with your child and the school.

LEARNING DISABILITIES THROUGH CHILDHOOD

The search for early indications or warning signals for learning disabilities among preschool and primary grade children has been frustrating. The skills that are impaired in children with learning disabilities are often difficult to identify during early childhood. The few indications that are known so far are excessively slow development of coordination in large muscle groups (legs, torso) or small muscle groups (hands, fingers), fidgetiness, and delayed reading readiness. Though they occur in learning disabled young children, distractibility and letter reversals are not clear indicators because they are also common in nonimpaired young children.

In the early grades the indicators are severe distractibility in a wide variety of settings, reversals of letters and numbers through second grade, sloppy work, difficulty following directions, poor handwriting, poor spelling, poor reading comprehension, poor math performance, poor language arts performance, difficulty understanding concepts, poor planning skills, and inaccurate copying from the board.

When an ADHD child in the primary grades responds well to one-on-one attention from the teacher, a common mistake is to conclude the child is simply poorly motivated or trying to get attention. Unless there is evidence of great psychological turmoil or abuse in the home, such a conclusion is incorrect. Unfortunately, it is made often and postpones home-based assistance and assignment to special education classes that can alter an ADHD child's attitude and performance. The labels applied most frequently by well-meaning school personnel to ADHD children are "unmotivated," "immature," "underachieving," "bright but not working to potential," and "won't settle down."

Sometimes a well-meaning teacher will not recognize a child's hyperactivity or learning disabilities, even though there may be definite problems in the classroom. The teacher may describe disruptive behaviors without realizing they constitute the symptoms of ADHD. During a conference, for example, the teacher might say that your child would get along better if he would sit still longer, write more legibly, slow down and take his time, not talk so much, or not hit the other children.

ADHD-ld and Delinquency

As a group, the learning disabled are followers rather than leaders. If they become involved in any adolescent delinquency, they are more likely to get caught than their nonlearning disabled ADHD counterparts. Once apprehended, they might not understand what they are supposed to do or say, express their side of the story convincingly or accurately, or answer questions appropriately. For the same offenses, ADHD-ld adolescents have higher rates of adjudication, being more than twice as likely as nonimpaired adolescents to be judged delinquent by the courts. According to a recent study, about one-third of the boys ruled delinquent by U.S. courts have learning disabilities; about one-half of that group have ADHD-ld.

ADD Without Hyperactivity (ADD-noH)

Since the early 1980s there has been considerable interest in the difference between ADHD and attention deficit disorder without hyperactivity (ADD-noH). Surveys indicate the latter occurs about one-fourth to one-half as often as ADHD.

Children who have many ADHD symptoms but few or none that directly reflect an abnormal amount of fidgetiness or impulsivity seem generally to reflect a more restrained personality than is typical for ADHD children. They tend to have few conduct problems and rarely become involved in delinquent behavior or drug abuse in adolescence. They are socially withdrawn, shy, and unpopular with peers.

Their overall school performance is poor, they often have learning disabilities, and they are at high risk for academic problems and retention. Their difficulties tend to cluster around mental confusion factors, such as difficulty concentrating and finishing a task, poor organization of schoolwork, daydreaming, inattention, problems following instructions, absentmindedness and forgetfulness, drowsiness (not because of medication overdosage), and being slow moving.

Their energy seems to be directed inward, in contrast to the outward-flowing energy of the hyperactive child. Compared with hyperactive attention disordered children, these children are more likely to

- lie rather than fight;
- be diagnosed as having a phobia, depression, or anxiety;
- be tense and nervous;
- plod through work and be generally slow acting;
- be self-doubting and critical of their appearance;
- avoid fights and be nonaggressive;
- show inhibited, but not bizarre, behavior;
- feel guilty and remorseful.

Their low overall satisfaction and low happiness are distinctive characteristics, and they are more likely to become depressed than ADHD children. Self-critical and lacking in confidence, they tend to appear anxious and worried. Since their self-doubts include their appearance and strength, they are less likely than their classmates to participate in sports.

Despite these difficulties, ADD-noH children are better liked by teachers and classmates than their hyperactive ADHD counterparts.

THE EXTENT OF LEARNING DISABILITIES

About 10 million school-age children in the United States have learning disabilities, and about one-third of these children are from families with at least one other learning disabled member. Learning disabilities affect more boys than girls, and these children often have a history of complications during pregnancy or delivery, head injury, infection, or exposure to toxins. The parallels between ADHD and learning disabilities suggest that they stem from similar biochemical imbalances within the brain.

Learning disabilities are a subset of learning impairments, somewhat analogous to donuts being a subset of baked goods. Learning impairments are any difficulties consistently experienced by schoolchildren, whether or not they require special educational services or placements. The available research on the overlapping occurrence of learning disabilities and ADHD shows that about 30% of U.S. children have significant learning impairments. About one-third of those children—roughly 10% of the school population—have ADHD.

From 5 to 10% of the learning impaired group are classified as learning disabled by school districts. About 30 to 50% of those classified as learning disabled also suffer from attention deficit and hyperactivity.

These overlapping characteristics are less confusing if you imagine a series of concentric circles arranged somewhat like the rings on a target. Each circle is larger than the next. The target has five rings representing, from the largest to the smallest, (1) all children, (2) exceptional children, (3) educationally or learning impaired children, (4) learning disabled children, and (5) the ADHD-ld subgroup of learning disabled children.

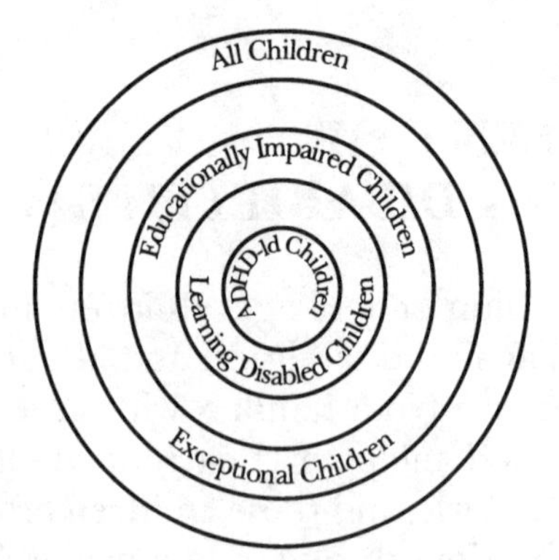

Among ADHD children, best estimates indicate 50% are said to be underachieving or underperforming in school. About 10 to 40% of ADHD children have learning disabilities. The ADHD-ld subgroup occurs in as many as one-third of ADHD children and comprises as many as one-half of learning disabled students.

Though not necessarily a guarantee of access to the benefits of Public Law 94-142 or to special school services, ADHD is tantamount to a learning disability that merits the least restrictive environment with appropriate educational services and access to special education programs.

Educationally, ADHD children have just as many difficulties as learning disabled children. Their problems remain the most significant and unresolved in our educational system. They underachieve because they do not understand or follow instructions and because they have difficulty storing and retrieving information once they have learned it. Numerous surveys comparing ADHD students with their non-ADHD classmates have consistently shown them with lower retention rates, failing grades, and the need for special placement.

From preschool through high school, the observations of teachers about these children consistently indicate nine distinctive classroom characteristics. ADHD children and adolescents show more of these traits, and in greater severity, than non-ADHD students.

- Being out of seat too frequently
- Deviating from what the rest of the class is supposed to be doing
- Not following the teacher's instructions or orders
- Talking out of turn or calling out
- Being aggressive toward classmates
- Having too short an attention span and being too distractible
- Bothering classmates by talking to them or intruding on their work efforts
- Being oblivious and daydreaming
- Turning in assignments late, incomplete, or sloppy

One of the most tragic ironies of special education is that it is often withheld until the child is severely behind academically, almost to the point of no return. Finally a discouraged, depressed, disheartened child with only the slightest remnant of self-confidence about academic ability is given special instruction in a too-little-too-late attempt to make up for years of being underserviced by the schools. For the ADHD child whose learning problems are not quite severe enough to warrant special education placement, the gap between the child's potential and actual achievement gradually widens and discouragement sets in. The school district may offer no relief except the continuing threat of lower grades. The end result is a student whose motivation is too low to redeem.

Every major component of the ADHD syndrome interferes with classroom behavior. Problems sustaining attention, distractibility, and deficits in selective attention interfere with academic work. Impulsivity leads to academic blunders, frequent errors, and disrupted relationships with classmates. Even for those of above-average intelligence, their ability to absorb and display knowledge by academic performance is impaired.

Although their seatwork or homework may be incomplete and they contribute little to classroom discussion, ADHD children of above-average intelligence are often at grade level on achievement tests. They are able to pick up enough knowledge to score satisfactorily on such tests, and their high intelligence compensates for their distractibility. But adding unfinished seatwork to homework to be done at home often results in academic overload.

ADHD children with average or below-average intelligence are at an even greater disadvantage. They may underachieve because of difficulties with concentration, study habits, planning, and focusing attention as well as specific gaps in knowledge. Learning disabled ADHD children (ADHD-ld) not only must overcome academic impairments that afflict about one-half of all ADHD students but must also compensate for specific learning disabilities. Those with serious perceptual dysfunctions have difficulties in several subjects at school; those with lesser dysfunctions do well in many subjects but show unusual weakness and difficulty in one or two classes most relevant to their handicapping conditions. ADHD-ld children with visual problems often have difficulty with written language, while those with auditory problems have difficulty with reading-related subjects like spelling.

The symptoms of the ADHD child, and more so those of the ADHD-ld child, impinge strongly on subjects like math, reading, and written expression. The child might try to perform three-place multiplication by progressing from left to right, subtract when adding is called for, subtract up instead of down, or assume all problems call for the identical mathematical operation asked for in the example, without noticing whether to add or subtract within each problem.

They don't learn the core skills, so are increasingly impaired under the weight of the accelerated demands and expectations at the higher grade levels. Many of the one-in-four high-school students who drop out before graduation are ADHD-ld adolescents who have not succeeded in special programs. They are less likely than ADHD peers to be able to obtain and hold employment after high school.

A developmental lag in the mental organization and problem-solving ability needed in a particular subject or skill area, such as a discrepancy between the child's reading or math level and the expected level for a child of the same age and intelligence level, is referred to as a specific developmental disability.

Children of average intelligence should be reading at a grade level that is five years behind their age. For example, an 8-year-old should be reading at the third-grade level, a 9-year-old, at the fourth-grade level, and so on. A 10-year-old with an average IQ who reads at the first-grade level rather than at the fifth-grade level would be four years behind the expected reading level and would be considered learning disabled.

The following are the most common areas of academic difficulty for ADHD children, especially for those in the ADHD-ld subgroup. Many of these areas represent communication disorders; common names for specific disorders are indicated in parentheses. Many of these terms are also listed in the Glossary.

- *Reading:* comprehending and decoding of printed letters, letter combinations, and words; understanding words or numbers; reading words accurately (alexia and dyslexia); understanding written directions

- *Math:* performing calculations with and without paper and pencil; solving thought problems with concepts such as size, volume, or number of objects; keeping rows and columns of numbers separate; correctly placing decimals; understanding abstract concepts like times, dividing into, square root and negative numbers
- *Writing:* performing the mechanics of cursive writing or printing (dysgraphia)
- *Attention focusing:* sustaining attention, blocking out distractions, persisting in tasks, avoiding daydreaming
- *Thought processing:* understanding, organizing, prioritizing, symbolizing, and remembering; restating thoughts and concepts in similar words
- *Visual memory:* remembering what something looks like, especially letters and numbers; remembering sequences visually; remembering written symbols used to communicate information
- *Organization:* sequencing—composing sentences and paragraphs within a logical order (first to last, prior to later, cause to effect); selecting important information and discarding unnecessary data; understanding the length of time necessary for an activity; understanding the concepts of past, present, and future; labeling, classifying, and sorting information; recognizing parts of a whole; recognizing a whole when most, but not all, of the parts are present; breaking down a whole into its parts; recognizing degrees of comparison such as big-bigger or smaller-smallest
- *Prioritizing:* selecting the main idea in reading, listening, or writing; emphasizing what is important to include in written compositions; discarding unimportant ideas; drawing conclusions independently
- *Bridging:* remembering more than two events or instructions at once; understanding similarities and differences; relating one fact or event to another

- *Encoding:* selecting the correct words with which to express ideas; producing several concepts and statements when asked to describe or talk about something (expressive language dysfunction); using correct syntax
- *Decoding:* comprehending what is read; semantics —pairing of words with their meanings; receptive vocabulary and receptive language skills—understanding words read or heard (aphasia); understanding comparisons, poetry, and other abstract concepts; connecting cause and effect; recognizing oneness of objects, symbols, and words with separate identities; understanding marks, sounds, or patterns representing an object or an idea, for example, a question mark
- *Neatness:* having orderly handwriting, keeping arithmetic columns vertical, turning in papers without smudges or erasures
- *Recall:* remembering isolated facts, names, or dates, especially in subjects like math, science, history, and foreign languages; remembering to bring materials and completed work to class
- *Spatial relationships:* knowing left from right and understanding left-to-right progression; visual perception skills such as recognizing whether an object is facing left or right, up or down; understanding and giving meaning to figure-ground perception and size, shape, and color
- *Relationships between sounds:* listening; discriminating one sound from another; discriminating and perceiving auditory input; sound blending; remembering sounds in sequence, such as a melody or a long word like *Mississippi;* rhythm timing; grasping phonics principles
- *Perceptual-motor coordination:* kinesthetic awareness of position of limbs and torso; fine-motor and gross-motor coordination; visual tracking; eye-hand coordination; motor performance skills, such as acro-

batics; responding to stimuli on a computer screen; legible handwriting; maintaining the place when reading
- *Selective attention:* distinguishing important from unimportant facts and activities; outlining essays and lecture notes; studying from textbooks

Do not attempt, however, to diagnose your child's problems from this or any other list. If you suspect any of these difficulties, you should seek professional advice since a breakdown in any of these areas interferes with the learning process and may signal the presence of developmental or learning disabilities.

GETTING HELP FOR LEARNING DISABILITIES

Special Education

Any good special education program starts with a comprehensive psychoeducational evaluation to pinpoint the child's learning style. A well-done psychoeducational evaluation identifies difficulties in any of the seventeen areas listed above. It should involve psychometrics—formal diagnostic tests—that are valid and appropriate for your child's age and academic level. The evaluation should include measures of intelligence quotient (IQ), achievement (knowledge level), and aptitude (potential for learning certain skills) as well as your child's social and emotional adjustment, classroom behavior, and level of school survival skills. (See the discussion of TAPIC later in this chapter.)

The results from the formal tests will often be presented to you as a comparison between your child and other children through norms developed specifically for each test. Percentile scores are the most common method; the score represents the percentage of similar children who score lower than your child on the same test. Grade equivalents are another common method; your child's performance is categorized as typical for students of a certain grade level. For example, if your child provides the same number of correct answers as average students in their second month of fourth grade, your child's grade equivalent for that particular test performance would be 4.2. An IQ is simply a ratio between your child's mental age and chronological age, expressed as a percentage. A 10-year-old child whose mental age is fourteen would have an IQ of about 140.

The classroom teacher can submit rating scales or checklists summarizing your child's adjustment—for example, the Taylor Social/Emotional/Academic Adjustment Checklist (see Appendix B).

Speech and language problems often involve difficulty with specific speech sounds but can include more severe impairments. A specialist in speech disorders can assess receptive (hearing) and expressive (speaking) language skills, including speech articulation, speech fluency, voice characteristics, and a host of other factors relating to your child's ability to communicate.

ADHD children often have trouble with small or large muscle coordination, though seldom with both. An occupational therapist can evaluate your child's coordination, including the ability to integrate different mental and muscle-group processes, and can suggest specific exercises, if necessary.

Some schools have special activities programs for children with learning problems that focus on a particular area such as music, dance, art, or sports. Activity-oriented groups can help your child increase self-confidence and expand social skills. Encourage the school to offer enrollment to your child in these types of nonacademic activities to counterbalance the pressure of the more mentally demanding aspects of the curriculum.

Make sure the teacher has a copy of the psychoeducational report and follows its recommendations. Have a conference and include the examiner if necessary to guarantee clear, specific recommendations that fit your child and can be used by the teacher. Diagnostic prescriptive teaching—incorporating specialized techniques to assist a child—is called for after the teacher has received the psychoeducational evaluation report. The report should specify whether the academic tasks your child is being asked to do are sufficiently fine-tuned to your child's readiness. Not only should the teacher develop a plan of action based on the report, but you should also apply the information at home to help strengthen your child's academic and study skills.

However noble the goals of special education, don't exaggerate them. Special education will not normalize your child, but will minimize the effects of learning difficulties so that she can function on a par with *average* students, not the most successful students.

Proper placement in school is a crucial factor for the ADHD child, and it influences how successful biochemical treatment will be. Don't expect your child to sit still and focus her attention in a class far above her readiness level. The evaluation should recommend suitable class placement, with specific recommendations for mainstream and resource classes, and should discuss eligibility for the special services available within the school district.

Some ADHD children, especially those in the learning disabled subgroup, may need the extra help available in a resource class because of difficulty with some of the demands of a regular class. The gap between academic goals and a student's social, emotional, and mental status is sometimes bridged by a special service, the resource room.

The resource room is designed to assist children who have academic difficulties; classes are taught by specially trained teachers. The children come to the resource room individually or in small groups, and visits to the resource room are usually one or two hours per school day, though longer periods might be arranged if necessary. In schools in which students change classes, they can visit the resource room relatively unnoticed by their schoolmates.

The emphasis in the resource room includes training in problem-solving skills that can be applied to subjects taught in the mainstream classroom. The resource room does not imitate the mainstream classroom, but takes a more creative approach. It addresses specific ADHD symptoms individually as they interfere with classroom learning. Specialized materials are introduced and each child's progress is continuously monitored, with a careful matching of instruction to the student's readiness.

In concert with the popular deemphasis on labeling and categorizing children, mainstreaming represents a significant turning point in public education. Its goal is to maximally integrate each child's educational experience into a regular classroom setting. It might range from special instruction with a small circle of classmates to spending a substantial portion of the school day in a resource room.

Consider these four factors when you negotiate with the school about how much and with whom to mainstream your child. Mainstreaming will work better if your ADHD child

1. wants to be in the regular classroom for most or all of the day;
2. has the minimum reading, writing, and note taking skills to participate successfully in the regular classroom;
3. is likely to be accepted by classmates; and
4. is willing to take advantage of friendship opportunities and other positive social growth experiences.

And if your child's teacher will

1. follow the classroom approach given in this book or similar guidelines from some other reputable source;

2. have a small enough class to allow the needed individual attention to your child;
3. have the necessary energy and a positive attitude;
4. have support staff and specialists with whom to consult if problems occur;
5. have a cooperative relationship with you and be willing to receive as well as give counsel;
6. maintain good coordination with the resource teacher;
7. support your biochemical treatment approach.

Special Services Through Public Law 94-142

You might be able to secure some extra help for your child through the legal provisions of Public Law 94-142. A landmark civil rights act, this law is intended to guarantee a fair and equal education for every child. All school districts in the United States are required to develop Individualized Education Programs (IEPs) for every special-needs child. This law mandates that the ideal special education program be as unrestrictive and as close to a mainstream classroom as possible. Mainstreaming capitalizes on each child's strengths and addresses educational needs in a setting that minimizes isolation and stereotyping of those with handicapping conditions. Its purpose is to save time, money, and other resources and to reduce social and emotional problems among students.

The age range is from three through twenty-one except where state laws provide a more restricted range. Public Law 94-142 includes the following provisions:

- Entitlement of all children with educationally relevant handicaps to an evaluation involving any of several professional disciplines

- Development of an individualized education plan (IEP) specifying goals, objectives, and needed services for each handicapped child
- Allowance for as much time as possible spent in the least restrictive setting, usually the mainstream classroom
- The right of parents to an independent outside evaluation or second opinion
- The right of parents to be notified and involved in the evaluation process and to approve the final IEP
- Vigorous identification of at-risk children
- An annual review of the child's program and progress
- No discrimination because of social or economic background, and all written and oral information to be in the native language of the child and parents
- Protection of confidentiality and due process rights of handicapped children and their parents
- Submission by each state and local school district of an annual program plan for implementation, including the policies and procedures for providing special education
- Federal funds to assist state and local districts with the services required by this law

The IEP must indicate the child's level of academic performance, annual goals and short-term objectives, special education and related services needed, the extent of mainstreaming, start-up dates and duration of the various services, and impartial criteria for evaluating progress. Although the IEP is not a legal contract, the school district is required by law to provide all the services described in it for a specified time period. Federal regulations don't require the school staff to guarantee that your child attains the goals; the only obligations are that the district make a good faith effort to assist the child toward the goals and revise the IEP annually.

This law relies strongly on dialogue between parents

and school professionals and assumes joint decision making for the child's benefit. It lists seven basic areas of academic disability: basic reading skills, reading comprehension, mathematics calculation, mathematics reasoning, oral expression, listening comprehension, and written expression. The last three are especially reflective of the difficulties of ADHD children.

Like much legislation, the intentions behind Public Law 94-142 are more impressive than the follow-through. In most states, ADHD children do not automatically qualify for its services, and many school districts violate its provisions.

Even districts that act in good faith are somewhat bound by its narrow and restrictive definition of learning disabilities; thus, many ADHD children with severe learning problems are denied its protections. School districts vary greatly, for example, in how they define the discrepancy between achievement and intellectual ability, and their definitions often exclude ADHD children who have obvious and severe learning problems. A child's difficulty concentrating can artificially lower the results of an intelligence test. Comparing the child's suppressed academic achievement with an inaccurate IQ leads to the conclusion that the child is performing at an appropriate level for a child with that apparent IQ. The net result is that the child is not considered learning disabled and receives no special help.

There are three stages for obtaining specialized services: identification, evaluation, and placement. During the identification phase, qualified professionals observe your child and meet to decide whether the difficulties noted fulfill the criteria specified in the law. During the evaluation phase, professionals under the auspices of the school conduct a psychoeducational evaluation and any other relevant assessments. During the placement phase, you and the school staff decide on the best class placement and prepare an IEP.

Feel free to contact the school even if your child is a

preschooler. Since the law provides incentives for the education of 3- to 5-year-olds, your public school officials should be able to help you find appropriate services or offer some services themselves. Inform the principal or other qualified personnel of your child's special needs and indicate all aspects of your child's disorder that might qualify him or her for assistance under Public Law 94-142.

Local school systems and states vary in their definitions of the chronic illnesses serious enough to impede progress in a regular education program. There is no uniform definition of how to determine the level of severity that makes a child eligible for special services. Children who have obvious severe medical conditions along with ADHD are likely to qualify. Among ADHD children, those who have the sensitive-allergic or other obvious severe accompanying conditions are most likely to qualify. Because this disorder is not included in this law as a specific criterion for receiving special services, the majority of ADHD students who receive services under its provisions qualify by being labeled learning disabled or emotionally disturbed. Those labeled emotionally disturbed often are incorrectly diagnosed; many simply have ADHD without an accompanying mental or emotional condition.

Despite numerous evaluations and reports shared among helping professionals, a lack of coordination in the entire system for delivery of services can still occur. You might need to be the central liaison and advocate to coordinate the services for your child.

Help During Transition Periods

Any switch in schools can be difficult because of the flood of new situations and new people your child must contend with. The transition is even more difficult when the class scheduling of the two schools is different. Clearly, the greatest such challenge for ADHD children is a transfer from a small elementary school, which has supported and nurtured the child's abilities, to a large middle school or junior high school. Besides the many new faces, large secondary schools have complicated class rotation schedules, time pressure between classes, confusing lunchtime procedures, and significantly reduced individual attention to learning problems.

During these periods, your child needs a transition plan. Make arrangements ahead of time for your child and you to establish a relationship with a counselor, homeroom teacher, or another supportive adult at the new school.

By securing a thorough evaluation of your child's academic needs, you lay the groundwork for more effective help at school. Follow this with a thorough first conference with the teacher at the beginning of the school year. Stay involved through frequent courteous meetings and communications with the teacher. Through these avenues you can help ensure that the school program your child receives will best fit his readiness.

The budgets for many special education programs have been cut so severely that the eligibility requirements are very narrow, admitting only those students who are severely deficient.

Many ADHD children don't receive special services until their problems are too severe to be resolved. The solution is never to leave the matter entirely in the hands of the schools. Expect to spend some time during evenings and weekends helping your child compensate for learning problems as well as training and supervising homework and study skills. For the ADHD child there are no substitutes for early diagnosis of academic problems, extensive tutoring, carefully orchestrated classroom techniques, and careful guidance through the educational process by concerned parents.

PARENT/TEACHER COOPERATION

Of all the available support systems, the classroom teacher is the key figure in determining your child's school success. Everything you can do to develop a positive, trusting relationship with the teacher is beneficial. Working together, you may be able to discover how best to help your child.

Because of limited experience or training in handling hyperactive students, the teacher might not feel comfortable dealing with your child. She may represent a special challenge, so be patient and tolerant. Give as much guidance as possible to help the teacher understand potential causes of any problem behavior. An occasional teacher who is not willing to accept instruction from a parent may accept it from an authoritative written source. The goal is to have the teacher become familiar with your child's characteristics. Supply written materials, including relevant sections from this book, if the teacher appears likely to respond well to such an approach.

In maintaining the delicate balance between your firmness on behalf of your child and your understanding of the teacher's frustrations, show an awareness of the rights of other students in the class. Don't automatically interpret hesitancy on the teacher's part as an effort to avoid helping your child. Help the teacher balance your child's individualized needs against the requirements of the other children in the classroom.

It is important to avoid an apologetic "I'm sure you know best" attitude. State clearly and strongly what you expect for your child. The teacher is more likely to respect you and cooperate if you are polite, self-assured, and firm.

Make clear your intentions to assist the teacher in every way possible. Mention the types of support you are prepared to give on the home front (see Chapter 12) and assure the teacher of your readiness to communicate at any time. If you approach the school and the teacher as adversaries, they are likely to accept that role. If you approach them as potential allies, you will usually find them cooperative and willing to work for the benefit of your child.

If extreme conflict arises with the teacher, basic issues must be resolved before progress can be made. If the teacher makes excuses to sidestep the obligation to deal appropriately with your child, talk with the school principal or counselor and arrange for a joint conference or request a classroom reassignment for your child.

Maintaining Contact with the Teacher

The importance of maintaining close communication is illustrated by an experience related by the parent of an ADHD child.

> At school they don't seem to understand Ryan's problems. At first they thought he was being abused in some way and called social services. They thought the only reason a boy would be so angry and obnoxious was that he was abused. I was so hurt when the principal did this.

I have observed that a history of difficulty with ADHD children has prepared teachers and parents to be somewhat on guard about the support each is willing to give to the other. Let your involvement and concern be your calling card, and approach the teacher as a willing partner in a joint venture for the benefit of your child.

Communication between you and the teacher will usually occur by five methods: school visits by you, home visits by the teacher, conferences, telephone calls, and notes. Each method has its strengths and weaknesses.

School Visits. Depending on the circumstances, you may want to serve as an aide in your child's classroom. This arrangement may help the teacher by providing time for him or her to give your child the special attention that he needs. It also keeps your child on the teacher's mind and makes it less likely that the teacher will be unfair or lax in meeting his or her obligations toward your child. Visiting the classroom to observe your child, without actually volunteering your services to the school, is another type of school visit that may be beneficial.

Home Visits. Seeing your family in its home setting can give the teacher a better understanding of your child, especially if she behaves much differently at home than at school. It may be helpful for the teacher to gain a new perspective by seeing how she acts in a different setting.

Conferences. Conferences are vital. They provide a chance for you and the teacher to examine your roles in helping your child. Each conference should be prearranged and should be prepared for by all persons involved. The teacher's preparation should include a review of your child's past academic work, recent summaries of his attitude and behavior, and examples of current work.

Your preparation should include checking to see that you have received all report cards for the current year; that you have a copy of the school's current handbook dealing with suspension, promotion, attendance, special education programs, and similar information; that you know how to get answers to your questions if the handbook is unavailable or insufficient; that you have answered all correspondence from teacher and principal; that you have written a list of questions to ask the teacher; that you have noted your child's statement about his enjoyment of school, his participation in school activities, and the quality of his work. Bring written notes and leave them with the teacher if necessary, so that he or she can review them later.

During the conference find out whether your child is

at grade level in all of the major subjects. Discuss whether recent achievement testing has been done. Find out what areas need more work. Inspect samples of your child's deskwork and find out what homework she should be bringing home. Ask about any changes in learning or classroom behavior. Finally, review the need for any additional special services and ask the teacher how you can be of most help.

The first few minutes of conferences are crucial. Your actions and the teacher's actions tend to reflect underlying attitudes. If the teacher starts the conference with a list of the latest complaints about how your child is ruining school for classmates, the teacher's attitude needs to be dealt with immediately. In the same way, your warmth and friendliness toward the teacher must be made apparent in the first few moments of the conference to help set the tone for a cooperative relationship.

Telephone Calls. Telephone contact is fast and convenient. It has the additional advantage of being direct, so you and the teacher can communicate without interruption and in privacy. It is best if done after school hours by prearrangement, so that the teacher is freer to talk. If you call the school in the morning, it may be advisable to leave the message with the school secretary rather than to try conversing at length with the teacher. Use the phone to relay a quick warning to the teacher in the morning if your child is having a bad day, so that he or she can adjust expectations and activities for your child. After-school telephone calls can be used to personally express appreciation to the teacher whenever your child comes home particularly happy or encouraged about what occurred at school that day.

Notes. Brief written notes can flow between home and school. The teacher can send special instructions for the child, explanations of homework assignments, or descriptions of classroom events. You can use notes to inform the teacher about special family situations, behavior changes you have noticed or other matters.

It is important not to overdo communicating with the teacher. Reasonably frequent communication will probably help the teacher understand your child. An excess of letters and phone calls, however, may cause harmful attitudes to develop; the teacher may start thinking of you as an overprotective parent more to be avoided than paid attention to.

Communication from the school personnel to you should include allowing you easy access to the resource room, informing you about programs, explaining the purpose and approach used in any of their services, reporting why a particular material is or isn't being taught and why your child does or does not learn it. A newsletter, bulletin board, or parent brochure helps maintain good communication and indicates a responsive school administration.

Your child's academic success may require ongoing collaboration among you, helping professionals, and school personnel. The physician, the psychologist, and the teacher can each make valid and accurate observations within one particular setting. Each can also enlarge the view of the other. Close contact among school personnel about various aspects of managing your child's school experience also helps. Give the school realistic expectations about your child. Left without adequate information, the school staff are likely to make their own interpretations, which could lead to unrealistic approaches. Become aware of what each staff person does with your child. As your child goes through school, you will attend many meetings, make and receive many phone calls, and accumulate many documents. A comprehensive, well-organized notebook or accordion file will help you identify patterns and discrepancies in your child's learning and behavioral characteristics, keep track of progress, prepare for meetings, and obtain an appropriate educational program with little delay if you move to a new school district. The file furnishes documentation to justify your request for services or to hold the school district accountable for its obligations.

Review your child's school file and request one copy of everything in it. Also request copies of reports completed by professionals outside the school district and sent to the school. You might want to include your child's medical, developmental, and academic history; applicable special education laws; names, addresses, and phone numbers of relevant organizations; observations and notes about your child's academic strengths and weaknesses; report cards and progress reports; samples of schoolwork that illustrate points of special difficulty or strength; a record of problems encountered in school and the attempted solutions; evaluation reports; copies of your child's Individualized Education Program (IEP); notes and results of IEP meetings; questions asked and answers received at school conferences; notes of visits to special education programs; notes of phone calls or personal contact with school personnel; letters sent and received; calendar of the school year indicating dates of meetings and conferences; photocopied articles or sections of books relevant to your child's situation; and letters you have sent to teachers after conferences that summarize the points discussed.

Handling the First Parent/Teacher Conference

At the beginning of the school year, convey your desire for excellent results for your child and a harmonious cooperative effort between home and school. Don't assume the new teacher has read all of your child's school records. Even if the teacher reviews the records, be prepared to explain any special academic and social needs as well as the coordination of the treatment program. Bring the teacher up to date on any changes since the end of the past school year.

As further evidence of your interest in your child's progress, use the Taylor Academic Problem Identification Checklist (TAPIC) to pinpoint areas of special need (see Appendix B), based on your knowledge of your child's school adjustment in the previous school year. Highlighting particular difficulties is a convenient method of indicating where the teacher may need to make accommodations. Show the results to the teacher at the start of the school year and ask for help in improving performance in the problem areas.

The classroom teacher can deliver better services to your child if he or she can rely on the advice and assistance of others. In assessing your child's unique learning style and in developing specific strategies for strengthening those areas that require special attention, teamwork and the opportunity to brainstorm with other teachers are essential.

In addition, aides, team teachers, interns, student assistants, and tutors who can work one-on-one with your child are extremely helpful. The school might be able to arrange a peer tutor to help your child understand directions and assignments, read important directions and instructions, drill on key memorized lists, summarize important principles from the teacher's lecture or textbooks, coach on note taking, and assist with textbook and workbook assignments.

Be specific in stating your requests and concerns. Instead of saying "My child can't stand pressure," say "When my child has a long assignment, she starts to become very forgetful and disorganized and responds well if the teacher checks on her every fifteen minutes or so."

Expect to inform each teacher about your child's unique learning and behavior styles. Even among teachers who have received inservice training about ADHD students, there is no universal understanding of exactly how to approach each child. Try to avoid general labels such as learning disabled or hyperactive. The interpretation varies from one teacher to the next.

Although able to recognize hyperactivity and other symptoms of ADHD, the teacher has never had *your* child in class before. Suggest the activities in which your child functions best, and request that these activities be included in the classroom as often as possible. Tell the teacher which disciplinary techniques work best with your child. Discuss your child's hobbies, interests, and talents.

Make sure you give the teacher a clear understanding of your child's input and output capacities. *Input capacity* is the rate at which your child gains knowledge, understands lecture material, reads, and so forth. *Output capacity* refers to the number of pages of homework assignments, the number of pages per night, the number of correct homework answers, and so forth, which the child is able to complete. Both rates may need to be adjusted downward for your child as compared with the rates for non-ADHD classmates.

Chapter 11 presents a complete program of academic approaches that have been found effective for ADHD children and adolescents. Do everything you can to see that each of your child's teachers adheres as closely as possible to that program.

11

Ensuring the Best Teaching Efforts

There is definite validity to the concern commonly expressed by teachers that ADHD children in the mainstream classroom detract from their ability to provide quality teaching. Numerous studies have revealed that teachers give more negative feedback, punishment, and commands to ADHD students than to their classmates. This negative mind-set also spills over into their methods of responding to the non-ADHD students, so all students pay the price for disruptions in the classroom stemming from the ADHD student. This chapter details effective approaches teachers can use to minimize negative reactions to your child's presence and maximize the learning environment.

It contains guidelines to help *any teacher* become more successful in assisting *any ADHD child or adolescent.* Be willing to show this chapter to all interested teachers, administrators, and other school personnel who can influence the expectations placed on your child and the classroom approaches used by your child's teachers.

Effective, successful teachers of ADHD children and adolescents generally pursue six major goals: (1) learning to know the child as an individual; (2) assisting with the biochemical treatment program; (3) guarding the child's self-esteem; (4) helping the child improve relationships; (5) using humane, preventive discipline; and (6) adjusting academic tasks to fit the child.

In classrooms where teachers don't address these areas, ADHD children usually show increased resistance, decreased interest in schoolwork, frequent conflicts with other children, and low grades.

LEARNING TO KNOW THE ADHD CHILD

One of the most frustrating, discouraging, and damaging roadblocks to success in the classroom is a teacher who denies the existence of ADHD. Accepting the reality of your child's disorder is the first step the teacher must take to properly educate your child. Teachers should regard your child as a precious human being, as lovable as any other child, and the ADHD symptoms as a challenge, an opportunity to expand their teaching skills to reach a child with special needs.

When your child does poorly, the teacher should be self-critical, questioning his or her teaching methods and academic demands. There should be no easy, superficial jumping to conclusions or labels like lazy or unteachable. Instead, the teacher should ask questions: "What am I doing that might be slowing this student's progress? Was the material too demanding? Should it have been broken into smaller steps? Should I have checked more often on this student's progress? Did the activity offer too many choices? Was perception fragmented because of the child's distractibility?"

The effective teacher will want to obtain a brief history from you about your child's interests, favorite activities, special talents, and other personal bits of information. The teacher will particularly want to know about the situations that tend to trigger negative reactions, so that he or she can avoid exposing your child to them. What your child's other teachers have found to be effective disciplinary as well as instructional techniques will also be important.

The teacher will want to know how your child relates to the rest of his family, particularly to brothers and sisters who attend the same school. Your child's place within the family structure will be an important piece of information for the teacher, who may want to interview him to obtain a full picture of how he sees the family and the world at large.

Despite her loud voice and talkativeness, your child may not have developed the ability to clearly express and communicate her feelings to others. Through self-expressive art forms, the teacher can gain insight into your child's current emotional state that may not otherwise be apparent. If your child seems to be angry one day, for example, the teacher may offer some paint or other art medium with the instruction "Paint a picture about why you are mad" or "Draw a picture that shows someone who feels the way you do today."

The teacher will want to learn your child's particular styles of dealing with potentially threatening or stressful tasks, so that he or she can find ways to stimulate his wholehearted participation in the class. The teacher will be interested in what you have noticed about his avoidance techniques as well as what you have heard about them from previous teachers.

If your child has developed a fear of failure, gives up quickly, or refuses to try tasks that look challenging, she has probably also developed some other telltale signs that indicate she is afraid to take risks. When the quality of her work will be judged, your child may be tempted to give up or may not try to do the work. Common comments among hyperactive children who display this type of misbehavior are: "I can't do this now"; "I already know how to do this"; "I haven't been able to do it before, so why try now?"; "I'll do it at home . . . tomorrow . . . later . . . in a little bit . . . as soon as I finish this other thing"; and "I did it last year, so why do I have to do it again this year?" The teacher will be alert for such indications of discouragement.

Your child may try to avoid academic stress by finding excuses to leave the classroom. Getting drinks from the water fountain, going to the bathroom, wandering the halls, going to the library, going to his locker, visiting a counselor, and hunting for items like bandages and facial tissue are common excuses. Inside the classroom, some popular excuses for avoiding work are breaking pencils, combing hair, and looking for papers. The teacher will note any such actions by him and discuss them with you.

ASSISTING WITH THE BIOCHEMICAL TREATMENT PROGRAM

Of all the professionals able to help ADHD children, teachers are among the least utilized. Surveys consistently show they feel underused and isolated by physicians and parents in helping to determine the best type and level of medication treatment. ADHD children perceive teachers, probably accurately, as being relatively uninvolved in decisions pertaining to their medication. This lack of coordination among teachers, parents, and physicians is a consistent stumbling block to successful treatment.

Helping with Diagnosis

In the diagnostic phase, the teacher should fill out an untitled Taylor Hyperactivity Screening Checklist (THSC) if the physician prefers that the teacher not know the purpose of the questionnaire. Using this form and the Taylor Social/Emotional/Academic Adjustment Checklist (see Appendix B), the teacher who sees your child in a regular classroom setting for several hours daily will generally be able to provide a helpful overall portrayal of your child's school adjustment. A resource room teacher whose contact with your child is more limited and involves fewer total stresses might also be able to supply useful information, particularly if behavior differs in the two classrooms.

In a secondary school in which your child has several teachers, at least three weeks will probably be required before the teachers become sufficiently familiar with your child to be able to submit valid checklists. For obtaining school information to assist in diagnosis, arrange with the counselor to send each teacher the Taylor S/E/A Adjustment Checklist and an untitled version of the THSC.

Monitoring Medication Effects

When medications are first prescribed, give the teacher a small supply of TSMER forms (see Appendix B) with dates for mailing them already inserted. The teacher should send a TSMER to you or to the physician weekly to assist in establishing the correct daily regimen, then less frequently as requested by the physician. To monitor medication effects if your child has several teachers each day, have the school counselor distribute and collect the TSMER forms.

School administrators often want information included in the student's file about medications or dietary arrangements at school. Be prepared to answer the following questions:

1. What are the names and phone numbers of the physician and the pharmacist?
2. How does the child's medication affect behavior?
3. What are its side effects, if any?
4. What procedure should the teacher follow if the child arrives at school without having taken medication that morning?
5. Should the teacher confront the child privately if he or she suspects the child has not taken medication that morning?
6. Is adult supervision necessary when the child takes medication at school, for example during the noon hour?
7. At what times of day is the medication to be taken?

Reminding About Medication Times

There is wide variation among school districts about the responsibilities for medication treatment. To avoid misunderstandings with school personnel who may not have known or approved of your child's bringing medications to school, take a weekly or monthly supply of medication to school, preferably in its original container and with the physician's instructions for its use. School districts vary in their policies about supervising children's medications, though the general principle is that only a nurse may insert medication into a child's mouth. Therefore, in most instances, the role of school personnel is to make the bottle of pills available to the child, then witness the taking of medication or call the parent if the child refuses.

The most severe and frequent medication-related conflicts between parents of hyperactive children and school personnel revolve around forgetting to take the noon medication. Sometimes school personnel mistakenly conclude that the child's forgetting to take medication is a purposeful act of rebellion. In the vast majority of instances, however, such forgetting is a direct reflection of medication wear-off and has nothing to do with the child's attitude about cooperating with treatment.

Even when they understand that the faulty memory for the noon medication is proof of the need for it, some school personnel might balk at the idea of being asked to remind your child. The most common statement parents receive in such instances is "We believe children as old as yours should have learned to take responsibility for their own actions, including their medication." There are three methods for solving this conflict.

The simplest is to switch to a long-lasting medication that eliminates the need for a noon dosage. The second is to appeal to the teacher to give your child a simple, unobtrusive signal, such as "Remember our secret." The third is to provide additional structure and reminders that do not involve school personnel.

It is best if your child coordinates taking the medication with another activity, such as going by the office on the way to lunch or recess. A simple and effective procedure is to get your child to associate taking the medication with eating—he uses his mouth for both activities. He should use a simple self-reminder: "I can't eat until I take my pill first" or "I take my pill when I eat my lunch."

Another method is to put a brightly colored piece of paper in your child's notebook that has nothing written on it, or that has the words *our secret* on it. The bright color is a code that reminds your child to take a pill at noon. Your child mentally translates the colored paper into the self-reminder "Take my pill at noon."

Overcoming Problem Behaviors

If your child is unusually disruptive, the teacher might suspect that medication was skipped. The teacher should note the behavior problems and any other factors that might explain the sudden deterioration in behavior. Tell the teacher to call you at the end of any school day during which a symptom-reactive state has apparently occurred. Find the source of the problem and solve it, either by adjusting the medication or some other means. If S-R states become too severe to manage and medication is not yet adjusted well enough to eliminate them, be on call to pick up your child at any time during the school day.

If your child's behavior is markedly worse at school than at home, try to observe a typical school day. Compare observations with the teacher to isolate problem behaviors, then work together to find solutions.

Sometimes medications wear off in the early afternoon, and the child returns to a symptom-reactive state for the last school period. Here are some solutions that have worked for many ADHD children in this circumstance:

Protein Supplement. Arrange a high-protein snack such as cheese or peanut butter and crackers about thirty minutes before the symptom-reactive state ordinarily occurs.

Low Dosage of Medication. Arrange a low dosage of the medication about thirty minutes before the symptom-reactive state is likely to occur. Taking medication at other than during a busy lunch hour or recess may cause embarrassment. Consider having your child assigned as "office helper" for a brief period in early afternoon, for example, thereby having an unquestioned reason for going to the office each day.

Medication Schedule. To help medication effects extend later into the afternoon, provide a higher dosage in the morning. If a wear-off of the medication occurs two to three hours after the noon dosage, that dosage level is probably too low and should be adjusted.

CLASS SCHEDULE. If no other adjustments seem to work, ask that the more demanding academic subjects be scheduled in the morning to coincide with the more potent effect of medications.

Monitoring and Reminding with the Feingold Program

The teacher should use the TSMER form to record progress in symptom control at school if your child is on the Feingold Program. Party snacks, foods used in teaching, and school lunches are the most likely potential sources of disruption. The teacher should remain alert for such moments and make a quick phone call to you if necessary to check on the suitability of a food or beverage. If your child refuses served foods, classmates have an open license for teasing. Provide approved snack items to be stored in a refrigerator at school for use at such times.

When an S-R state occurs at school, the teacher should note when it started. The source is most probably through skin contact or inhaled chemicals if the child has not been exposed to an offending chemical through foods or beverages. Careful review of the environmental conditions or classroom projects to which the child was exposed at home in the morning and during school hours will uncover the source of the difficulty. (Appendix E lists school-related chemicals that are the most troublesome for ADHD children.)

GUARDING THE CHILD'S SELF-ESTEEM

Diagnostic terms such as ADHD, hyperactive, attention-disordered, learning disabled, and similar labels should never be announced in front of the class, or spoken of within hearing range of the students by anyone. Classmates should not know about the medication treatment. If someone discovers the pill-taking routine and brings it up during class, the teacher should avoid the issue and should inform you about what happened. The confidentiality of your child's condition and treatment should be defended and honored. There should be no public reminders to take medication, and the public address system should never be used to call your child to the office for medication. The teacher should earn your child's trust by preventing embarrassment and supporting the treatment effort.

If instructions must be stated slowly for your child, the teacher should direct the instruction to the entire class to avoid singling out your child.

The successful teacher knows that every child needs to feel successful and will, therefore, create opportunities for your child to achieve a sense of satisfaction and accomplishment. Placing colorful hand-drawn smiles, stars, or stickers on your child's papers can acknowledge special effort, or the teacher may send a personal letter of encouragement to your child. Such a letter would be treasured and would serve as an excellent way for the teacher to help maintain your child's interest and involvement in class activities. The teacher's verbal acknowledgment of your child's effort should ideally be similar to the encouragement methods described in Chapter 6.

Touch is very important in giving any child the sense of being nurtured, cared for, and worthwhile. The teacher should try to greet your child each day and find unobtrusive ways to touch him briefly, perhaps with a light pat on the shoulder.

Effective teachers know the best ways to teach responsibility are to expect it and to create situations in which it can be shown. They will assign responsibilities with the expectation that your child will be able to carry them out or will at least try hard to do so. Even if the child is not completely successful, the teacher should respond in a supportive and encouraging way.

The teacher should not display the classroom work of only a handful of favored students. Instead, *all* students' work should be displayed around the room, including your child's work.

The successful teacher should use your child's strengths as the foundation for his classroom participation. The most successful teaching approaches maximize these strengths to help compensate for weaknesses while simultaneously attempting to strengthen the weak areas. The multimodal approach, discussed later in this chapter, is excellent for accomplishing both objectives.

There are many additional ways for the teacher to use your child's interests and talents to increase self-esteem. For example, the teacher can acknowledge your child's hobby by having her share with classmates the steps that were necessary to complete the project. Your child can write a report about some aspects of the hobby—its history in social studies class, its impact on nature in science class, or its measurements in math class. Make sure the teacher knows about these special areas for bolstering your child's feelings of success. An excellent example of this support was given by a teacher of an ADHD boy in my practice who enjoyed making backyard items in his home workshop. The teacher thoughtfully invited him to make a presentation to the class on his bird feeders and birdhouses as part of a science unit. On another occasion, he spoke about their construction and demonstrated tool safety as part of a safety and health unit.

HELPING THE CHILD IMPROVE RELATIONSHIPS

Learning disabled ADHD children and adolescents generally have impaired social competence. They use socially unacceptable behaviors when interacting with others, are less able than their peers to solve social problems and predict the consequences of their behavior, are more likely to misinterpret body language, are less likely to adjust to their listeners when carrying on a conversation, and are less likely to take into account the thoughts and feelings of others.

Several surveys have shown that compared to their nonimpaired peers, learning disabled children are less well liked and more rejected; they show more anxiety, withdrawal, depression, and low self-esteem. Learning disabled adolescents participate less in extracurricular activities. ADHD-ld children and adolescents generally have trouble with complex social skills such as persuading, negotiating, adjusting to criticism, giving uncritical feedback, and resisting peer pressure.

The teacher needs to anticipate and prevent problems, rather than merely react to them. The kind-but-firm combination is best, socially and academically, for ADHD children. Teachers who are high in warmth but low on structure often cannot provide the needed supervision and organization to help hyperactive children avoid classroom problems. Teachers who are harsh and authoritarian discourage the zeal for learning and spark a rebellious attitude.

The teacher should try to involve your child in a social awareness program, small group discussions, self-concept exploration, or similar experiences. This process—called affective education—can include pamphlets, tape recordings, and other devices to educate students in the basic principles of interpersonal relationships, conflict solving, and self-esteem. In addition to direct instruction, the creative teacher should also be a role model who demonstrates effective social skills. The teacher can develop a group spirit and a sense of cohesiveness among the students by minimizing competition and emphasizing projects involving cooperation.

When intervention is necessary at a difficult moment,

the teacher will avoid labeling or condemning an action. By privately explaining your child's hyperactivity to individual classmates who are temporarily frustrated or angry, the teacher can help them better accept her. Relationships can remain smooth with well-placed statements such as: "It is sometimes hard for Melanie to sit still and to avoid talking to you, even when she knows you are trying to concentrate."

There are many opportunities at school for pairing your child with suitable prospective new friends. The teacher should coordinate with you on fostering constructive relationships.

Helping undo the wake effect is a further step in bolstering your child's social standing with classmates. The teacher can instruct the entire class in social relationship skills, including the destructiveness of ridicule, scapegoating, exclusion, name calling, boasting, and similar tactics. The teacher can teach these skills without isolating your child or using him as an example.

Many school counselors conduct groups for children who are having relationship difficulties. Such a group, if well administered, can be of great assistance.

USING HUMANE, PREVENTIVE DISCIPLINE

Successful teachers place a great deal of emphasis on preventing misbehavior and use the classroom's structure and procedures for that purpose. Such teachers know that effective classroom discipline must rest on a positive, happy atmosphere and a spirit of caring and cooperation between teacher and students.

The seats should be movable so the student's desks can be rapidly rearranged whenever a disruption threatens to take place. The teacher should also have spare pencils, paper, and facial tissues handy for minor upsets in routine.

There should be a neutral time-out area where your child can go to calm down. The area might have games, art supplies, or other materials to help overcome pent-up feelings and to occupy him whenever he is unable to participate in the regular classroom activity. When time-out is needed, the required area can be in a corner of the classroom; but it might also be elsewhere, such as just outside the classroom on a small bench or chair. It is most effective when there is a minimum of conversation between your child and the teacher at the time; but there should be a brief discussion after school, and the teacher should inform you about the incident.

There should be provisions for music that the teacher can turn on and off as a behavior control measure. Or the teacher may use the lights for behavior control, primarily as a signal for a change in activity.

The effective teacher will realize the importance of routine and will write a schedule on the blackboard, for example, outlining each day's activities.

The thinking teacher will not overwhelm your child with the responsibility of making too many choices in a short period of time. Instead, he or she will allow your child to make choices gradually, starting with a simple choice between only two options.

The teacher should know that your child must always be permitted to finish speaking when she has started to say something, even if the teacher would like her to stop. Recognizing that this rigidity is not a defiance of authority but is, instead, a symptom of your child's hyperactivity, the teacher will wait politely until she has finished talking, so she will not experience needless frustration in being interrupted.

The teacher will emphasize cuing and reminding as ways to prevent problems from developing. Rather than giving a loud reprimand, the teacher should touch your child's arm or shoulder while giving a softly spoken, direct message that specifically indicates what your child is to stop or start doing. Research clearly indicates that a mild reminder is much more effective than ignoring the first occurrence of misbehavior.

A secret signal system can be developed for the teacher's use in reminding your child to get back on task. The best signal is three light taps on his desk. Arrange this private code among you, the teacher, and your child. He is to interpret the three taps as equivalent to the teacher's saying, "Get back to work; stop fiddling around." Point out that the code is a special way to avoid embarrassing him. As a way to return this favor, your child is to cooperate completely with the signal whenever the teacher gives it.

Providing periodic opportunity to discharge built-up energy is a key to successful classroom behavior management. The teacher should understand that sustained sitting can lead to problems if not alternated with more vigorous activity, and should find opportunities for movement, rather than trying to force your child to stifle that need. Helpful methods that have worked in some schools include allowing the child to assist the cafeteria, custodial, or office staff for short periods or allowing a quick run around the playground. The opportunity to go to the gymnasium to bounce on tumbling mats or throw baskets can also help a great deal in preventing misbehavior. Such an arrangement needs to be coordinated with all involved school personnel, of course, but is quite successful in many schools.

Similarly, highly organized, very predictable, and tightly structured classroom procedures need to be balanced by occasional periods for rest, vigorous activity, and play. For this reason it is very important that ADHD children be allowed to participate in recess. Restricting your child at lunchtime or recess is not a wise disciplinary tactic. Your child needs an active recess period to compensate for the stress of self-restraint throughout the rest of the day.

If your child is especially disorganized about coming to class prepared, turning papers in on time, or self-control of classroom behavior, consider using the Taylor Classroom Daily Report. The teacher enters the relevant information, signs it, and sends it home with your child at the end of the day. If you wish to confer about anything on the form, simply initial at the indicated location. The form can be returned daily by your child to the teacher to verify you have examined it, or it can be used simply for one-way communication from the teacher to you. This procedure requires extra effort and deserves your frank recognition. Thank the teacher and keep him or her apprised of its helpfulness.

ADJUSTING ACADEMIC TASKS TO FIT THE CHILD

Multimodal Learning

An especially effective technique involves using more than one of your child's senses in the learning experience. Combinations of sight, hearing, touch, movement (kinesthesis), taste, and smell can be involved simultaneously to create an integrated experience. This use of several senses at the same time permits learning to take place faster and more effectively than by using just one sense at a time. For certain limited learning situations, this approach is the preferred method.

This process, called multimodal learning, can be illustrated in teaching a first-grade child the sound of the letter *M*. A typical multimodal approach would be to have the child say "mmm" after hearing the teacher say it, as

The Taylor Classroom Daily Report

Student ______________________________ Date __________

	Yes	*No*	*Comments*
BEHAVIOR—Did my child:			
Arrive on time?			
Bring needed materials?			
Remain on task?			
Participate appropriately?			
Behave correctly?			
SCHOOLWORK—Did my child:			
Complete seatwork today?			
Turn in homework on time?			
Was the homework neat?			
Was it complete?			
Did it have the proper heading?			
Was it according to directions?			

Overdue or incomplete work still out:

Homework given today:

Additional comments:

I request a telephone call from you if initialed: ______

_________________________ _________________________

Teacher Parent

the child traces with his fingertip on a large piece of sandpaper a large letter *M*, which is painted on the sandpaper. The child *hears* the teacher and himself say the sound of the letter; *moves* his hand, arm, and mouth; *sees* the large letter on the sandpaper; and *feels* the sandpaper with his fingertip. Even though your child may have poor coordination, a multimodal approach involving movement will be helpful. Multimodal learning is the ideal, but it may not be practical in some classrooms because of other demands made on the teacher.

By writing the assignment on the blackboard for the children to copy, the successful teacher can reinforce verbal instructions. Parents can also use the blackboard at home. Using a typewriter or word processor at home or at school can be a helpful multimodal experience, especially if your child repeats aloud what she is typing.

Individualized Instruction

One-on-one teaching is often very effective with a hyperactive child, but unfortunately it usually has to be severely rationed in most school systems. The principle is nevertheless valid, and a successful teacher will try to arrange some method of one-on-one teaching for your child. Your child will make more progress if he has five minutes of individual attention and help, and then spends the remaining twenty-five minutes working by himself, than if he had to work as part of the class (lecture method) for thirty minutes. Providing one-on-one instruction for your child will be much easier if aides are helping the teacher.

Neither too much nor too little help will be offered by the truly effective teacher. The need to repeat such admonitions as "figure it out" or "try harder" may indicate that your child has already reached her frustration level because of the difficulty of the work. At such moments, one-on-one attention and instruction should be given.

Help from the teacher should be available, but withheld until your child makes an earnest attempt to learn through her own efforts. Providing individualized instruction does not always mean forcing your child to work alone. Assignments can be given so your child's work is part of a coordinated class activity.

Individualized Curriculum

The curriculum should be individualized to concentrate on the most important courses and topics. To create your child's curriculum, the teacher will want to measure abilities such as reading, cursive writing, spelling, mathematics, and other relevant areas. Ideally, the teacher will also want to hear your ideas about curriculum adjustment.

The effective teacher should try to teach at approximately your child's achievement level. An extremely easy assignment may not be challenging, or even satisfying. Tasks that are too challenging are also not satisfying and may quickly lead him to stop trying. Curriculum planning should provide opportunities to exercise his abilities without becoming frustrated. In this way your child's self-confidence can be developed and he can experience the joy of accomplishment and the momentum of success. It is important to dilute challenging material with enough other work so the total experience is not too stressful.

Individualized Assignments

Introducing one step at a time and dividing the assigned work into units, such as three ten-minute assignments rather than one thirty-minute assignment, allows your child to complete each unit before moving ahead to the next one. Each succeeding unit should involve a slightly more difficult or advanced stage of learning, so that the learning process can be graduated.

This procedure makes each task achievable and lets your child concentrate fully on each one before taking on the next. She will be able to organize her thinking and concentration for each step without being distracted and overwhelmed by concerns about the total cluster of new concepts involved in the complete lesson. The task, therefore, will seem less difficult, less confusing, and less frightening than if it had been presented as one large assignment.

The creative teacher will avoid overloading your child by introducing a few concepts at a time. After each new group of concepts is introduced, it should be reviewed, so that the child can be tested to see if he has really acquired, absorbed, and retained the new knowledge. A few more concepts can then be introduced. The next review may be cumulative, including previously learned material as well as the most recently introduced. New knowledge is thus presented, reviewed, absorbed, tested, and integrated step-by-step with previously learned material.

The teacher should allow your child to complete one activity before starting another. For example, your child might be asked to first copy *all* the arithmetic problems, then solve them.

The course of progress should be from simple tasks to complex ones, from mastery to challenge and be geared to your child's particular needs. Homework loads vary greatly between districts and among schools within districts. A rough general guideline is a half-hour daily in fourth grade, expanding to two-and-a-half hours in high school. A heavier homework load is probably too severe for most ADHD children and adolescents.

Physical Education

One part of your child's curriculum that merits special attention is physical education. For early adolescent hyperative children, gym class is often one of the most troublesome and embarrassing times of the school day. The requirements of physical education classes—disrobing, wearing uniforms, displaying physical coordination—can be very difficult challenges. Your child needs opportunities to release energy, and a physical education class is such an opportunity; but many physical education courses offer little more than competitive team sports.

In a truly effective and creative physical education program, your child can experience release of energy, control of breathing, improvement of muscle coordination, sharpened sense of balance, and knowledge of exercise and nutrition principles. These results can occur if the physical education curriculum includes such activities as dance, relaxation training, structured exercise programs, posture and body movement training, and individual sports such as swimming, bowling, tennis, skating, golf, racquetball, handball, and archery.

Classroom Size and Structure

Small classes or high adult-to-student ratios are more conducive to learning than crowded classrooms. Anything out of place can be distracting to your child and can preoccupy him. Ideally, there should be a special section set aside where classroom supplies, particularly those used by your child, would always be in the same place; the blackboard should be cleaned at the start of each day; there should be no mobiles dangling from the ceiling and no clusters of brightly colored pictures on the wall.

The teacher should be calm and unhurried, avoiding quick or extreme movements of the hands, fingers, or pencils. Pointers should be moved slowly and smoothly, rather than in rapid starting and stopping motions.

Your child's desk should be in an area relatively free from distractions and where supervision is easy, so she can be given instructions quickly. Depending on the physical arrangement of the classroom, her desk might be next to the desks of quiet children, next to the teacher's desk, or in a corner, separated by a partition to narrow her immediate range of vision. It might face a wall rather than the classroom and should be away from windows, doors, and high traffic areas. For a child on the Feingold Program, it is best to avoid sitting next to a heating duct or a source of offending chemical inhalants.

If the desk is in a corner, a bookcase, a filing cabinet, a blanket draped over a rope, sides of a large shipping carton or specially constructed opaque screens might be used to isolate it. If a large object provides too much isolation, the teacher should try to construct and attach a border around the desk, such as from cardboard and approximately fourteen inches high, to help reduce your child's visual distractions while at the desk. It might become your child's "office" where she can work peacefully. Under no circumstances should this special seating arrangement be used as punishment, although sometimes other children might use it as a time-out area. Your child may have to be taught the need for this arrangement: that it is intended to allow her to concentrate more fully on classwork, and that it will enhance her enjoyment and participation in the class. The teacher should explain these concepts to the other children without embarrassing or labeling your child.

Although a screened desk may seem at first to hinder any child's sense of belonging, the opposite is usually true if the arrangement is handled properly. This special plan allows a much higher level of academic success and therefore enthusiasm for school than a standard arrangement. Academic success paves the way for social success, and behavior is better controlled and more tolerable when the seating arrangement controls distractibility.

Sometimes your child may be so distracted by the background and format of a page in a book that the ability to concentrate on the word or idea being taught is lost. The teacher should help by isolating the item from its background and writing the word or phrase on the blackboard or on a separate piece of paper. Nonessential material should be covered, and your child should be encouraged to use a pointer, marker, or hand-held cardboard border. Reading machines might also be used.

Your child's desk should be uncluttered. The only items on it should be those necessary to complete each assignment as it is given. At other times, the desk should be cleared of all objects, with the possible exception of a brightly colored contrast mat, which can help limit his visual field during desk work.

Though the guidelines given in this chapter may seem lofty, they are generally reachable by any concerned teacher. Even when your child is in a symptom-reactive state, most are applicable and can help the teacher prevent the situation from becoming a major interference to the class. Helping an ADHD child in the classroom is an exciting and fulfilling challenge that represents teaching at its finest.

12

Encouraging Academic Success

Once you have assured your child of maximum assistance at school, you yourself can do much to help ensure success. This chapter describes the study skills and homework monitoring methods parents have found most effective for ADHD children and adolescents.

The best learning is interesting, relevant, and fun. Encourage your child to undertake creative projects. Select materials and activities for play that have an educational component. Play educational games and extract the instructional elements out of board and card games. Read to your child and find other ways to show that learning is an exciting process.

Discuss ideas at home, sharing opinions about social and political trends that affect your community and your family. Show an interest in books, read informational magazines, and use encyclopedias and other reference materials. Attend educational programs and use the library often.

Share your joy and excitement about what your child is

learning. Use mealtime for answering questions and discussing what he is learning at school. Avoid an authoritarian attitude when inquiring about how he is doing. Keep the conversation friendly and low key, and convey your expectations and assumptions of his success. Academic success is the inevitable outcome of consistent effort; it is a process, not a static state. Emphasize the process of learning and studying rather than the product of high grades.

STARTING EACH DAY WELL

When asked what parental support they most want, teachers in elementary and middle schools consistently put providing a good breakfast at or near the top of the list. For ADHD children, nutrition is an especially important aspect of their daily functioning. Research shows that children who miss breakfast perform poorly at school in the morning. Breakfast should supply about 40% of your child's daily nutritional needs. By breakfast time, your child has already been without food for about twelve hours. For ADHD children, protein consumption is somewhat more crucial than for most other people. There is nothing wrong with a bowl of cereal, but try to accompany it with some cheese, an egg, or meat. Consult your physician about any special nutritional concerns.

STRENGTHENING CLASSROOM SKILLS

Basic to your child's ability to stay organized is a notebook. Discourage her from using a collection of pocket portfolios; all of those pockets become convenient hiding places for assignments that are incomplete, supposed to be given to you, not turned in, forgotten, or lost. The standard three-ring notebook is a far better choice. Allow a spring clip, an envelope taped to the front cover, or a small plastic pouch punched to fit the notebook rings as the only place for holding loose papers.

One of the most frequent teacher complaints about ADHD children is that they talk to other students when they should be listening to the classroom instruction. A self-reminder can prevent this problem: "I mustn't talk when I'm listening." Listening is central to active participation, and most hyperactive children have difficulty with it. Good listening means focusing attention, understanding, mentally processing, and thinking about what the teacher is saying. It can be improved with careful practice.

Sitting near the teacher rather than toward the back of the room is one of the best ways to improve listening. Encourage your child to choose a seat that allows close eye contact with the teacher, preferably near the teacher's desk. This location is one of the best from the teacher's point of view also, so you shouldn't have difficulty arranging it for all classes with assigned seating.

Remembering what the teacher said is another key ingredient. On average, adult students remember only 25% of what they hear immediately after hearing it. A month later, if it hasn't been repeated, they remember only 2%. Hyperactive children are much less able than average adults to recall what they have heard. Even their immediate memory for simple two-part or three-part requests tends to be faulty. Don't assume that your child can rely on memory without the advantage of writing down important parts of what is being taught at school. Efficient note taking improves memory and is absolutely essential if your child is to survive academically. It is even more complicated than refining listening skills, because note taking starts where listening leaves off and involves several additional skills. Outlining is the most efficient method because it requires few words, simplifies learning by focusing on main ideas, relieves concern about spelling or punctuation, and minimizes handwriting.

Teach your child these note-taking strategies. *Find the major and minor points* and try to form a mental image of what is being said. Particularly note (1) anything teachers write on the board, (2) the main ideas of what they say, (3) definitions and lists, (4) information they repeat, and (5) anything they refer to in the text. Also include at least one example of what is being taught—for example, a mathematics problem—even though the child thinks he knows the points.

Use common abbreviations and symbols. This facet of good note taking is crucial in math classes. Show your child how to represent an increase with an upward-pointing arrow, "less than" and "more than" by a caret pointing to the left or right, and other useful symbols. Your child should include brief sentences in the notes if possible. "Pilgrims wanted freedom of religion" is much more helpful than "Pilgrims—freedom—religion."

Write on only one side of the paper; date notes and any supplementary material. Also consider having your child tape record any especially significant or difficult lectures and listen to the recording while reviewing her notes.

SUPERVISING AND ASSISTING WITH HOMEWORK

Establish a quiet, protected place for study. The chair should be straight-backed with just a little padding. Purchase or make a special study desk or table. You may want to glue a small corkboard border on the edge of the desk to keep your child's attention on the desktop and block out noises and visual interference. Provide supplies:

paper, pencils, pens, erasers, correction tape or fluid if a typewriter is used, ruler, clock, assignment book, three-by-five cards, stapler, paper clips, folders, and items for specific classes such as compass and protractor for geometry. Store all of these study materials in one place, such as a desk drawer or shelf. Arrange good lighting; inadequate lighting can cause mental fatigue and dramatically lower the energy for studying. Have a special place for the finished work where it will not be forgotten the next morning, such as on top of the notebook, in a backpack or book bag, or inside the notebook.

Some parents purchase extra copies of textbooks to keep at home. Up-to-date reference books should be available, including English grammar aids like a thesaurus and a college-level dictionary.

At each study session make sure your child is neither hungry nor tired. The study desk should be free of all items except those needed that evening. Sitting upright maintains mental alertness much better than leaning back, lying on the floor, or reclining. Protect her from all outside interferences and distractions, including phone calls, music, television, radio, and visits from friends. It is important that family and friends respect the study time. Inform friends she can accept telephone calls before or after the regular study hours. Take messages (or if necessary to get friends to comply, refuse to do so) during the scheduled study time. Consider a Do Not Disturb sign for the study room and control household noises during this time.

Bad habits are cruel masters; good habits are loyal servants. Schedule a regular study time and try to keep it constant throughout the week. Becoming accustomed to studying at a regular time while in elementary school enables your child to study regularly as homework loads increase. If he has not yet established good homework habits, start with short sessions of as little as fifteen minutes per night. This routine needs to overcome the attractive options and distractions at home that would otherwise sidetrack his efforts. The best time is shortly after school; the second best time is immediately after the evening meal. Refer to the clock: "It is 4:00 now; homework time!"

Set goals for the amount of work to accomplish in each study session if the assignment is a long-term project, but strictly enforce a fifteen-minute effort per night. Suggest a goal, but allow your child to influence the final decision. Your child should spend the entire period studying and should complete the assigned work. If the amount of homework is less than usual on any particular night, use the designated time for other learning activities, such as reading, using workbooks, practicing on the typewriter or computer, doing religious study, listening to educational or religious tapes, working with flashcards, memorizing vocabulary and spelling words, reading the newspaper, or reading educational or news magazines. To keep up with the lessons, encourage a review of the material presented in class each day as well as reading or scanning the material upcoming the next day.

Help plan the study time so that both of you have a clear idea of what is to be accomplished. This arrangement sustains work habits and prevents rushing through the work at school to evade homework that evening. To avoid missing any assignments, ask the teacher to send a schedule of all upcoming assignments once each week, preferably on Friday.

Gradually lengthen the sessions as the ability to do the homework increases. Check periodically to make sure the assignments are being done correctly. Be available to assist, but don't stand over your child's shoulder. Some ADHD children require more structure and profit from the parent's actually remaining in the same room during study time.

Observe the rule of 50–10: fifty minutes of studying earns a ten-minute break. For many ADHD children, the rule of 25–5 works better: a five-minute break after every twenty-five minutes of studying.

The actual completion of the assignments is the most desired route to academic success. Give suggestions and support, but don't do the entire task. Do the first problem or part of the assignment as a model, then stand by as your child tackles the second item or part. If a homework assignment seems particularly troublesome, assist by breaking it down into smaller segments. Or alter the sequence of steps for approaching the task, by recommending doing a certain part of the work before proceeding to other parts.

Long-term assignments are especially troublesome. If the teacher will not agree to turning in segments of the work, make sure your child works at least fifteen minutes nightly on them and builds steadily toward completion of the task. The Master Chart (described in Chapter 13) will help greatly. Check regularly to see that your child has entered all long-term assignments and upcoming tests on it.

Make sure your child understands the assignment directions. Have her read the directions and essential portions of the text to you, then ask a question or two about the directions and the text to confirm that she understands what she has just read. Summarize important textbook passages, and have her repeat them to you. Rephrase the instructions in your own words if necessary, and ask specific questions to guide her reading. If study questions are already provided and you need to give assistance, point out the paragraphs where the answers are but do not point to the answers themselves.

Clever encouragements can help maintain a positive attitude about using the daily study time wisely. Keep a chart of the total number of items your child learns, for example, vocabulary words, countries or states and their capitals, spelling words, foreign-language words, and math facts. Temperature on a thermometer that slowly rises or a picture of a train that gradually approaches the station are novel methods to add impact to charting your child's progress.

The ability to type is no longer a skill reserved for only a few. Your child should learn to type and to use a computer keyboard. Current educational software is faster and more efficient than other instructional aids like workbooks and flashcards. If your child has a history of school difficulties, think seriously of purchasing or borrowing a microcomputer for home use. Numerous computer programs ensure successful learning and thereby bolster sagging self-confidence.

The computer embodies many of the characteristics of a skilled special educator. It gives your child undivided attention, individualizes instruction to any readiness or skill level, responds with positive and encouraging feedback, accommodates any working pace, teaches skills in small steps, provides incentives for learning, repeats a task or question until the principle involved is learned, informs continuously and immediately about progress being made, is fun and entertaining, minimizes failure and frustration, and measures areas of relative strength and difficulty.

To assist with a reading problem, borrow a program that provides multisensory instruction and reinforces word-decoding skills with auditory and visual prompts. If your child has trouble remembering math facts, a program can strengthen his memory and math facility. A program that requires a pause before a response can compensate for impulsiveness and hyperactivity. This feature trains him in self-reminders of the stop-and-think variety.

Many educators are using computers with students who have a broad spectrum of learning problems. If your school district has introduced microcomputers into its classrooms, your child should be allowed to use them. This use should not, however, be confined merely to practice and drill. Programs that enhance cognitive skills and thinking processes should also be made available.

Even though skills gained in homework are important, do not allow homework to monopolize all your child's evenings. Be sure to balance your child's daily life. Get her involved in evening activities requiring vigorous physical movement and less mental discipline than schoolwork. Parents generally report that hobbies, social and cultural events, arts and crafts, civic and church groups, and athletics are especially helpful.

Troubleshooting Problems

Resistance to homework is often expressed with statements such as "I don't have any"; "School is dumb"; "I'd rather watch TV." Your child might do homework for only one subject, complain that the teacher assigns too much, or try to lure you into doing it. Discover the source of homework avoidance. Is it a form of rebellion against you, too heavy an assignment load from school, a reflection of difficulty with study habits or planning ability, assignments far behind or far ahead of your child's readiness and skill level, or some other cause? Ask your child how you can help make homework more manageable for him.

Sometimes an absence of interest in homework reflects an underlying personality clash or conflict with the teacher. ADHD children are often unpopular among school faculty, and such conflicts occur frequently. Consider this possibility if you can't find a substantial reason for your child's problems with the assignments themselves.

If your child has difficulties handling homework, suspect a breakdown in one or more of the following steps:

1. Writes down the assignment.
2. Understands the assignment.
3. Checks to see what to bring home at the end of the school day.
4. Arrives home with the assignment and needed materials.
5. Starts to do the homework.

6. Completes the homework.
7. Checks the homework for neatness and accuracy.
8. Puts completed homework in the notebook.
9. Takes the homework back to school.
10. Keeps track of it until the proper class.
11. Turns it in.

During the first grading period of the school year, closely monitor your child's homework efforts. Get an accurate feeling for the pace, difficulty level, and total homework load. If you suspect problems, keep a record of the actual homework time. Assess how well your child is handling each of the eleven steps; then negotiate with the teacher for any needed changes in the assignments or the arrangements for monitoring homework performance.

Compensating for Distractibility

Their distractibility causes some ADHD children and adolescents to fritter away an hour or two of homework time, then ask to watch television or do other things. Here are nine methods parents have found most helpful for facilitating concentration and lessening the effects of distractibility.

1. The stopwatch. Tell your child he must produce a certain number of minutes of *on-task* study during the study period. He is to stop the watch whenever he goes to the bathroom, gets a drink of water, looks out the window, yawns, or does anything other than homework. Emphasize that wasting time simply extends the period he has to remain studying.
2. Irregular check-in. At irregular intervals of a few minutes each, check on what your child is doing during the designated study period. If you discover she is busily involved in schoolwork, she earns a point. Arrange a pleasant reward after she earns a certain number of points.

3. Self-monitoring. Suggest a useful self-reminder, such as "I need to get back on task" or "Always get back on task as soon as I can," whenever he catches himself being careless.
4. Segmented tasks. Keep the tasks as short as possible and arrange a pause to review each segment, perhaps submitting the work to you.
5. Work before play. No other activity is permitted until the study time has met the criteria you have set.
6. Staggered tasks. Shift to a less demanding task for a brief period. Varying the tasks and alternating hard and easy or liked and disliked subjects lets the child focus better on the task at hand.
7. Distraction control. Remove sources of distraction such as music or television.
8. Sequenced tasks. Some children respond better if the more difficult tasks come early in the session; others need the boost in self-confidence provided by completing smaller assignments before moving on to the larger ones.
9. Increased meaning. Magnify the meaning and relevance of the assignment by explaining its usefulness and direct applicability to your child's life, either for the present or the future.

Increasing Comprehension

Many processes are involved in using new information. Applying several of these to what he is studying will greatly increase your child's comprehension. The processes include defining, labeling, describing, explaining, summarizing, breaking into parts, noticing relationships between parts, outlining, joining parts to form a new whole, composing, creating, evaluating, supporting with relevant information, and justifying.

Try to build on as many as your child seems able and willing to perform.

You can accomplish this enhancement by having your child read aloud, underline words and phrases, write comments, outline chapters, describe what was read, paraphrase important passages, find arguments for and against key points, write down all listed items (including lists that are hidden in regular paragraphs), draw pictures reflecting the content of the material, and imagine what it would have been like to be present at the scene described in the reading passages.

Asking the newspaper reporter's classic questions—who, what, where, when, why, and how—helps develop a clear mental picture of any homework assignment and is especially useful with long reading passages. To further strengthen this approach, have your child play the Newspaper Reporter Game from the Fun Idea List (see Chapter 13). Have her circle answers to the six key questions from current articles in newspapers, then show you the circled points.

PREPARING FOR TESTS

In reviewing for tests, typed notes are easier to study than handwritten lecture notes. Typing the notes forces your child to rethink the material and aids understanding. Reading aloud is a more efficient way to remember the information than silently reading the notes.

Several short review periods provide better preparation for a test than one long cramming session. Your child will score higher by reviewing notes daily for a week or so before the test. Arrange for expanded study times as the dates for important exams approach. A good plan is to devote at least fifteen minutes of study on each of the last five days before any major test.

Active review and rehearsal provide the best memory strengthening. Ask your child to tell you about the material and read to you from class notes. Rehearse the test by composing one test question for each paragraph in the assigned readings. Put the questions on three-by-five cards, and keep reviewing them until he has learned all the answers. A similar technique is to have him compose the questions and give you a test on the topics covered.

Another useful method is joint study with a classmate. One child reads to the other from one set of notes while the child who is listening follows along by reading the other set of class notes.

Discourage your child from simply trying to remember unconnected facts or lists. Help your child examine the underlying issues, concepts, and relationships to find correlations. For lists, self-quizzing is a useful technique, facilitated by a cassette recorder or flashcards. When using a cassette, your child records vocabulary words and their definitions, spelling words and their spellings, states and their capitals, historical events and their dates, or any similar facts. There should be a brief pause between each entry and its matching answer; for example, "Vitamin A . . . carrots." Then your child can self-quiz by listening to the first item of each pair, answering out loud during the pause, and comparing the response with the correct answer.

When using flashcards, your child writes the first item of each pair on one side of a three-by-five card and its matching answer on the other side. An advantage of the flashcard method is that easily mastered items can be put into the learned-well pile, while the others remain in the review-again pile. Gradually the review-again pile shrinks as the facts are thoroughly memorized.

Have your child get to sleep early the night before a test and review early on the morning of the test. This is much more reliable than studying into the wee hours the night before, then taking the test after inadequate sleep and no breakfast that morning. Even when they are receiving medication, sleep and nutritional factors are the two most common sources of day-to-day variation in the mental functioning of hyperactive children.

USING TUTORING TO ADVANTAGE

An increasingly popular method among teachers of ADHD students in mainstream and self-contained classrooms is peer monitoring. A reliable agemate or slightly older child functions as a teacher's aide to help your child interpret and apply instructions, tutors and assists with individual assignments, and advises about any needed improvements in behavior.

If peer monitoring cannot be arranged, consider spending a few minutes each night at home in a minitutoring program. Most teachers are delighted if parents review material with their children at home. After you are familiar with the teacher's approach, review and reinforce his or her efforts at home. Closely coordinate your lessons with the classroom instruction. Such a joint effort brings you meaningfully into the educational process and helps your child perceive home and school as integrated parts of the educational enterprise. Although not suitable for every parent of an ADHD child, ten- to fifteen-minute sessions with flashcards or other interesting drills can add a meaningful dimension to the learning process.

If you think that tutoring your child will cause too much strain on your relationship, hire an outside tutor. Currently employed or retired teachers, graduate students, college students, and high-school students are often willing to tutor. The tutor can employ games, flashcards, and similar activities that encourage academic skills without creating the tension that often accompanies book work. Monitor your child's progress and occasionally sit in on the tutoring sessions.

REINFORCING PARTICULAR SKILLS

Reading

The best remedial reading program for most ADHD children is multifaceted; it emphasizes phonics, involves overlearning at each difficulty level, and ensures mastery at one level before proceeding to the next level.

Poor readers have difficulty understanding what they read by how it sounds. Skilled readers, on the other hand, depend on how the written material looks as well as how it sounds. ADHD children who have difficulty reading usually profit from training in phonics and breaking words into syllables and common letter combinations. Although becoming familiar with configuration—how words look—might help a little, the major victory in learning to read is knowing how the letters and words sound. Your child needs to know the sounds of the individual letters, the sounds of common letter combinations, and the rules for piecing together the parts of words.

Individualized instruction in phonics is superior to small group instruction. If your child is having trouble, placement in the slow reading circle might not be sufficient remedial reading. Follow your child's progress and ask for more help from the school if there is little improvement. At the same time, I recommend providing supplemental phonics instruction at home. The best methods are to play with phonics flashcards for ten minutes each evening and to have your child read to you. Whenever your child makes a reading error, tactfully explain the phonics principles or letter sounds involved. Give your child a sense of having learned something important and having conquered a new word. Maintain a My New Words list to help your child celebrate these successes.

Handwriting

If difficulties with handwriting hamper your child's school performance, four basic adjustments are possible. One method is to negotiate with the teacher regarding the form of the work. Perhaps assignments could be presented orally, through tape recordings, by transcription expressed in your handwriting, or with a typewriter or word processor. Another method is to arrange for fewer assignments though all these would still require handwriting. The third method involves tutoring and practicing handwriting skills, letter by letter, at home. Have your child write extra large letters, approximately five inches by eight inches. Pay careful attention to the sequence of strokes or letter parts, and follow the sequence being taught at school. Gradually reduce the size of the letters until they are the correct size for normal handwriting. Drill for about five minutes each evening until the handwriting improves. The last method, which asks the least of the teacher, is to allow increased time for completing written assignments.

Better handwriting is the most frequently cited academic change reported by teachers of ADHD children who start the Feingold Program or prescribed medication. Therefore, adjusting the biochemical treatment is often an integral part of helping an ADHD child improve handwriting.

Spelling

Help your child learn the meaning of the spelling words by explaining how each word can be used. Be willing to split the study session into two or three short segments, alternating with other homework. For an especially difficult or unusual word, look up its root (often Latin, Greek, or Old English) that helps explain its spelling.

Devise simple nonsense statements to help recall a letter sequence. If your child is having trouble remembering the *a* comes before the *u* in *gauge,* give an example such as: "Two people are riding in a car. One thinks they might run out of gas. The other says, '*Aw, you* (A,U) are wrong—look at the gauge!'

Incorporate the sounds of the words into the studying by helping your child learn to pronounce each word correctly. If a word obeys common phonics principles, refer to them: the *e* at the end of a word is usually silent, every syllable requires a vowel, *i* before *e* except after *c,* and so forth.

Combine several channels of learning by using the multimodal approach mentioned in Chapter 11. Have your child trace the letters (sense of touch and muscle control), see the tracing (visual), say the letters out loud (vocal), and hear the word and letters spoken (auditory).

Another method is to play the Spelling Teacher Game. Let your child teach you the words on the list by pronouncing them and then spelling them out loud. You can even have a mock oral or written test, in which you purposely make some errors for your child to catch.

Math

If your child has trouble with word problems, part of the difficulty could relate to reading comprehension problems. Explore that possibility before you conclude the fault lies in difficulty with mathematics concepts.

Perceptual problems can pose a special challenge. Poor figure-ground perception would cause your child to have trouble deciphering which parts of the math problem have been included as a distraction and which parts are important for obtaining the answer. Other perceptual problems include lining the numbers straight down the paper, keeping the decimals in the correct position, subtracting downward rather than upward, progressing from right to left when multiplying, and so forth. The best solution to these problems is to arrange with the teacher to have your child use graph paper for all mathematics assignments. To prevent orientation errors (up-down, left-right), teach your child some simple self-reminders, "Make sure things add *up*" and "Subtract means go *down* like a sub(marine)."

Memory problems also plague mathematics efforts. Often ADHD children have not memorized the necessary addition, subtraction, multiplication, and division facts or the decimal equivalents of fractions. One of the best ways to strengthen this area is to play a game of rhythmic chanting to the sound of a drum or hand clap: "3 times 2 is 6; 3 times 3 is 9; 3 times 4 is 12," and so forth. Because money is based on the decimal system, coins and dollars provide convenient and effective examples of fractions and percentages. A quarter, for example, is 25% of a dollar as well as one-fourth of a dollar.

The abstract concepts that abound in mathematics sometimes represent formidable stumbling blocks to the ADHD student. Ideas such as square root, infinity, negative numbers, ratios, and logical proofs can confuse any child who tends to think in concrete and literal terms. The best approach is to find a factual example of the abstract concept. Have a box with many small parts in it, such as miniature plastic building blocks, pennies, checkers, marbles, or buttons. Use these items to illustrate and explain any abstract concept that seems to stifle your child's understanding of how to do a mathematics assignment. By translating numbers into actual objects, you can teach your child to manipulate and count.

CONSIDERING OTHER EDUCATIONAL OPTIONS

Although a time-consuming process, selecting a private school is an option preferred by many parents of ADHD children. A comprehensive psychoeducational evaluation is a helpful first step (see Chapter 10). Obtain a directory of private schools from a library and carefully investigate each prospective school. Be frank and assertive when inquiring about any school's ability to meet your child's educational needs. Make lists of these needs and then compare what each school offers with your criteria. On-site visits are much better than catalog shopping for private schools.

Home schooling is another option that has gained popularity. Approximately 12,000 to 20,000 ADHD children in the United States are currently being educated at home. If you have the necessary time, patience, and ability and the public and private schools seem unlikely to adequately serve your child's needs, home schooling may be a viable option. Concerns about limiting your child's social experiences, frequently given as an objection, shouldn't prevent you from considering it. Many home-schooled children experience gains—not losses—in social contacts, both in the quality of supervised contact and the number of new friends. Any decrease in daily social contact can be compensated for by following the friendship-building suggestions in this book and by involving your child in character-building activities offered by church and community groups and athletics. The basic requirement for home schooling is that your child can demonstrate an increase in knowledge level each year that is equivalent to the average increase shown by children of similar age in the public school system in your community.

Specific requirements as to the number of hours of instruction and the subjects to be taught vary from one community to another. The best way to ensure success is to purchase texts and workbooks specifically published for home schooling or obtain copies of the materials used in the public schools in your community. You will need to register with your local school district or the office that keeps records of home-schooled children.

Although academic adjustment and achievement are prominent issues and certainly merit intense concern, don't sacrifice the bonds of family love to enforce academic goals. Even if your child continues to have difficulties with arithmetic and handwriting, the long-term results are not extremely damaging. Typewriters and personal computers are suitable substitutes for penmanship, and hand-held calculators can overcome many arithmetic deficiencies.

By teaching good study habits, monitoring homework, investigating alternative education, and providing specific help for those subjects that seem particularly troublesome, you can help your child gain increased academic skill and confidence. With consistent effort, you can make education much more fulfilling and exciting for your child.

13

PREVENTING AND COUNTERACTING MISBEHAVIOR

Typically, parents of ADHD children exhaust their supply of disciplinary techniques in a desperate attempt to stop the relentlessly continuing misbehavior. They try everything from talking quietly to spanking severely, but nothing works for long. Rewarding, ignoring, explaining, pleading, punishing, depriving of privileges, and every other tactic all seem to have the same fate —ineffectiveness.

The bottom line is that nothing works until the biochemical cause of the ADHD is stopped or muted through medication or the Feingold Program, aided by the child's advancing age and maturity (probably through the action of hormones). It is at once a great frustration and a great relief when parents learn that their discipline attempts had little or nothing to do with their child's continuing misbehavior. The important next step is to be realistic about discipline and stop overdoing it. Harshness and severity do very little except make things worse.

If I were to summarize in one sentence what my experience has taught me over the past two decades of assisting parents of ADHD children with discipline, it would be "Get the emphasis off after-the-fact discipline and put it into prevention and supervision."

THE THREE S's TO PREVENT MISBEHAVIOR

Refocus your disciplinary efforts away from motivating your child and onto encouraging the desired behavior. Plan activities several hours ahead, hunting for stumbling blocks or situations that increase the risk of misbehavior, and then supervise the occasion to prevent problems from occurring. Think of how to structure to prevent misbehavior and of the supervision and support that would be most helpful. If your small hyperactive child is going to sit in the audience at an evening program, for example, consider whether to bring something such as a coloring book or a snack to prevent boredom, squirming, and chatter. Don't just take the child along, then get upset when hyperactivity symptoms flare up during the program.

These three key principles can help save your sanity as you learn to cope with hyperactive behavior.

1. Structure. Carefully place and arrange objects ahead of time and follow orderly processes and routines to prevent problems from occurring.
2. Supervision. During any activity, check periodically to make sure your child is proceeding correctly; deal with problems while they are still manageable.
3. Support. To ensure continued success, provide instruction on any changes needed next time and offer encouragement.

Structure

External order compensates for the internal chaos ADHD children experience. Establish routines at every potential high-stress event—arising, mealtimes, doing chores, after-school hours, and preparing for bed in the evening. Maintain the routines as much as possible. Explain why significant temporary changes in routine are necessary, and take him through any permanent changes step-by-step.

Structuring to prevent problems requires the thoughtful placement of objects. Don't leave money on the dresser in an unlocked bedroom while you are away; don't have food available that is apt to trigger an S-R state in your child. Set out clothing needed for the next day; have schoolbooks in a special place so they won't be forgotten in the morning. There is no end to the number of helpful ways you can simplify your life and minimize your child's problems.

Part of structuring to prevent problems is minimizing the chance of bad days (described in Chapter 3). Inadequate sleep is probably the most common and the most controllable factor for preventing bad days. Although children vary in their need for sleep, most toddlers require ten to twelve hours nightly. By the time they enter first grade, they should be sleeping ten or eleven hours nightly. Elementary-school students should get about ten hours of sleep, and the ideal duration of sleep lowers to nine hours for adolescents.

Structure can be more easily imposed if daily routines are specifically stated in writing and conspicuously posted.

Charts provide constant reminders and are silent and efficient substitutes for your memory and your tongue. Put the steps your child is supposed to follow onto charts, using pictures if she is too young to read. I have found the three charts listed here especially useful for families with hyperactive children.

Chore Charts. Simple chore charts (described more fully later in this chapter) let each family member know instantly who is supposed to do what chore each day or week.

The Master Chart. Make a Master Chart for each month and mount it on a wall in your child's room to remind him of deadlines and appointments. Include all waking hours in large blocks of paper, with school-related tasks; long-term assignments; test dates; appointments; extracurricular programs, meetings, events, and activities; visits during the evenings and weekends; and similar information. Have him pencil in class hours, mealtimes, travel times, work hours, and regular activities. This chart should be reviewed at your weekly Personal Private Interview (PPI) (described later in this chapter).

The Daily Activities Chart. Decide with your child what are the important daily activities and assign a certain amount of time for each. Start with the skeleton of each day, divided into half-hour segments. Write down the proposed daily schedule on a large chart and mount it on the child's bedroom wall or closet door. Fill in the spaces with the activities for the day. Consider including coming home from school as well as household chores, after-school snacks, homework, extracurricular activities, recreation, personal time, entertainment, socializing, mealtimes, and church or Scout activities. Here is a sample of the afternoon and evening portion of the Daily Activity Chart.

3:00–3:30	Arrive home, snack, and rest
3:30–4:00	Homework
4:00–4:20	Break
4:20–4:50	Homework
4:50–5:15	Practice piano
5:15–6:00	Play outside
6:00–6:40	Dinner and clean-up

6:40–7:20	Homework and flashcards
7:20–7:30	Tidy room
7:30–9:00	Free time
9:00–9:10	Bedtime
9:10	In bed, tuck-in, and tapes

Your child needs to be contented with the schedule, preferably having participated with you in its development. Modify it from time to time as her situation or family needs change. Use the PPI to discuss temporary changes in the daily schedule. Have alternative plans available when weather or transportation problems prevent outdoor activities or away-from-home events.

Supplement the structure of charts by thoughtfully arranging your child's day to prevent flare-ups of misbehavior. Try to keep the child's stimulation level low by having her play with only one friend at a time, rather than with a large group of children. Be willing to allow a larger play group as she shows increased ability to play easily with more children, but don't expose her needlessly to large groups.

Try to keep your child occupied with one thing at a time, for example, one toy at a time from a closed toy box. When he is working at a table, clear it of all objects except the one with which he is working. Turn off a television or radio that is creating needless background noise. Designate a room or part of a room as your child's special place where he can do arts and crafts work, play with toys, and busy himself safely and without overstimulation.

Some hyperactive children are bothered by their sense of a lack of predictability in their responses and actions. Constancy becomes important to them, and they are reassured when the events at home are scheduled and predictable. If your home is orderly, with things in their proper places, your child will be less likely to become overstimulated or confused. Make changes slowly and gradually whenever possible. Deviations in routines or furniture arrangements should be announced ahead of time. When routines and scheduled activities are changed without advance warning, your child might need some special help. Explain the situation rather than leaving him surprised and confused, and avoid sudden terminations of his activities. It is better to say "Five more turns" to bring a game to a close than to announce suddenly that the game is over.

Time your requests to conform with your child's daily schedule, taking mood fluctuations into account. When you schedule an activity, consider your child's readiness at different times of day. If he is calmer in the morning than in the afternoon, for example, take him shopping with you during the morning.

Simple chores can be completed in short periods of time and a small timer may help give the child a sense of the passage of a few minutes. An instruction such as "You have ten minutes to pick up the toys" or "You have five minutes to finish watching TV" can be reinforced with the timer.

Touch her rather than giving only verbal direction from a distance. Avoid showering her with commands. Help structure the situation by directing and beginning her movement toward the desired activity. If you want toys to be picked up, for example, stand next to her, pick up one toy, put it into the toy container, pick up another toy, hand it to her and say, "You pick up the rest of the toys now; I'll be back in five minutes to make sure they're all put away."

Make a definite statement rather than asking a question. Avoid an apologetic "Okay?" at the end of your statement. Don't haggle or negotiate about petty issues like an extra television program or trying a new food. Take a firm position, state clearly and concisely what you want, and stick by it.

Word your requests in positive terms. In a theater, say "Whisper," rather than "Shhh, don't talk so loud." Say "Please carry your coat" rather than "Don't drag your coat."

Your child may have trouble understanding more than

one request at a time. Make sure that you have his full attention, then state your request in simple, clear, one-concept statements. Have him repeat the request to you if necessary. Speaking slowly is also helpful, as is writing the request. Smaller children can be helped by pictorial lists to help them understand any words they may not yet be able to read.

Sometimes your child may need a demonstration of new or difficult activities that she is being asked to engage in. Be willing to show her what to do, in addition to telling her.

Summers can be especially difficult for school-age children. Arrange activities to minimize the likelihood of misbehavior during summertime by keeping your SOCs on: *structured* activities, rather than unstructured time; *outdoor* rather than indoor activities; activities with *companions* rather than leaving the child to play alone.

Not only during summertime but also throughout the year, developing a Fun Idea List and a Fun Idea Drawer (see Appendix F) can be extremely useful for preventing discipline problems. They enable you to find pockets of time to develop into quality experiences for your child.

Especially for ADHD children, boredom is one of the major contributors to misbehavior. At the first feeling of boredom, your child can consult the Fun Idea List for something to do. Whenever you suspect restlessness or discontent, suggest a quick trip to the list for some ideas about a fun activity. Invite your child to use the special phrase "I'm bored" whenever boredom sets in. Whenever he approaches you with this phrase, you agree to stop what you are doing and help him get started with something from the Fun Idea List. I have found the "I'm bored" phrase very helpful in preventing arguments and misbehavior. The few moments spent helping your child find something constructive to do pay off richly, not only by providing a delightful point of contact between you, but by preventing squabbles and bickering and improving peace and harmony within your family.

The Fun Idea List should be mounted low enough to be easily seen and should include various categories of activities: indoor and outdoor, quiet and active, alone and with other children. In just a few minutes you can come up with dozens of ideas, and you can supplement your list with ideas from library books on children's activities. Add new activities to the Fun Idea List as you think of them, so that the list consistently matches your child's interests throughout the growing years. Detailed suggestions for the Fun Idea List and Fun Idea Drawer can be found in Appendix F.

Two other methods that I have found extremely helpful are the Concerns Notebook and the Personal Private Interview. Have the interview in a private place such as the bedroom; schedule weekly meetings at first. Your role is similar to that of a newspaper reporter. You want to discuss how your child is doing in the major areas of day-to-day living. Review academic performance and needs, social life, material needs, medical needs, and your child's roles within the family including chores and responsibilities.

In preparation, each of you should have a Concerns Notebook. You note critical incidents or other information you wish to talk over, and your child enters gripes, issues, questions, and conflicts she wants to discuss. It is important that your Concerns Notebooks not appear to be ordinary notebooks. An attractive, clever picture of a worried person, cartoon figure, or funny animal and a title such as "These Are My Concerns" can be photocopied onto the corner of sheets of writing paper and punched for insertion into the notebook. Your child should help design it.

Parents of ADHD children who have used this method marvel at its simplicity and effectiveness at keeping all of their children's problems small and manageable. Issues never fester unnoticed, but instead are dealt with in an open and direct atmosphere of mutual respect and frankness. Hyperactive children and adolescents who can bring their concerns to parents with confidence that they will be listened to and respected do not need to resort to misbehavior or tantrums.

Respond to the expressed concerns with decisive action toward a change for the better, so that your child experiences direct benefits from sharing concerns with you in this calm format. You want the entire procedure to teach assertion and negotiation. There is no need, however, to give a final answer to his requests during the interview unless it is convenient to do so. Simply arrange a date by which you will have a response ready, then allow yourself sufficient time to gather information, explore alternatives, discuss the issues with those involved, secure the necessary money to support your response, and make all similar preparations so that you can give a helpful, empathic, and suitable answer. Make your response at least partially fulfill what he has asked for, or provide suitable explanations for your inability or unwillingness to do so. The PPI is not a blank check; it is an assurance that you will address the expressed issues.

A distinct advantage of PPIs is that they provide a dependable way to monitor your child's cooperation about the various behavior modifications you request. She quickly learns she will have to face you at the next meeting to explain how well she did at changing her behavior. Limit such requests to one per interview, however, so that the bulk of the time is devoted to the interviewing process.

An additional advantage of the Concerns Notebook is that it can assist when you must have instant obedience. Introduce this system ahead of time: (1) child complies with the parent's request; (2) child writes down frustrations about the event in the Concerns Notebook; (3) child shares the concern at the next PPI. In this way, the Concerns Notebook can control behavior and eliminate nagging. If you simply must have instant obedience and there is no time to deal with the issue, say: "Write it down in your Concerns Notebook and I'll talk with you about it. But right now do as I ask." Then keep your word and deal with the issue at the next PPI, including making amends if your child has a legitimate complaint about how things occurred during the crisis.

Supervision

ADHD children tend to lie, omit information if not asked directly for it, selectively perceive and remember facts and sequences of events, and use poor judgment and poor observational skills about self and others. The net result is lowered trustworthiness. My experience has been that parents often simply cannot afford to believe what their child tells them, even though they wish they could. They sense their intimacy with the child is disrupted as a result.

Use close supervision and don't rely simply on the honor system. Outline the expected activities, routines, and assignments; then check for compliance. Use routines and the rules to enforce them as ways to prevent problems from developing. Clearly state behavior guidelines. Decide in advance how you and the child will both know when a rule is being observed or when it has been broken. Suppose the rule is that homework must be completed, checked, and corrected before the TV is turned on. The method for enforcing the rule is to have your child bring the checked and corrected homework to you, then after you have examined it, you allow the television to be turned on.

Rules should be phrased in positive terms. Be sure to provide *specific directions:* instead of "Be nice to your sister," say "Show her how to dress her doll"; *segmented assignments:* break complicated tasks into smaller units and give time limits for each unit, if necessary; *written rules:* write specific instructions and post them so there is no doubt about what is supposed to be done and when; *age-specific rules:* keep rules reasonably in tune with your child's age, judgment, memory, and activity level; *important rules:* make rules that really matter when health, safety, social learning, personal development, or family issues are at stake; and *realistic rules:* make enforceable requests, such as "Don't take your brother's sweater without asking" rather than "Don't do anything that your brother doesn't like."

You can influence your child's decision making through your example, reasonable rules, calm discussion, and Personal Private Interviews. Don't expect, however, to be able to control all his decisions even with the best supervisory techniques.

Support

Confronting your child should be a two-sided instructive process; he should learn about better behavior choices, and you should learn more about his underlying needs and readinesses so you can adjust your expectations and help prevent future misbehavior. The I CARE sequence is one highly effective method of confronting and correcting a misbehaving child. The first letter of each segment is the key to giving support and encouragement.

Let's suppose that your hyperactive son, Matt, is bothering his little sister Melissa again:

INTERRUPT. Be willing to interfere with or interrupt and break up the process. When you separate combatting children and send them off in different directions, the negative behavior comes to a screeching halt, and your child must face a new set of issues having to do with your presence and your involvement.

Use the codeword *huddle* as you call your child aside for a quick talk. Be calm in your approach and agree with him ahead of time that either of you can call a huddle whenever there is something amiss. "Matt [You go up to Matt and gently pull him away from Melissa], this is the third time you have made her cry in the last hour. I can tell Melissa's bugging you and you're bugging her."

Cool Off. Send your child to a time-out place such as the bedroom for a few minutes before discussing the event. Relabel the time-out procedure if needed to gain your child's cooperation. Refer to the time-out place as your child's quiet place, relaxing place, or calming-down place and the period of time as a quiet time, relaxing time, or calming-down time. If your child bites, scratches, lashes out, and refuses to go, gently nudge, escort, or carry him to the bedroom. Tell him you will be back shortly, after he has calmed down and remained quiet for two minutes. Urge your child to write down concerns, or lie on the bed to calm down.

At the same time, take advantage of the moment to gather your composure and do your own cooling off. Then when you and the child both seem ready, enter the room and sit next to your child.

Affirm. Start with empathy for your child's feelings and convey your concern. Empathy includes (1) listening ("Tell me more about how you feel"); (2) understanding ("I understand how you feel"); (3) accepting ("I accept your feeling as real and valid from your point of view"); (4) identifying ("I would feel that way too"); (5) caring ("I wish you happiness and don't want you to have this painful feeling"); and (6) desire to help ("How can I help you so you'll feel better?"). The universal empathy statement to make to your child when you can't think of what else to say is "This is a hard time for you, isn't it?"

Express faith and confidence in your child's judgment and ability to understand what you are saying and willingness to cooperate with you. Accompany the confrontation with honest appreciation for the helpful and constructive things he does. Include as much affectionate touching or holding as he will allow during this step. If touching or holding seems unacceptable, proceed with the conversation while simply sitting nearby.

> This is a hard time for you, isn't it, Matt! Are you mad at Melissa about something? [Matt answers yes.] Well, I want you to feel happy about being home with her today, not feel bugged by her. What is going on? [Matt explains.] I know you can be so kind to her when you want to! You often help her color the pictures in her coloring book, and she likes it when you read to her. Your daddy and I love you a lot, Matt, and we want you to be a happy boy.

Redirect. Having intervened to break up the processes contributing to misbehavior, steer your child in a new direction, perhaps toward reentering the situation with a new mind-set. This is an especially prudent moment to use the Fun Idea List for instant access to other activities if boredom, fatigue, loneliness, or irritability are taking their toll. Often it is better to save this step until after you have proceeded through step E, Educate.

> Since you seem to be having a hard time enjoying being with Melissa today, let's take a look at the Fun Idea List and get you started on something interesting.

Educate. Explain in very concrete terms the exact domino effects of the misbehavior—the natural consequences likely to develop as others react:

> Now Melissa doesn't want to be with you because she feels hurt that you threw her toys and insisted that she play your game. She will probably want to play with you in a little bit, but she's not going to want to continue playing with you if she can't have a more pleasant time with you.

The events that occurred in the few minutes preceding the incident provide important clues to the reasons for the misbehavior. Find legitimate channels for meeting whatever needs seem to be reflected by the misbehavior. Ask what can be learned from the event and what can be changed so that next time can be better. Label the misbehavior as a mistake, and clearly give better alternatives for next time: "What could you say next time when she asks you to play but you don't want to play what she suggests?"

If your child answers "You should make Melissa act differently," respond with "Yes, but what can *you* do to help make things turn out better?" Use the think-of-another-way approach: "Don't downgrade yourself. Think about what caused you to lose your self-control. What is another way you could handle this situation next time, that would work out better for you as well as for your sister?"

This step is the hallmark of the I CARE method. It is a much more effective confrontation than the usual harsh, angry dialogue that ends up creating more problems than it solves. It is best to have all of your disciplinary interventions be instructive. It is easy to develop the habit of exaggerating and overemphasizing the point you want to make in an effort to "reach" the child. The E, however, stands for Educate, not Lecture.

In discussing better choices of behavior for next time, stimulate strong moral values for these choices. Clear, polarized options help ADHD children order their thinking about moral choices. Left to their own devices, most are too suggestible, too impulsive, and too deficient in thinking of future consequences to process complicated moral decisions without some well-defined anchor points. Be firm and blunt, simplifying the moral choices so that they are between good and bad, smart and dumb, or kind and mean behavior. The older your child, the less polarized these labels should be. It is much easier to loosen overly high standards as children mature and gain life experience than to tighten standards that have been too lax. Of course avoid labeling the children themselves as bad, dumb, or mean.

Part of the educational aspect of discipline is that you demonstrate and describe the desired behavior. Have your child imitate or practice the correct behavior if necessary.

Sometimes you will not have the opportunity to use the entire I CARE method. Under those circumstances, provide temporary emotional support through empathy and touch, and maintain a thread of communication to prevent total withdrawal. Be an impartial referee between your child and the circumstances or other children. Help her become accurately aware of what happened and which of her actions contributed to making things worse.

Make clear, concise, directive statements. Approach so you can talk in a normal volume from a courteous distance. Stand within arm's length and pretend to touch him every time you speak. This imagined contact will help you develop the useful habit of approaching and standing near before giving directive messages. Try not to steer or direct your child with words from far away. In general, keep the amount of verbal directives low. Stoop, kneel down, or sit facing a young child. Wait until he is quiet, obtain eye contact, then give your instructions in simple terms. Don't assume he will understand and remember your message; ask him to repeat it, if such a request does not cause conflict.

For a very contrary ADHD child who simply won't listen, I have found that making a special "deal" sometimes bridges the gap. I call it the ticket-to-talk method. Introduce it as a way for your child to feel less nagged at by you. The deal is that you agree to give no more than three sentences of instruction or correction. In exchange for being relieved of "lectures," she agrees to "really listen" and take to heart what you are saying. Although it is not the best parent-child communication, it is useful to prevent a deadlock and keep some communication flowing. Severe communication problems require the assistance of a skilled counselor.

NATURAL AND LOGICAL CONSEQUENCES

Logical and natural consequences are especially helpful because they provide the needed firmness to teach ADHD children the direct, specific, domino effects of their behavior. You can then stand by as a helpful ally without adding insult to your child's already fragile self-esteem.

Natural Consequences

Natural consequences do not involve intervention by other people. They are the natural sequence of events following misbehavior. They are not manufactured by parents; instead they are simply allowed to occur. The natural consequence of your child's grabbing a small dog's fur is being nipped by the dog; of running on an icy sidewalk, a skinned knee; of experimental puffing on a cigar, coughing and choking; of grabbing playmates' toys, being rejected by playmates. Natural consequences are spontaneous ways of learning about life and can be powerful teachers.

When you want a natural consequence to become a corrective influence on your child, do not intervene. Temporarily divorce yourself from the situation and be patient and quiet. Be your child's ally and avoid giving I-told-you-so speeches afterward. If she brings up the event for discussion, express hope that she will change her actions in some way next time so that things work out more pleasantly for all concerned. Treat the experience as you would any mistake—an opportunity to learn and improve.

In many instances, however, a natural consequence would not be the most efficient learning method. It might take too long to materialize, or it might jeopardize the child's health or safety. Sometimes an overriding concern, such as financial cost, must be given consideration. For example, the natural consequence of allowing a bicycle to stay out in the rain is that it will rust; however, losing the use of the bicycle may be too disruptive to the child and to the family. The natural consequence of his coming to the table with dirty hands is that he may become ill, and the natural consequence of his playing carelessly in the street is that he may be hit by a car. Obviously, adult intervention is needed in these instances.

Logical Consequences

When it seems inappropriate to permit a natural consequence, you can intervene in a humane, sensitive, and loving way. The consequence of the misbehavior can be logically related to it. Logical consequences are known ahead of time by all concerned. You guide them and he experiences them as logical in nature. If the conflict involves your child's tracking in mud, you can inform him ahead of time that he is to leave his muddy shoes on the porch from now on or he will have to mop up the kitchen if mud is tracked in.

Explain to your child the new actions you will take in response to his misbehavior. Tell your child what you will do, and let him decide what he will do. After your initial explanation, there is no need for nagging about your new policies. Use logical consequences without continuing to explain or justify them to him.

When your child starts to misbehave, put the emphasis on controlling yourself rather than on controlling her. Stop cooperating with her. Don't do her any favors relevant to the misbehavior. In this way you can let her know that you do not endorse the misbehavior. Control what you will give to, do for, or permit for your child. Wash only those items of clothing that she has placed in the correct laundry containers. Do not serve her meal if she comes to the table with dirty hands until they are washed.

Set a time limit for your child's combined work and play. Let him determine how much time he will have left to spend at play by the amount of time he takes to do his work. The longer he takes to do the dishes, for example, the less time there will be for you to read a story, because both activities must be accomplished by bedtime. The more your child delays you by badgering you about something, the less time you will spend playing with him afterward. The longer he delays his bedtime preparations, the less time you will spend tucking him in.

A guideline should be that work must come before play. Prohibit play until chores are done. If work is done before play, he will enjoy both activities more than if he had reversed the sequence. Work will be done quickly because he will be eager to begin his play, which he will enjoy more because he will have earned it: "You may go out to play after you have done the dishes and I have looked at them" and "As soon as you show me that your homework is done, you may watch television."

Withdraw a privilege he abuses and give him a chance to regain it later when he shows that he can handle it responsibly. Let the consequence do the teaching. For example, temporarily deny him the use of his bicycle if he rides it carelessly, or forbid his use of the telephone temporarily if he has not used it properly.

Do not insist or even expect her to accept the consequences in any specific attitude or any special style. She might react to the consequence in any of a variety of ways: she might be angry, she might be quiet, she might pout, or she might be resigned to it. The benefits can be lost if you become emotionally involved with her style of accepting the consequence.

It is important that logical consequences be used firmly, dramatically, quickly, and calmly. Your child should not be given a second chance or an opportunity to manipulate his way out of facing the consequence at the time of his misbehavior. You should remain firm and consistent without feeling guilty or sorry for him. The consequence should be fair, humane, and justified and not delivered with vengeance. When a similar situation occurs in the future, he will have another opportunity to choose a better course of action. "Next time you'll have another chance" is sufficient in response to any plea he may make for a second chance.

Although logical consequences will not make you the helpful ally that you could be when you allow natural consequences, you will at least not be the adversary that you become when authoritarian punishments are used. Remain calm and exercise your parental responsibility of putting your child in touch with her ability to make decisions. Do not take actions that would make her feel worthless, incapable, or unacceptable. Your proper attitude should be one of mild regret that she has chosen to act in a way that has led to these consequences.

Never refer to logical consequences with I-told-you-this-would-happen speeches. Try to replace nagging with one directive message; then combine the message with an enforcing action. Actions are the salad and words the condiment of effective parenting of ADHD children.

A conditional yes and a no with possibilities should be your guide to answering requests. "Yes, you may go over to Derek's house, as long as you call and ask his mother's permission and are home by 8:00"; "No, you may not go over to Derek's house tonight, but we will see about inviting Derek over this weekend."

If your child is completely out of control in a dangerous situation, you will have to restrain him physically. Approach him from behind, so that your stomach is pressing against his back. Stand behind him, cross his arms across his chest, and envelop him from behind with your arms. Maintain your grip until he has calmed down and speak softly to him to subdue his frenzied state. Another method that some parents have found helpful in an emergency for stopping out-of-control behavior is sending the child into a cool (not cold) shower.

The repayment or pay-back consequence is an important social skill. Far more relevant and effective as a disciplinary maneuver than ordinary punishments, this approach allows the child to have a meaningful part in setting things right after a judgment error. It is an integral part of the Six A's of Apology. If there is a monetary value to damage done through misbehavior, the child helps replace the loss directly by paying for it or indirectly by performing labor services to you or to the offended person.

OVERCOMING COMMON DISCIPLINARY PROBLEMS

Household Chores

Hyperactive children become unhappy and misbehave when they are idle. Household chores provide opportunities for learning self-discipline, promptness, neatness, reliability, and the importance of being helpful.

Organization and supervision of chores are doubly important in families with a hyperactive child. Give instructions for each chore, and be sure to do some chores along with your child. Unexpected tasks can spark an uncooperative attitude in hyperactive children. If household chores are natural and expected parts of the daily routine, conflicts diminish.

A regular family chore time works the best. The set time can be daily, weekly, or both. As the entire family pitches in, the child associates work with pleasure and family unity. Try a brief tidy-up period before bedtime each day and on Saturday morning.

Develop a system to distribute chores among family members, a method of supervision and inspection, and the motivation or incentives you want to use. The goal of these arrangements is to get all family members, including your hyperactive child, involved in keeping everything clean, usable, and in its place.

Present a list of chores for your children to choose from, or simply assign tasks. Rotating chores daily, weekly, or monthly is usually helpful. Post the chore assignments on a chart to avoid complaints. An effective chart informs everyone of who is supposed to do what, when, and for how many days. Include names of family members, chores to be done, and the times (days, weeks, or months) during which a specific child does a specific chore. For a very young child, use pictures rather than words. Various designs can be used for keeping track of each family member's assignments.

Pictures of several chores on a large piece of thick cardboard make a simple and highly effective chore chart. Several colored dots or other color-coded movable objects, such as cardboard tags, can be moved from chore to chore; they can hang on small nails or rest in small pockets glued onto the chart. Each child is assigned a color, and everyone—even a nonreader—knows instantly who is assigned which chores that day or week.

A floor-plan chart is also effective because of its simplicity. Paint the floor plan onto a large piece of wood or stiff cardboard, with two hooks sticking out at each room and hall. Write chore assignments and your children's names on small tags, then pair a chore tag with a child's tag on the two hooks at each chore location.

The pocket method involves preparing a series of pockets either by sewing cloth (or stapling or gluing a horizontal strip of cardboard) onto a heavy cardboard or wood backing. Staple, glue, or sew every few inches, to make pockets along the strip. Label each pocket with a chore, and write each family member's name on a separate strip of paper. To rotate chores, simply insert the paper strips into new pockets.

The box system is a pleasant, light-hearted venture that motivates your children to take care of their things and keep them in their proper locations. It is particularly helpful for a hyperactive child. What is fetched out and used must be put back. Have shelves, bins, or boxes available for easy toy storage. Items that are not picked up are put into a special box or hamper. Decide how long the objects are to be stored, what types of items are to be put into the box, who will be allowed to put things into it, and how items can be redeemed. To add interest, give the box a name such as the Saturday Box or the Clean-up Box. A typical arrangement is to auction off unclaimed items if the child does not want them anymore or doesn't pay the fine for them. A nickel per item is a suitable fine. Accumulated fines are used for a family fun project.

Don't let your child get by with "I didn't do it, so I shouldn't have to clean it up." Explain how chores help the family and why they are a shared part of family-living—this home is *our* home, this family is *our* family, and these dishes are *our* dishes. The person doing dishes did not eat off all the dinnerware, use all of the utensils, or drink from all the cups.

Teach your child that the consequences will be unpleasant if obligations are not met. Stay as outwardly uninvolved as possible; avoid nagging and reminding. Supervise from a distance and randomly check on performance unless more stringent monitoring is needed. If you use too much pressure, a contrary hyperactive child will not feel a personal sense of ownership of the chore, including the pride of accomplishment. The issue might then become a power struggle over your right to assign the chore. Use the I CARE method if grumbling occurs as chore time approaches. Repeated balking and grumbling about chores by a hyperactive child usually indicates that the biochemical treatment needs to be adjusted, the proper attitude of helpfulness needs to be developed more, or the chore should be simplified and divided into smaller units.

Clear, direct expressions of appreciation and thanks for chores completed go a long way toward training hyperactive children to be helpful. Comment on the large amount of effort shown. Nobody likes to try hard only to have others dismiss the effort by not seeming to notice or value it. (See Offering Encouragement, Chapter 6.)

Bowel and Bladder Control

If daytime wetting or soiling occurs, the child should be responsible for changing clothes and depositing the soiled items in the laundry basket or washing machine. The whole procedure should be routine and devoid of psychological implications. At a calm time, review the activities preceding the elimination control problem, checking for any other motive or mechanism aside from insufficient awareness of internal body signals that is part of the ADHD syndrome.

The child who wets the bed should help change the sheets and should bathe the next morning. Disallowing liquids before bed is an unnecessary and usually profitless restriction. The child will manufacture urine out of whatever food has been ingested, whether or not accompanied by liquid before bedtime. A small sip of liquid will not affect the bedwetting but might help contribute to a smoother tuck-in and a more contented child at bedtime. Milk allergy, particularly in ADHD-sa children, can aggravate bedwetting. The possibility of a physical cause of bowel or bladder problems is remote but should nevertheless be investigated by the physician.

Urinary alarm systems using a moisture-sensitive pad are available from major retailers. When moistened with urine, the alarm buzzes. There are two types: one mounted under the sheet, and the other in specially designed underpants that can be worn underneath pajamas. The underpants are more comfortable and convenient than the under-the-sheet type. These alarms tend to be quite effective for most bedwetting children.

Bowel and bladder control generally improve with successful biochemical treatment. I have found the antidepressants to be somewhat more consistent than stimulants in enhancing ADHD children's bowel and bladder control. A nasal spray developed in the late 1980s also helps prevent bedwetting in hyperactive children.

Traveling

Keeping an ADHD child occupied and stimulated is the key to successful long-distance car travel. Plan ten-minute stops after each two hours of travel. The stop should include a restroom visit, exercise for everyone, and washing of hands and faces, if needed. Have some special activities planned ahead of time, such as jumping rope, blowing bubbles, or tossing a large ball.

Let the whole family help plan vacation trips, making a list of possible things to do or see. Plan a variety of activities and alternate them for a change of pace. Be careful not to overschedule your child. When you arrive at the destination, settle in your overnight lodgings rather than trying to cram busy sightseeing activities after a day of travel.

Let each child pick her own clothes and fill a sack or backpack with items for self-entertainment. If you are traveling with a young child on public transportation such as an airplane or bus, bring a favorite teddy bear or doll, blanket, snacks, and coloring or drawing materials.

Use snacks advantageously. A mouth chewing on a fruit strip or licking a large caramel sucker has a hard time whining. Periodically providing snack food can facilitate extended periods of peace and quiet during your travel. Although care must be taken not to ruin appetite or cause an unnecessary S-R state, snack food has its place in traveling. Of course, select the most wholesome variety that will occupy your child's attention and that she will enjoy.

Verbal activities that keep your child's mind focused on the conversation also help. Play word games, counting games, and quiz games to prevent quarreling, complaining, harassing, and whining that might otherwise ruin the trip. Use an almanac to generate quiz questions.

Encourage activities to keep little hands busy. Here are some items that help release pent-up energy during long hours of travel. They should not, however, be expected to take the place of periodic rest and exercise stops. Be careful not to include any that might trigger a reaction if your child is observing the Feingold Program.

adhesive strip bandages	new crayons
telescope or binoculars	handicraft supplies
tape recorder	magnetic board
maps of the trip route	clipboard
reading materials	folding lap trays
pads and pencils	paper plates to color
"magic" slates	sticker books
drawing supplies	peg games

Grocery Shopping

As in most situations, the key is prevention. Provide something that occupies your child during the shopping excursion. If tantrums occur, sit with him in the car briefly as a time-out maneuver and use the I CARE sequence to help set things right.

Two basic strategies can be used to help ensure a tantrum-free visit to the supermarket. The first is to give her a large fruit such as a banana from the produce section. Your child remains silent and occupied, and you retain your composure. The second is to actively involve her in the shopping process, such as by having her fetch the items you specify, stack them in the cart, or help search for them.

Consider playing Food Bingo. As an activity from the Fun Idea List, have your child make Food Bingo cards by cutting out pictures of food items from magazines and pasting them on a piece of cardboard that has been divided into twenty-five squares. Take a Food Bingo card and a pencil or crayon along on the shopping trip. Your child marks off each item as you move down the aisles. As soon as all the items are marked off, she wins a small treat. This game holds the interest of ADHD children quite well and also keeps siblings from squabbling if you have them play it simultaneously.

Untidy Bedroom

Most ADHD children and adolescents prefer to decorate their rooms in an Early Tornado theme. There is no point in generating unnecessary conflict, so try to avoid power struggles about the appearance of the bedroom. Closing the door so others do not have to experience the room by sight, sound, or smell is probably the simplest solution, though it doesn't teach much in the way of self-care.

To encourage a cleaner, tidier bedroom, use structure to advantage by devising a place for everything. Use plastic dishpans as bins and provide plenty of shelves and drawers as well as small sturdy cardboard storage boxes (available from business supply stores). Color-code the bins and boxes for different purposes—building blocks in the red bin, clean underwear in the white drawer, doll clothes in the pink box, for example.

Have a minimum of furniture. The fewer items of furniture, the more easily your child will locate toys and other items within the room. If only one child is using the room, a bunk bed provides an excellent storage area that quickly transforms into a bed for overnight guests. A hamper (cover and decorate it with your child), a wastebasket, and adequate shelving are essential structural aids. Consider converting half the closet into shelves.

Develop a routine for picking up and cleaning the bedroom. The suggestions given earlier for getting cooperation with household chores generally apply for this responsibility.

Television

Predictably, television watching is one of the few periods in which most ADHD children become more controlled. Watching television tends to drain energy from the viewer, so a bland, nonviolent program can be helpful just before bedtime as a calming influence on your child.

Control the television set, however, so that it does not control the family. Plan your daily routine so television watching does not cut into the many important activities that should be occupying your child's time and interests. Put a reasonable time limit on the total hours your child watches, as well as the time of day or night during which the watching takes place. The best arrangement, according to many parents of hyperactive children, is to post a list of each week's approved programs. If conflicts arise over which program to watch at a specific time, arrange a simple rotation schedule so each child gets a turn at determining what to watch. Put the schedule on the Daily Activities Chart.

If aggressiveness is a problem, be doubly diligent in reasonably censoring the television messages coming into your home. Various research studies have demonstrated that children become more accepting of aggression and more physically aggressive themselves after watching violence on television, regardless of whether the characters are cartoon figures or human performers.

Lying

Lying is one of the most difficult misbehaviors to correct, in part because it prevents a frank discussion of what really happened. It also gives the child a great amount of illegitimate power because you can't *make* him tell the truth, and the lying can provide a cover-up for almost any kind of misdeed. Many hyperactive children become so skilled at lying that they lose their awareness of what is real and what is fantasy. If your child lies to evade consequences or avoid a responsibility or chore, there are several actions you can take.

Discuss. Discussing the lie helps put your child in a more objective, emotionally removed position. Explain that all lies are of two basic types—to claim to be *more* than you are or *less* than you are:

> Some lies say you are more than you are, like bragging about something you have or something you did. And other lies say you are less than you are, like saying you didn't do something wrong or didn't take something that belonged to someone else. Which type of lie was this, the first or the second?

Explore your child's thoughts that led to the lie. Get him to state his motives and intentions behind the lie—what he was trying to accomplish or avoid.

Empathize. Make it safe emotionally for your child to convey these feelings to you by showing empathy. Use as many as you can of the six ways of expressing empathy from the I CARE discussion earlier in this chapter.

Explain the Negative Impact. Having shown empathy for your child's logic and motives, label them as mistakes. If the lying occurred as a cover-up for a misdeed, two mistakes have occurred—the misbehavior itself and the cover-up attempt:

> You made two mistakes here. The first was thinking the best way to make the other boys like you was to tell them your teacher intends to give you the prize. The second was to think you needed to lie and deny you said that when the teacher asked you about it.

Gently explain the undesirable domino effects of each mistake—the natural consequences most likely to occur if the mistake is repeated—for example: "Now it will be harder for the boys to like you, rather than easier. You tell me why." [Child answers.] "And it will also be harder for the teacher to trust you. Why?"

Explain the Positive Impact of Truthfulness. Outline the natural consequences of developing a reputation as an untrustworthy person—people will learn not to trust him, a reputation as a liar will be hard to change, people will stop telling him their secrets, and so forth. Keep this and the preceding explanation in simple, concrete terms with a clear cause-and-effect sequence.

Encourage Apology. Review the Six A's of Apology to clear up any damaged feelings or relationships over the incident.

Get a Commitment for Change. Help your child think of what to change so he can make wiser choices next time. Arrange that in return for an agreement not to lie about future incidents, only logical consequences will apply; that is, simple compensation or repayment.

Stealing

The best preventative for stealing is biochemical treatment. If your child attempts to label the actions as merely taking, taking without returning, borrowing, borrowing without returning, or taking and not asking, label the actions as stealing and emphasize the importance of the event as an example of the type of judgment that must improve. Discuss the matter calmly without turning the conversation into a sermon. Avoid dire long-term threats or predictions. Realistically explain the domino effects of stealing—others will not trust him, friendships will be broken, and so forth. Reduce opportunities and increase the probability that he will be caught if stealing occurs again.

Just as a carpenter must have a variety of tools available to accomplish the goals of the trade, you must also have many tools for the important stewardship and privilege you have of raising your child. No good carpenter would use a screwdriver in a situation that calls for a hacksaw. In the same way, you should carefully select the approach that best fits your child and the situation. If you emphasize structure, supervision, and support, you will become calmer, more confident, and more effective as your child's leader. Good discipline is not harsh, nor does it involve a long string of deprivations. By implementing the three S's to prevent misbehavior, using natural and logical consequences, and overcoming common disciplinary problems, you can train your child in a positive way that maintains an atmosphere of mutual respect.

14

Providing Positive Play Experiences

A large part of your relationship with your child consists of the play experiences you make available. Play, which occupies much of most children's days, teaches them a great deal about their social relationships, place within the family and peer groups, various academic skills, and numerous other talents that are useful throughout life. Play is, in some ways, children's work, providing opportunities for creativity and fantasy through pretending and for the discharge of large amounts of energy through movement and activity. Children's play activities have an important role in developing their innate capabilities into effective life skills.

STRUCTURING YOUR CHILD'S PLAY

Like any other aspect of your child's life, play activities require your intervention. Without becoming overinvolved, you can use play to help keep your child occupied and enrich his life. An important parental function is structuring, and sometimes supervising, his play so he has access to stimulating and wholesome means by which he can channel his energy and activity. It is unrealistic and nonproductive to put him in the difficult position of having to use several consecutive hours of playtime in random, haphazard actions merely to stave off boredom. He will benefit from play only if he is appropriately supervised.

Often the easiest way to help your child start a play activity is to arrange the setting ahead of time. Laying out the necessary materials and saying something like "Here are some papers for you to cut out and put together" is better than asking an open-ended question like "What would you like to do now?" Provide an apron and some clean-up rags as part of the preparation if the activity involves the possibility of spilling things.

Group settings are generally more stimulating than solitary play. Often a hyperactive child will do well for a limited period of time in group play but will gradually become overstimulated and bothersome to playmates as the playtime continues. Try to ease her into play groups for short periods at first. As her play becomes more cooperative, gradually increase the playtime and the number of playmates. By careful observation you can determine how long your child can play with friends. End the play sessions before they deteriorate because of your child's increased excitability.

Integrating your child into group play activities is a rewarding but challenging task. Occasionally observe the situation from a distance to determine how she is getting along with other children. Listening only to her explanation of what went wrong with the play experience will give a one-sided picture. If she says, for example, "They won't let me play and they hit me and told me to get out," the statement may be true; however, she may not have reported what she was doing to aggravate her playmates.

You can help your child best if you know exactly what aspect of her behavior the group objects to.

Cooperative group play can work better if all of the children understand basic principles of courtesy. A few moments of supervision at the beginning can provide the needed instruction. Teach your child, and the playmates if necessary, that possession of a piece of equipment is determined by its use—whoever is using it keeps it until finished with it. Throwing heavy or sharp-edged toys and taking toys apart, or any other acts of destruction, are not allowed. Pushing or hurting each other is forbidden. The children should be asked to share.

Learning the principles of cooperative group play is difficult. It is easy to become discouraged and frustrated at his slow rate of improvement in learning to get along. Unfortunately, parents usually show their disappointment more automatically and more vividly than they acknowledge their recognition of his progress. Acknowledge even his small gains and improvements, and be very specific in describing them to him. "It was very nice of you to let Billy take a turn right after you" emphasizes improvement while "I see you still can't shoot baskets very well" stresses defeat. The actions that constitute being a good sport are hard for a hyperactive child to understand. Such basic courtesies as waiting for his turn, sharing, talking politely, accepting without argument that he is out for the moment, and appreciation of the skills of others may be hard at first. Under your specific instruction and supervision, however, he can slowly develop good play habits that will serve him well throughout his life.

YOUR CHILD'S PLAY ENVIRONMENT

Hyperactive children generally need a lot of space to move around, tumble, explore, run, and discharge their large amounts of energy. Those who live in an apartment without an adequate play area or in a neighborhood without a large yard or nearby park or school playground may not be able to release enough energy. The result can sometimes be increased misbehavior and irritability, among other problems.

In addition to providing a large outdoor play area, many parents have found that a high fence or other protective partition helps assure them of the child's whereabouts and safety. The hyperactive child's unbridled curiosity and poorly developed sense of danger make a physical barrier surrounding the play area even more necessary. Neighborhood improvements that increase the child's area for safe and free movement, such as sidewalks, are also desirable. In the country, hyperactive children usually enjoy roaming through large plots of land. Make sure it is safe to wander in these open areas.

In the home, the hyperactive child needs a safe place for being very active. The best location would be a playroom in which the furniture is inexpensive and sturdy. It should contain various items for quiet as well as for active play. A corner can be set aside as a bouncing and tumbling place by placing one mattress on top of another on the floor. In a home without a playroom, a bouncing and tumbling place in a basement, attached garage, porch, or other defined area will serve equally well.

Despite intentions to the contrary, most parents of hyperactive children find that the bedroom ends up being a playroom, too. Furnish the room with pieces that can stand heavy wear and tear and expect some physically rough treatment to the room and its contents through the years. The walls should be drab so they do not overstimulate or frighten the child, especially at night; try to avoid loud or bright colors, stripes, and mirrors. The hyperactive child will probably need to have either the playroom or the bedroom as a time-out place for moments when she must be separated from others in order to reestablish cooperative behavior.

Your child should be encouraged to display her artistic creations. Arrange a place on a wall or shelf to show her work. Provide a set of shelves or drawers that are clearly labeled and easy to use, so that she can store her playthings without clutter.

THE IMPORTANCE OF A REGULAR FAMILY PLAYTIME

In addition to the opportunity to play alone and the opportunity to play with other children, your hyperactive child needs to play with you. The importance of special parent-child playtimes cannot be overemphasized. It is crucial for family harmony. At these times permit the child in you to respond to your child, so that a new and special bond can form, one that strengthens and expands the other loving and caring feelings that connect the two of you. Parents who make a special place in their weekly schedule for a regular playtime with their children usually find the experience surprisingly reassuring and fulfilling, even when other aspects of their relations with their children are less positive or pleasant.

Being able to have fun with your hyperactive child is essential to enjoying his company, regardless of any other feelings you may have toward him. A regular playtime has a number of other important rewards. It allows regularly available high-quality time for interacting with him. It can be a pleasant change from conflict-laden interactions and can also counterbalance the less intense experiences that occur when parents have busy schedules.

By allowing yourself to enter wholeheartedly into a play experience, you can temporarily abandon outside concerns and can focus on your home and family, using the opportunity to train your child in important skills.

Keeping a regular playtime also permits you to give a fair share of yourself to your child. You can then do more things for yourself, your spouse, and the other children in the family without feeling apologetic or guilty. Regular playtime also serves as a periodic reminder that fun is an important aspect of family life and of love for each other. Siblings will be far less jealous of the attention given their hyperactive sibling if they know that they, too, have their own special place with you. Finally, regular play increases the loving feelings between you and your hyperactive child, strengthening the bonds of emotional caring, closeness, and mutual understanding. Just a casual walk through the neighborhood may provide an opportunity for genuine psychological intimacy.

Certain activities are much more beneficial than others at playtime. In general, competitive games involving a winner and a loser are destructive and dangerous for the hyperactive child as well as the other children in the family. Cooperative games teach children the value of group effort and the importance of helping each other rather than trying to oppose and defeat each other.

Playing together in situations the child will face in the future is educational. Giving a party, playing store, and similar experiences provide rich learning opportunities as well as fulfilling forms of togetherness. Accompanying your child in active physical play such as climbing, digging, tussling, and organized sports can also be enjoyable.

ACTIVITIES TO IMPROVE YOUR CHILD'S LEARNING SKILLS

In addition to providing entertainment, many activities can be instructional and can help build basic learning skills.

Auditory Skills

The abilities to hear well and to remember and organize what is heard can be strengthened by having your child close his eyes and try to identify the objects that you are holding by the sounds they make (toothbrush against cardboard, small electric motor, pencil on paper). Have him try to find an object with his eyes closed, locating it by the sound that it makes (bell, whistle). Someone can wear a tinkling bell while your blindfolded child tries to catch him or her. A tape recorder, used under your supervision, can provide hours of entertainment and be an aid in self-expression.

Letter sounds can be used for many interesting activities. Riddle chaining is done by having your child make up a riddle whose answer starts with the last sound of the preceding answer. For example, "I say meow; what am I?" (ca*t*); "I am tall and have leaves; what am I?" (*t*ree); "I am a very thin fish; what am I?" (*ee*l).

Tell a story and leave out a word, pausing so your child can fill in the correct and obvious word (" 'Twas the night before Christmas and all through the . . .").

"Wouldn't it be funny if . . ." is a source of much amusement when the child takes turns with other family members in completing the statements with silly rhymes. ("Wouldn't it be funny if bees had fleas? . . . if sharks stayed in parks? . . . if flowers counted the hours?")

Say several words beginning with the same sound. Occasionally include a different beginning sound and have your child clap her hands when she hears the different sound.

Your child can tap out variations in rhythm and loudness that you first beat or tap out; hand claps work well for this entertaining exercise. While she has her eyes closed, have her tell you how many times you have tapped with a pencil and on what object, or just have her identify sounds she hears when sitting quietly.

Visual Skills

Have your child look carefully at a picture or drawing with a number of details in it; then have him draw it from memory, practicing until he can remember everything he sees in the picture.

Place several objects on a table; ask your child to turn away while you remove two of the objects; then have him try to guess what is missing.

Draw a picture but leave out one part; then let your child fill it in with crayon.

Using pictures of familiar objects, cut out one or two pieces from each and have your child identify what is missing and replace the missing parts.

Have your child join dots to form patterns of increasing difficulty; then have him also draw letters, numbers, and objects that are outlined in dots.

Using two checkerboards, make a pattern with four checkers on your board and have your child duplicate it on hers, gradually increasing the number of checkers. Eventually ask her to try to duplicate the pattern from memory after she looks briefly at yours.

Have your child sort and arrange a collection of miscellaneous small objects by size, then by shape, color, and composition. Change the order in which pictures or objects are arranged, and have her put them back in correct sequence.

Cover a word with a card; then move the card slowly to the right so that the letters your child will read appear in proper sequence. Do the same for sentences, sliding the card so that words appear from left to right at a comfortable pace. Make the sentences fun to read by including loving messages or humor in them.

Coordination

Construct a balance board by placing a board about two feet long on a horizontal cylinder, and have your child balance himself by placing his feet near each end of the board.

Play family Follow-the-Leader, and include lots of skipping, jumping, crawling, and use of right and left feet and hands.

Have your child walk while balancing a bean bag on his head or while pressing it between his knees; then have him hop, sit, lie down, or run with the bean bag in those positions.

Play family Charades and act out sentences, ideas, or activities: going fishing, opening a jar.

Play Simon Says as a family, or play it with your child in front of a full-length mirror.

Do rhythms and dances as a family, such as stamping your feet, slapping your sides, Hokey Pokey, Farmer in the Dell, and so on.

Have your child walk and skip backward with you.

Have your child close her eyes and write in large letters on an extra-large sheet of paper or a small blackboard.

Cutting with scissors is an excellent activity. Start with large simple shapes and gradually have her cut out more complicated and smaller shapes. Ball and jacks is another good activity, as are large sewing cards.

Concept Formation

Start a scrapbook with your child. He can organize it into categories of his favorite things and collect pictures, news clippings, and so forth, about animals, sports, or other interests. At a simpler level, you can have him categorize a collection of pictures of various objects (cut out of magazines) into appropriate subgroups, such as animals, plants, or buildings.

Memory games are also useful. "Going on a picnic or trip, I will take . . ." is an entertaining activity for the entire family. Each person names all previously named items plus one more, so that the fifth person names the four previously mentioned objects in addition to adding a fifth object to the list.

Have your child memorize a short poem or nursery rhyme. Write it down and cut out the phrases; then scramble them and have her replace them in order.

Guessing games also allow the development of concept formation ability. Have the child try to guess what object you are thinking of, providing only slight clues such as color or approximate size.

Having your child feel objects in a bag to guess what they are will also improve concept formation ability.

GUIDELINES FOR SELECTING TOYS

Your child's toys should stimulate as many senses as possible. He will enjoy toys he can feel, move around, make sounds with, and that exercise his imagination. The complicated gadget that performs by itself while the child sits and looks at it is probably not a wise choice. He should be able to control the toy, rather than having the toy control him or operate without his participation.

Hyperactive children are usually attracted to items and activities involving self-expression rather than those requiring focused or channeled concentration and restricted movement. Fingerpaints, modeling compound, guns that shoot small balls or darts, slimy semifluid, and confetti, for example, may be attractive to your child; more restrictive items such as coloring books, small building pieces, table games, plastic target shooting machines, and plastic models may be uninteresting. You should strike a balance between toys that focus his attention and limit his responses and those that offer unlimited choices and great self-expression. Practicing focused attention is probably more beneficial in the long run because it is a skill that is useful at school and in adult life.

Toys for hyperactive children should be simple, durable, and safe. In many instances, it is better to provide a genuine item rather than a toy imitation. The added durability and realism of a genuine pocket radio, for example, make it preferable to a toy radio. A small glider that really flies makes more sense than a heavy, out-of-proportion imitation of an airplane that can only roll on the floor.

Toys should not be fragile and should have little or no glass. There should be no pinching or cutting parts. Avoid electrical toys and those with lots of moving parts. Toys that shoot or propel hard or potentially dangerous objects should not be purchased.

These guidelines are very general, and allowance must be made for your child's own uniqueness and readiness for certain activities as well as for the play environment. If your child is on the Feingold Program and an S-R state occurs during play, consider inhaled (such as fumes from glue or paint) or skin-contact (such as from colorings in modeling dough) sources of chemical exposure from play materials. Coordinate your Fun Idea List and Fun Idea Drawer with toy selection.

Some Toys for Quiet Play

Toys for a hyperactive child's quiet play are often artistic in nature. She will enjoy making art paper designs using blunt scissors, tape, or paste. In general, chalk and pencil are probably preferable to paint, ink, wax crayons, and felt markers. Although chalk creates dust, it is only a temporary nuisance and can easily be washed from clothes and walls. Paint-with-water books, in which the paint is already in the paper and just has to be brushed with water, avoid the hazards of real paint while giving your child the experience of painting.

Modeling clay and modeling dough can be meaningful forms of expressive play. You can use cookie cutters, rolling pins, and other utensils to help your child make things from these materials.

Art projects should allow for quick success and easy completion, for the hyperactive child is not a patient worker. For example, snap-together rather than glue-together plastic models are usually a wiser choice. After any art project is completed, your child may suddenly lose interest in it unless his work is displayed on a wall or shelf. As time goes on, you can encourage your child to use more care and have more patience with art projects.

Consider also sets of tiny people; age-specific crossword or jigsaw puzzles; a sandbox for writing, digging, and building; small metal trucks for sand and dirt play; and wind-up and self-propelled vehicles. Soap-bubble blowing can also be a pleasant indoor or outdoor activity.

Depending on your child's age, playing with a record player, portable radio, walkie-talkie, or portable tape recorder might also be enjoyable.

Many items can be stacked and used for building: cardboard or plastic blocks, cardboard boxes, plastic bowls with lids, margarine or food containers with lids, and oatmeal boxes. In general, commercially available wooden and plastic building toys have been found to be satisfactory for hyperactive children when matched to ability level and supervised.

Some Toys for Active Play

Appropriate toys for punching and pounding for hyperactive children include sturdy punching bags, innertubes nailed to outdoor walls, and pillows. I have found the large three-foot duffel punching bag far superior to the small basketball-sized version. You can make a homemade version with a large pillow case or duffel bag filled with several pieces of cloth, such as discarded bedding.

Some commercially available inflatable punching toys are not sufficiently sturdy to withstand the energetic and heavy use a hyperactive child may give them.

Climbing, tunneling, and tumbling are important parts of your child's play needs, and such activities enhance coordination. A large plastic trash can with holes cut in the sides can provide lots of fun. Make holes large enough so he doesn't get stuck. A simple tent made with bedspreads, sheets, or blankets draped over a card table or other piece of furniture can keep a hyperactive child happy. Large cardboard shipping cartons can become play caves but make sure there are air holes. Hopscotch markings chalked on cement and a basketball hoop placed low stimulate play that helps develop coordination.

Riding and moving toys may be useful. Plastic balls, plastic flying discs, and similar items can be used in safe and enjoyable lawn games.

With appropriate structure and supervision, water play can be an enjoyable experience for your child. Running through a sprinkler or playing with the hose on hot days can be fun. Hyperactive children especially enjoy water fights with squirt guns and cups, using buckets of water as "ammunition." The goal is to douse the other person without getting doused in return. A helpful rule is that neither team may destroy the other's water supply.

ADOLESCENT RECREATION

The importance of your companionship increases when your hyperactive child reaches adolescence. Attending outdoor sporting activities or spectator games together can be mutually enjoyable, as can arts and crafts in which both of you participate.

Peer relationships are very important. Adolescents

often want to participate in organized team sports and if they are not successful, they sometimes become so unpopular with their classmates and peers that they are not wanted on the teams. In such a situation, the adolescent needs help in regaining his popularity before he can join a team.

Individual outdoor sports are generally preferable to outdoor team sports. Activities such as running, swimming, biking, and skiing, for example, can develop his skills at a pace uniquely suited to his own readiness. There are no teammates to disappoint or seek approval from; there are no opponents to become angry at or feel inferior to. The adolescent competes against his own past record and thus improves his self-confidence and his skill level.

Suitable indoor recreation depends more on personal preferences and habits than on the presence or absence of hyperactivity. Hyperactive adolescents enjoy table games if they are not too complicated and if there is not too much emphasis on competition. The mild activity of table tennis or billiards also seems to be attractive to hyperactive adolescents.

Pay careful attention to structuring the play environment and selecting activities that match your child's readiness, energy level, and interests. Use play to enhance social skills and family relationships as well as to strengthen academic abilities and compensate for learning problems. Coordinate toy selection with the Fun Idea List and Fun Idea Drawer (Appendix F) so you are always ready to suggest wholesome activities. By following these suggestions, you can artfully integrate play into your total plan for helping your hyperactive child.

15

Joining or Starting a Support Group

A support group can be an important source of help for your family in many of the potential difficulties of raising an ADHD child. An effective way to overcome the frustrations of depending on bureaucracies to deliver all the needed special services is to work with other parents to bring about changes in community resources, health care, educational programs, and other related support systems for families of hyperactive children.

If existing support groups don't meet your needs, or none exist in your community, consider organizing one. Parents organized as a group can wield more power and attain more common goals than individuals working separately.

An effective support group meets regularly, usually in the evening. The meetings can be conducted by parents, a team of parents and helping professionals, or professionals. Meetings can include lectures, demonstrations, and question-and-answer or informal discussions. Professionals may offer informational presentations, or parents may offer practical care-giving suggestions. Parents are the primary conductors of the type of support group discussed here.

ORGANIZING A SUPPORT GROUP

Five steps are essential to organizing an effective support group for families with ADHD children: (1) determine goals and services, (2) arrange start-up meetings, (3) recruit skilled leaders, (4) expand the membership, and (5) take decisive action.

Determine Goals and Services

The goals and services of an efficient support group are almost limitless because the creativity and involvement of the leaders and members constantly expand its horizons. Here are some examples of the more common services that successful support groups provide.

Interaction. Members learn from other families' experiences and receive and share emotional support. Sharing reassures parents that their feelings are quite normal and their reactions appropriate; this awareness is a refreshing change from the mixed collection of criticisms typically received from outsiders. Knowing that they are not alone provides tremendous relief, particularly for the single parent. Chapter 9 details solutions for many of the stresses experienced by single parents of hyperactive children.

Discussion groups that allow participants to express concerns, ask questions and find answers, and share successful home and school arrangements offer empathy and support regarding family-related difficulties and the other issues nobody seems to understand except those who have faced similar trials.

Instruction. The group can arrange for qualified persons to present programs on topics relevant to the ADHD syndrome and its overlapping conditions' subgroups: prescribed medications, the Feingold Program, counseling services, parenting techniques, learning disabilities, conduct disorder problems, diagnostic procedures, family-strengthening activities, and others. Educational group meetings have the additional advantage of allowing parents to absorb complicated information by hearing topics discussed from differing points of view.

Standard parent education topics like encouragement and discipline are always popular. Sometimes the children can be the focus for presentations on topics such as anger control, friendship skills, stress reduction, or study habits.

Some school districts support and assist self-help parent organizations by supplying information, sending speakers, providing building space for meetings, and helping distribute announcements. Consider asking the school district to provide programs for your group; because school issues are always at the top of the list of difficulties for ADHD children, consider arranging programs on special educational and diagnostic procedures, tutoring skills, and other educational techniques to use at home to supplement classroom instruction.

Research. Because a large number of parents and children with a specific disorder and cluster of behavioral difficulties are available for study, an ADHD support group can assist in research. The focus can be on psychological issues, academic techniques, biochemical treatment, or any other aspect of life with hyperactive children and adolescents. The group can contact universities, known researchers in the field, and new researchers by referral from a national support organization. ADHD affects somewhere between 5 and 10% of U.S. schoolchildren but has received little research support compared to much rarer pediatric disorders. For every autistic child, for example, there are between 50 and 100 ADHD children.

Community Awareness. Group leaders can become acquainted with their local newspaper's key personnel. Other media sources such as radio and television talk programs may occasionally be interested in having a representative of the group participate. As the group makes the community more aware of the needs and characteristics of ADHD children, the families of recently diagnosed ADHD children can experience much greater understanding and help.

Special Services. Camping programs for learning disabled and hyperactive youngsters as well as those at-risk for delinquency are sponsored by various organizations throughout North America. Camps provide opportunities for ADHD children to succeed in a supportive learning environment as well as opportunities to develop meaningful new friendships. Consider conducting a survey of nearby camping programs and developing a special one if none of the local camps seems suitable.

The group can also organize special programs for the children who would not have easy access to other suitable activities. It can identify individual or family needs of member families and appropriate community resources to meet those needs. Once the group has identified and prioritized the needs of member families, a united effort can pave the way for better diagnostic services, medical care, behavior management counseling, social and emotional counseling, educational services, family recreation, and so forth.

Encourage the local school district to provide inservice training to familiarize teachers and administrators with the special characteristics of ADHD children and adolescents. If necessary, have the support group sponsor or provide this training of school personnel. At a minimum, send a representative from your group to every school board meeting and open forum.

Advocacy. Supplying advocates and advice-givers to individual families is another important function of a support group. Basic advocacy involves finding out what the family needs, outlining the options, assessing the family's chances of reaching the goals, and advising on courses of action. An experienced advocate can help member parents increase awareness of the needs of ADHD children and their families among professionals, schools, and agencies.

The group should inform parents of their rights and provide as much information as possible to help obtain effective services. It should train parents to be their own advocates, and it should intervene only if the parent is personally unable to obtain legitimate services.

The group can influence the directors and professional staffs of community resources to adopt desired approaches for helping member families, such as providing a summer camp for ADHD children. It can help parents prepare documentation to support requests for services on behalf of their children and can identify the correct appeals processes for services.

The group can investigate grievances about current services and can make certain the grievances are heard and complied with. The group can also assist parents in going to court if other avenues fail.

Information Gathering. Support groups share information among members and other support groups in various ways. For example, the group can arrange visits to out-of-district school programs and treatment facilities to observe any especially successful or creative services for ADHD children and adolescents. It can develop a lending library of resource materials, books, and videotaped and audiotaped lectures and organize a resource network with a newsletter, a telephone hotline, or a catalog of helpful local agencies and services.

Networking. A useful starting point is to organize within the school district boundaries, then link with similar organizations within neighboring districts. Share with other parent support groups solutions to negotiating within the local school district about obtaining special services for ADHD children.

Occasionally, some parents may need temporary child care away from their home or family. If the options for suitable child care are distant or nonexistent, the group can provide networking for trading temporary child care services between members.

Arrange Start-up Meetings

Launching a new support group takes effort but can be accomplished by anyone with enough determination. If possible, obtain the assistance at first from an umbrella organization, such as a church, public agency, private foundation, or local government group. A list of concerned parents, educators, mental health professionals, and physicians is a good basis for starting a group.

The Coordinating Council for Handicapped Children recommends three meetings for launching a support group: the organizational meeting, the public meeting, and the working meeting. Although a series of three specialized meetings is not suitable for every community, it provides an excellent starting point for understanding what these meetings should accomplish.

Get the word out for interested parents to contact you at a specified time and place. At this meeting, make plans for a large, more public meeting that will attract a large percentage of the parents of ADHD children in your community.

An interesting featured speaker and a selection of brief workshops is the most popular and successful type of program to offer. Promotional announcements should follow the guidelines given in *Dynamic Parenting* (see Selected Readings and Resources). Get the names and addresses of all who attend. At the next meeting, elect officers, develop a statement of goals, and start the relevant legal processes, such as obtaining a bulk mailing permit and incorporation.

Recruit Skilled Leaders

Leaders should be dedicated to the group's goals, good at motivating others to contribute their efforts, energizing to be around, positive and friendly, and willing to share monthly reports and to communicate with the membership. They should be open to suggestions and supportive of democratic decision making.

Leadership responsibilities include recruiting new members, building team spirit, developing other leaders, supporting fund-raising projects, carefully matching the skills of volunteers with their assignments, and following projects through to completion. Leaders need to pace the group's activities to avoid burnout or boredom of the membership and themselves. They should avoid giving too many duties to one or two faithful volunteers while others withdraw because they have too little to do. Members join the group and remain because of personal satisfaction and the desire to make a contribution in addition to the direct benefits of instruction or services received. Skilled leaders will maintain frequent contact with volunteers, listen to their suggestions, and reward them with appropriate acknowledgments and tokens of their service.

Expand the Membership

There is no substitute for a strong membership committee that encourages individual memberships as well as group memberships of civic and community agencies. Dues should be low. Develop a small information pamphlet describing the group. A newsletter is one of the most potent tools for ensuring the survival and growth of a support group; pay special attention to developing a readable newsletter that keeps members active and generates continual interest. Try to obtain membership of some professionals from each of the relevant disciplines but avoid letting the group get too top-heavy. Use the newsletter as a tool to keep the group prominent among the agencies and professionals in the community by asking a different administrator or helping professional to write an editorial or small informative article for each edition.

Take Decisive Action

One of the keys to a group's growth is making membership exciting by having real impact on the community as well as on the lives of member families. Complaints should become springboards for action. Leaders should ask for members' participation when a particular situation or problem is shared by several member families. Keep the focus on goals and avoid draining away resources on excessive parties, picnics, or trips.

GENERATING AND MAINTAINING ADEQUATE RESOURCES

Most support groups do not run an office, but operate instead as a core group of volunteers with minimal facilities. They often obtain supplies, funds, and services from local philanthropic and service organizations. Sometimes nonprofit groups are willing to donate funds to pay for a newsletter or the telephone and electricity bills, for example. Such help is particularly needed when a new support group is just forming and has not yet been able to establish a regular means of self-support. Many groups obtain the needed financial undergirding by selling seasonal items, such as Christmas trees, wreaths, and ornaments in December; fresh fruits (in containers sufficiently large for home canning) during the summer months; and baked goods at the major holidays. Among the most successful printed materials to sell are cookbooks and community calendars, which can be placed for sale by most merchants within the community. This type of fund-raising provides not only financial support but also public exposure.

The guidelines given in this chapter represent the combined experiences of leaders and members of support groups that vary greatly in funding, membership size, and focus. A strong, vital support group can flourish in your community, and you can play an important part in that growth.

Epilogue: A Final Word of Encouragement

This book summarizes the guidance and suggestions I typically offer when working with the families of hyperactive children. Many of them, such as the I CARE discipline sequence, the Concerns Notebook and PPI method, the A through G effects of biochemical treatment, the Fun Idea List and Drawer, the six A's of apology, and the charts and checklists, I have developed myself. In these pages, I have attempted to provide you with the information and tools for preventing or solving the types of problems you are most likely to confront as the parent of a hyperactive child or adolescent.

I do not want, however, to overwhelm or intimidate you with lists of potential difficulties. Although this book is devoted to correcting problems, that emphasis does not mean things never go right. There are many positive aspects to raising a hyperactive child. The vast majority of hyperactive individuals lead successful lives; and those fortunate enough to have parents like you, who are willing to read and follow guidelines such as those in this book, function well.

Please select those suggestions most relevant to your particular situation. Have confidence that improvement will come, and never let the negatives outweigh your awareness of the positives. Your gifts of time, resourcefulness, and commitment are priceless in helping your child achieve the best possible adjustment and success. Both of you are going to emerge as real winners!

APPENDIX A

STUDY AND DISCUSSION QUESTIONS

This book is designed to be exquisitely usable in support groups, discussion groups, and classes. Pretend an additional instruction, "Explain and elaborate on your answer," appears at the end of every question. Although geared to a group of parents, these questions can easily be adapted for use with college students, interns in the helping professions, or other groups.

CHAPTER 1

1. List at least four reasons why ADHD is so controversial.
2. Give an example from your personal experience of inconsistency among helping professionals with regard to diagnosis or treatment of your child.

3. What are the three most meaningful sentences for you in this chapter?
4. Of the mental difficulties listed, which two are the most significant for your child?
5. Of the physical difficulties listed, which two are the most significant for your child?
6. Of the emotional difficulties listed, which two are the most significant for your child?
7. Of the fetal, birth, early infancy, toddlerhood, and preschool indicators mentioned, which apply for your child?
8. What are your child's score and level of hyperactivity on the Taylor Hyperactivity Screening Checklist?
9. What surprised you most in this chapter?

CHAPTER 2

1. Rate your child's physician on a ten-point scale of helpfulness and effectiveness.
2. What are the three most meaningful sentences for you in this chapter?
3. If your physician would agree to read and follow the principles and instructions in any one paragraph from this chapter, which paragraph would you select?
4. Rate your child's and family's mental health professional on a ten-point scale of helpfulness and effectiveness.
5. What surprised you most in this chapter?
6. Give examples from your experience of trying to be a facilitator of professional help for your child (a) when you were too insistent; (b) when you were not insistent enough, and (c) when you were insistent without being pushy.

CHAPTER 3

1. Of the A through G effects, which have occurred most prominently for your child?
2. Rate your child's current medication on the Taylor Medication Effectiveness Report and compare it with ratings of other participants in this group.
3. If you have ever observed a slight overdose condition, an extreme overdose condition, or sensitivities/allergies in response to medication, report what you observed.
4. Using the guidelines given, track down the probable sources of a "bad day" your child has had and report results.
5. Discuss which methods for troubleshooting side effects have been successful for your child.
6. What surprised you most in this chapter?
7. What are the three most meaningful sentences for you in this chapter?
8. What are some of the advantages of using prescribed medication for ADHD individuals?
9. Suppose you are asked to discredit the medication treatment method. To make your case, cite at least five passages to exaggerate and to quote out of context.

CHAPTER 4

1. Of the objections by outsiders about medication treatment, which have been expressed to you?
2. What surprised you most in this chapter?

3. What are the three most meaningful sentences for you in this chapter?
4. Why is establishing a powerful pre-post contrast for the child emphasized?
5. Of the objections by ADHD children about medication treatment, which has your child expressed?
6. Discuss which aspects of the encouragement cycle apply for your child.
7. Take turns in your group role-playing being advised against continuing medication treatment by a critical outsider who expresses some of the objections given in this chapter. Give an assertive response to the criticism.
8. Of the child's responsibilities, list a few that your child is upholding well and cite instances that provide proof.
9. Suppose you are asked to discredit the medication treatment method. To make your case, which of the objections from outsiders do you think would be the most persuasive to include in a letter to the editor of your local newspaper? Why?

CHAPTER 5

1. Describe any sensitivities or allergies you know or suspect your child has.
2. What are the three most meaningful sentences for you in this chapter?
3. Describe your observations after a clear exposure of your child to any of the aggravating chemicals listed in Appendix E.
4. What is the most probable reason why the food industry has spent millions of dollars to persuade

people *not* to use a method that "doesn't work" anyway?

5. What does the claim that the Feingold Program works by suddenly giving the child "power and attention" show about the claimant's familiarity with hyperactive children?
6. Pretend you work for the Nutrition Foundation or the American Council on Science and Health (food industry proponents) and offer five statements to refute or dismiss the study that demonstrated 58% improvement with the Feingold Program—for example, "That was only one study."
7. Ask a dietitian, mental health professional, or physician about the validity of the Feingold Program, and try to get that person's opinion about why it works for *some* children. Share the results with the other participants in this group.
8. Why do most criticizers of the Feingold Program have little or no direct experience with it?
9. What surprised you most in this chapter?
10. Of the potential difficulties with the Feingold Program, which are most important for your situation?
11. What are the advantages of this method?

CHAPTER 6

1. Of the seven low self-esteem traits, which apply most severely to your child?
2. Report to the group your success at remedying your child's self-esteem.
3. Of the anger control methods given, which are most helpful for your child?

4. What are the three most meaningful sentences for you in this chapter?
5. Describe your child's regular exercise program or athletic participation and describe its benefits and drawbacks.
6. Of the responses to mistakes, which would be most helpful for your child to become convinced of?
7. What surprised you most in this chapter?
8. Contrast the approaches you have noticed other adults use with those given in this chapter for teaching your child to use mistakes wisely.
9. Directly apply at least three specific suggestions and techniques from this chapter for at least one week and report results.

CHAPTER 7

1. Explain why the statement "You should be more consistent" is unfair and misleading.
2. Why does this chapter emphasize the family roles for siblings of a hyperactive child?
3. What are the three most meaningful sentences for you in this chapter?
4. Which methods for reducing sibling rivalry have been most effective for your family?
5. Of the five most common social skills difficulties for ADHD children, which is the most difficult for your child?
6. Using the SCORED method, select one of your child's social skills that needs improvement and report results.
7. Give an example of how your child's reputation has led to unfortunate misunderstandings or problems.

8. Explain the six A's of apology to your child and report results after *you* have had an opportunity to use them as a model for your child to follow.
9. Which friendship skills have been most helpful for your child?
10. Which refusal skills have been most helpful for your child?
11. What surprised you most in this chapter?
12. Apply at least three specific techniques from this chapter for at least one week and report results.

CHAPTER 8

1. Of the five negative parental feelings, which was the most painful prior to finding a correct diagnosis for your child?
2. Share with the other participants several criticisms or other negative reactions you have received about (a) your child's behavior, (b) your parenting skills and actions, (c) the ADHD diagnosis, (d) the treatment method(s) you have attempted.
3. What are the three most meaningful sentences for you in this chapter?
4. Cite three extremely accurate sentences that describe exactly what you have experienced.
5. Have a group member role-play a well-meaning criticizer of the diagnosis of your child as hyperactive; role-play a sensitive, kind, but firm response. Repeat this exercise with several participants.
6. What surprised you most in this chapter?
7. In which areas mentioned in this chapter have you personally felt most guilty or inadequate?
8. What have been some of your major fears and worries regarding your family?

9. Directly apply at least three specific suggestions and techniques from this chapter for at least one week and report results.

CHAPTER 9

1. What are the three most meaningful sentences for you in this chapter?
2. Of the twelve destructive marital patterns, which two come closest to your situation?
3. In what ways do highly competitive persons make poor winners? poor losers?
4. Of the suggested methods of improving your marital relationship, which three have been most helpful for you?
5. Describe a specific instance in which the co-parenting method described in this chapter would have been helpful.
6. Of the suggestions given for rebuilding harmony, which two are most likely to succeed, or have succeeded best, in your family?
7. List at least three circumstances in which (a) you enjoy being with your child, (b) your child enjoys being with you, (c) your child enjoys doing something with the family, (d) the family enjoys doing something that includes the hyperactive child.
8. List at least three old habits you must break in order to respond supportively to decreases in your child's hyperactivity.
9. Cite at least one instance from your family experience that illustrates that children misbehave in part because they fear there is not enough love to go around in the family.
10. What surprised you most in this chapter?

11. Directly apply at least three specific suggestions and techniques from this chapter for at least one week and report results.
12. Of the advantages given for cooperative play, which seem to be the most important for helping your child?
13. Which of the six challenges of being the custodial parent apply most to you?

CHAPTER 10

1. Of the seventeen major areas of difficulty for ADHD children at school, which three seem to be most difficult for your child?
2. Share with other group members some approaches you have found successful in gaining the teacher's cooperation in jointly assisting your child academically.
3. What are the three most meaningful sentences for you in this chapter?
4. Inventory your child's academic problem areas using the Taylor Academic Problem Identification Checklist and compare the results with the inventories of other parents.
5. What surprised you most in this chapter?
6. Give an example from your personal experience of a truly helpful attitude or approach by a school administrator, counselor, or teacher.

CHAPTER 11

1. Of the six major goals for effective teaching of the ADHD child, in which area has your child experienced the least help from teachers?

2. Of the six major goals, which do you think would be the most challenging for your child's next teacher to accomplish?
3. What are the three most meaningful sentences for you in this chapter?
4. Use the Taylor Classroom Daily Report for at least a week and report results.
5. What surprised you most in this chapter?
6. Ask a cooperative teacher to read this chapter; then try to get an uncooperative teacher to do the same and report results.

CHAPTER 12

1. Why is notetaking difficult for most ADHD children?
2. What are the three most meaningful sentences for you in this chapter?
3. Of the many suggestions given for supervising and assisting your child with homework, which have been (or will be) easiest to incorporate and which have been (or will be) hardest? Why?
4. Where is your child most likely to break down in accomplishing the eleven homework steps?
5. Of the nine methods given for compensating for distractibility, which have been (or will be) easiest to incorporate and which have been (or will be) hardest? Why?
6. Why do you think this book devotes three chapters to the school adjustment of ADHD children?
7. What surprised you most in this chapter?

CHAPTER 13

1. Do you agree with the last sentence that good discipline maintains an atmosphere of mutual respect?
2. Although following the three S's involves considerable effort, why is it preferable to after-the-fact discipline?
3. Devise one of the three charts described, use it for a week, show it to the group, and share results.
4. Develop a Fun Idea List for your child, use it for a week, show it to the group, and share results.
5. What are the three most meaningful sentences for you in this chapter?
6. List at least five advantages of the Concerns Notebook.
7. Conduct two PPI meetings with your child and share results.
8. Use the I CARE method for one week and report results.
9. List five advantages of logical consequences over harsh punishments.
10. Apply the seven steps recommended as the best response to a child's lying, and report results.
11. What surprised you most in this chapter?

CHAPTER 14

1. What are the three most meaningful sentences for you in this chapter?
2. Which of the recommendations for vigorous outdoor play will your child enjoy the most?
3. Change the rules of a competitive game to make it more cooperative and report results.

4. What surprised you most in this chapter?
5. How can play be considered an important activity for a child?
6. Directly apply at least three specific suggestions and techniques from this chapter for at least one week and report results.
7. List and share with other parents the toys you have found appropriate for your hyperactive child during (a) quiet individual play, (b) vigorous individual play, and (c) vigorous group play.

CHAPTER 15

1. Do a survey of support groups in your area, regardless of their relevance to ADHD, and report results.
2. Briefly interview someone in any support group regarding how many of the goals and services listed in this chapter that support group actually engages in. Share results.
3. What are the three most meaningful sentences for you in this chapter?
4. What surprised you most in this chapter?

APPENDIX B

THE TAYLOR CHECKLISTS

THE TAYLOR HYPERACTIVITY SCREENING CHECKLIST

This highly accurate checklist (see Chapter 1) for helping diagnose true ADHD is an improved version of an original checklist I developed from interviews with parents of hyperactive children. From these interviews, I identified fifty-seven symptoms and gave the list of these symptoms to parents of fifty-one hyperactive children. Each hyperactive child was from a different family, and their ages ranged from two to fifteen. All had been diagnosed as hyperactive by physicians. The parents rated their children on each of the fifty-seven traits and its opposite.

Twenty-one of the most consistent symptoms were selected for the original version of the checklist. These traits were those in which the children were rated in the hyperactive direction by at least 67% of the parents (thirty-nine of fifty-one sets of parents), as well as those in which the children were rated in the nonhyperactive direction by less than 17% of the parents (nine or fewer from fifty-one sets of parents). In other words, those traits were consistently rated in the hyperactive direction and were shown to be valid for screening hyperactivity.

The accuracy and validity of the original checklist have been determined by administering it to additional groups. The children are from three different groups. The first group contained fifty-one hyperactive children whose scores were used in developing the checklist. The second group contained sixty-six hyperactive children seen in my professional practice. The third group consisted of twenty-two nonhyperactive siblings of the children from the first group.

Table B-1 shows the percentage of children with each of the traits from the right side of the checklist, which are hyperactivity traits. About four out of five hyperactive children were rated in the hyperactive direction on the checklist, while only one out of five nonhyperactive siblings without other disorders (22%) were rated in the hyperactive direction.

Table B-2 shows the percentage of children with each of the traits from the left side of the checklist, which are the normal opposites of the hyperactivity traits. Approximately three out of five nonhyperactive siblings without other disorders (61%) were rated in the nonhyperactive direction, while fewer than one in eight hyperactive children (about 12%) were rated in the nonhyperactive direction.

The improved version of the checklist that appears in Tables B-3 and B-4 incorporate the slight clarification of items that I have found most helpful, based on administering the checklist verbally to parents and to ADHD as well as non-ADHD individuals over several years. Because the research on its validity was done with the original version and there has been no comparable systematic

TABLE B-1
Percentages of Children Rated in the Hyperactive Direction (Column C*)

Item	*Group 1 (51 hyperactive children)*	*Group 2 (66 hyperactive children)*	*Group 3 (22 nonhyperactive children)*
1.	82	79	23
2.	82	71	14
3.	78	79	18
4.	82	77	9
5.	92	91	32
6.	76	82	14
7.	82	89	32
8.	94	92	41
9.	78	70	23
10.	86	91	36
11.	82	82	36
12.	80	68	9
13.	88	91	16
14.	84	79	23
15.	88	86	14
16.	67	82	18
17.	76	70	14
18.	90	86	32
19.	92	91	23
20.	71	70	32
21.	76	70	9
Average	82	81	22

*From the Taylor Hyperactivity Screening Checklist

study of the improved version, Tables B-3 and B-4 provide comparisons between the original and the improved versions for those items that have been altered. If they affect the accuracy of the checklist, these alterations would most assuredly increase it, so the validity figures obtained from the original version might be even more decisive if a similar research program were conducted on the improved version.

TABLE B-2
Percentages of Children Rated in the Nonhyperactive Direction (Column A*)

Item	*Group 1 (51 hyperactive children)*	*Group 2 (66 hyperactive children)*	*Group 3 (22 nonhyperactive children)*
1.	6	12	64
2.	4	21	59
3.	8	17	64
4.	8	18	86
5.	2	6	55
6.	6	9	82
7.	2	9	68
8.	2	5	41
9.	10	20	68
10.	2	6	50
11.	2	6	50
12.	16	27	59
13.	0	2	59
14.	6	18	64
15.	2	2	55
16.	6	9	68
17.	2	17	68
18.	4	5	36
19.	0	5	68
20.	6	24	64
21.	8	24	55
Average	5	12	61

*From the Taylor Hyperactivity Screening Checklist

TABLE B-3
Original Versus Improved Items in the Nonhyperactive Direction (Column A*)

Item	*Improved Wording*	*Original Wording*
1.	Quiet person	Quiet when sitting
8.	Slow to react, deliberate, not impulsive	Slow to react, thinks before acting
9.	Understands why parents/teacher/others are displeased after misbehavior	Understands why others are displeased after misbehavior
10.	Planful; thinks ahead to consequences before acting	Thinks ahead to later consequences
11.	Avoids other children's mischief	Avoids joining into others' mischief
14.	Constant mood with mild or slow mood changes; a calm person	Constant mood with mild or slow mood changes; calm
12.	Concerned about punishments and consequences; submissive	Concerned about punishments and consequences
15.	Easygoing; handles frustration without much anger; patient; can be teased	Easygoing, can accept frustration, can take no for an answer
16.	Emotions are reasonably controlled, are not extreme, and don't disrupt relationships	Emotions don't disrupt relationships, are reasonably restrained
17.	Cooperates with, obeys, and enforces the rules of work and play	Cooperates, obeys, and enforces rules
18.	Gives up when denied a requested privilege, item, or activity	Gives up when denied by parent or teacher

TABLE B-3 *(continued)*

Item	*Improved Wording*	*Original Wording*
19.	Concentrates and blocks out distractions when working on something of medium interest	Concentrates and blocks out distractions
20.	Follows through, has an organized approach to activities, finishes projects	Finishes one thing before starting another

TABLE B-4
Original Versus Improved Items in the Hyperactive Direction (Column C)

Item	*Improved Wording*	*Original Wording*
1.	Noisy and talkative person	Noisy and talkative when sitting
2.	Voice is generally too loud for the situation	Voice is generally too loud
4.	Flits around, runs ahead, needs to be called back, jumpy	Runs and jumps rather than walks
6.	Always has a body part moving; fidgets with hands or feet; squirmy	Always has something moving; fidgets with hands or feet; jumpy
7.	Has to be doing something to occupy self when sitting; quickly bored	Has to be doing something when sitting, to occupy self
8.	Too quick to react, impulsive, engages mouth and muscles before brain	Quick to react, reacts on impulse

TABLE B-4 ***(continued)***

Item	*Improved Wording*	*Original Wording*
9.	Feels picked on; is surprised and confused about why others are displeased; doesn't connect own actions to others' reactions	Expects others not to be displeased by misbehavior, or does not realize that misbehavior has occurred
10.	Does things without considering consequences ahead of time; careless; not planful	Does things without considering consequences; doesn't plan ahead
11.	Gets involved in mischief; attracted or curious about it, or starts it	Attracted by and gets drawn into others' mischief
12.	Pretends to have an "I don't care" attitude if threatened or punished; defiant	Pretends to have an "I don't care" attitude if threatened or punished; defiant
13.	Disobeys; needs supervision or reminding; forgetful	Disobeys and needs supervision or reminding
14.	Moody; unpredictable; quick to anger or tears	Rapid and extreme mood changes; happy one minute and hostile the next; moody
15.	Irritable, impatient, easily frustrated	Irritable, can't accept frustration, can't take no for an answer
16.	Emotions are extreme and poorly controlled; no "damper pedal" on emotion; explosive, tantrumy	Emotions are extreme rather than moderated; child seems ruled by them; very hostile or very affectionate

TABLE B-4 ***(continued)***

Item	*Improved Wording*	*Original Wording*
17.	Argues and gripes about the rules; wants to be the exception; oppositional	Wants rules changed, wants to be the exception
18.	Badgers, pesters, pushes; won't give up or take no for an answer	When denied, child pesters, harps on it, doesn't give up
19.	Easily distracted by noises or people nearby; short attention span	Gets distracted by noises, people, etc.
20.	Flits from activity to activity, starts things without finishing them; gets sidetracked	Starts many new things without finishing any
21.	Needles, teases, is mouthy, has to have the last word	Needles, teases, picks on others with words

THE TAYLOR ACADEMIC PROBLEM IDENTIFICATION CHECKLIST

Attendance

Attends scheduled classes

Arrives at school on time

Arrives at classes on time

Sits at assigned desk

Remains alert

Comprehension

Understands simple requests

Remembers what is heard

Remembers what is read

Remembers what is seen

Reads, understands, and follows simple written instructions

Understands and follows simple oral instructions

Understands and follows two- or three-step oral instructions

Attention Control

Completes tasks

Works alone for an acceptable length of time on seatwork

Academic Skills

Reads aloud with acceptable accuracy and speed

Reads silently with acceptable understanding and speed

Remembers the content of silent reading passages

Remembers the content of oral reading passages

Has an acceptable speaking vocabulary

Has an acceptable reading vocabulary

Correctly spells words

Has an acceptable hearing vocabulary

Uses correct language

Tells time on a nondigital timepiece

Emotional Control

Handles transitions between different activities cooperatively

Accepts the disciplinary consequences of negative behavior

Responds appropriately to teacher reminders/warnings

Doesn't argue or challenge rules

Displays self-confidence

Isn't easily discouraged

Social Skills

Obtains the teacher's help by correct means

Obtains the teacher's help at correct times

Is courteous and friendly toward teacher

Productivity

Has good study habits

Meets daily assignment due dates

Meets due dates for short-term (less than one week) assignments

Meets due dates for long-term assignments

Completes assignments

Submits neat, orderly, legible assignments

Shows interest in academic work

Is interested in grades and is motivated by the grading system

Brings needed materials to classes

Participates in class discussions

Tries hard on assigned seatwork

Perseveres on work

Takes pride in work done

Accepts challenges and follows through on hard assignments

Problem Solving

Organizes and approaches tasks efficiently

Uses good problem-solving and decision-making skills

Asks for help if stuck

Plans steps to reach academic goals

THE TAYLOR SOCIAL/ EMOTIONAL/ACADEMIC ADJUSTMENT CHECKLIST

Instructions to Teacher

This checklist provides a quick, accurate overview of the child's adjustment at school in social, emotional, and academic areas. Profile the scores in the matrix by circling the correct dot under each item. Each set of four dots represents the four alternatives; the more circled dots under the dashed line, the greater the child's difficulties in school adjustment. The sequence within each subcategory is: upper left, lower left, upper right, lower right. Thus, a rating of "Underachieves, does slipshod work" in the first subcategory would be indicated by circling the third dot under AC in the profiling matrix.

Student	Grade	School
Rater	Class	Date

ONLY ONE (✓) IN EACH SUBCATEGORY!

1. Academic Expression

Achievement concern

- ☐ Works near capacity; is concerned with quality; enthusiastic
- ☐ Usually tries; sometimes needs reminding
- ☐ Underachieves; does slipshod work
- ☐ Ignores assignments; doesn't bring materials

Creative initiative

- ☐ Contributes ideas; brings in outside materials; is curious
- ☐ Occasionally uses new ideas or materials
- ☐ Has little imagination; doesn't question; plods
- ☐ Copies others' ideas; follows; is apathetic

Independence

- ☐ Seeks only necessary help
- ☐ Is fairly self-sufficient
- ☐ Too frequently demands help
- ☐ Needs one-on-one help; doesn't function alone

2. Academic Response

Alertness

- ☐ Pays attention; is "tuned in"
- ☐ Follows most of class work
- ☐ Daydreams; often needs prompting
- ☐ Is oblivious; often not reachable

Attendance

- ☐ Nearly always present
- ☐ Recurring legitimate absences
- ☐ Excessive unexcused absences
- ☐ Rarely in attendance

Comprehension

- ☐ Retains and applies new ideas
- ☐ Knows enough to get by
- ☐ Understands little
- ☐ Rarely or never understands

Attention span

- ☐ Sustains concentration; is organized
- ☐ Is generally attentive
- ☐ Doesn't stay with tasks; needs reminding
- ☐ Is restless; has short attention span; is disorganized

ONLY ONE (✔) IN EACH SUBCATEGORY!

3. Emotional Adjustment

Self-confidence

- ☐ Realistically accepts own best efforts
- ☐ Occasionally is self-critical; responds to encouragement
- ☐ Is overly self-critical and perfectionistic
- ☐ Gives up; is fearful; won't try

Self-discipline

- ☐ Is cooperative and well behaved
- ☐ Requires minor prompting
- ☐ Often disturbs class or teacher
- ☐ Has constant discipline problems

Emotionality

- ☐ Stable, self-controlled, not excitable
- ☐ Occasionally upset for short periods
- ☐ Moody, impatient
- ☐ Unpredictable, explosive, quick to temper or tears

4. Social Adjustment

Peer relationships

- ☐ Popular, well-liked; many friends
- ☐ Generally accepted; some friends
- ☐ Withdrawn or annoying; few friends
- ☐ Alienated, rejected, or fights often

School staff relationships

- ☐ Friendly, well-liked
- ☐ Generally accepted
- ☐ Aggravating; tolerated, but not popular among staff
- ☐ Not liked or accepted

5. Strengths and Interests: ______________________________

____

____

____

6. Other Comments: ______________________________

____

____

____

1. Acad. Exp.			2. Acad. Resp.				3. Emo. Adj.			4. Soc. Adj.	
AC	CI	I	AL	AT	C	AS	S-C	S-D	E	PR	SSR
.	.	.	.	.	.	.	.	.	.	.	.
.	.	.	.	.	.	.	.	.	.	.	.
—	—	—	—	—	—	—	—	—	—	—	—
.	.	.	.	.	.	.	.	.	.	.	.
.	.	.	.	.	.	.	.	.	.	.	.

Appendix C
Support Groups

The organizations listed here provide information on diagnostic and treatment services, advocacy, and instructional literature for parents and professionals. Many also maintain lists of regional, state, and local chapters and groups.

U.S. GOVERNMENT INFORMATION SOURCES

Clearinghouse on Disability Information, Office of Special Education and Rehabilitative Services, U.S. Department of Education, Rm. 3132 Switzer Bldg., Washington, DC 20202-2524

National Information Center for Handicapped Children and Youth, PO Box 1492, Washington, DC 20013

National Institute of Child Health and Human Development, National Institutes of Health, Bethesda, MD 20892

NATIONAL SUPPORT GROUPS AND ADVOCACY ORGANIZATIONS

Allergy Information Association, 65 Tromley Drive, Suite 10, Etobicoke, Ontario M9B 5Y7

American Academy of Allergy & Immunology, 611 E. Wells Street, Milwaukee, WI 53202

American Allergy Association, PO Box 7273, Menlo Park, CA 94026

Asthma and Allergy Foundation of America, 1717 Massachusetts Avenue NW, Suite 305, Washington, DC 20036

Attention Deficit Disorder Assn. (ADDA), PO Box 488, West Newbury, MA 01985

Challenge, Inc., PO Box 2001, West Newbury, MA 01985

Children And Adults With Attention Deficit Disorder (CH.A.D.D.), 499 NW 70th Avenue, Suite 308, Plantation, Florida 33317

Council for Exceptional Children, 1920 Association Drive, Reston, VA 22091

Feingold Association of the U.S., PO Box 6550, Alexandria, VA 22306

Hyperactive Children's Support Group, c/o Sally Bunday, 71 Whyke Lane, Chichester, West Sussex, England PO19 2LD

Learning Disabilities Association of America, 4156 Library Road, Pittsburgh, PA 15234

National Center for Learning Disabilities, 99 Park Avenue, New York, NY 10016

National Federation of Parent Support Groups, PO Box 1082, Sandy, UT 84091

National Foundation for Asthma, Inc., PO Box 30069, Tucson, AZ 85751

National Institute of Dyslexia, 3200 Woodbine Road, Chevy Chase, MD 20815

Orton Dyslexia Society, 724 York Road, Baltimore, MD 21204

Tourette Syndrome Association, Inc., 42-40 Bell Boulevard, Bayside, NY 11361-2861

Appendix D

Chemical Exposure Studies

Here are two of several scientific studies that help indicate the validity of the Feingold Program.

In 1989, *Pediatrics* published "Dietary Replacement in Preschool-Aged Hyperactive Boys," a report on a ten-week study in which all food was provided for the families of twenty-four hyperactive boys.

Among the twenty-four hyperactive boys, 58% improved noticeably in overall behavior as a result of limited dietary manipulations that controlled for the power of suggestion (placebo effect) and expectation by parents of behavior changes. Decrease in the incidence of bad breath (an allergy sign) and lessening of sleep disturbances were also noted. Careful analysis of the data revealed that overall nutrition did not lead to the observed improvements; these results occurred clearly in response to a decrease in chemical exposure.

The scientifically designed experiment eliminated many of the flaws that were typical of food industry–supported studies. The dietary intervention involved eliminating artificial chemical flavorings and chemical dyes from food and beverages consumed by the families during the duration of the experiment. None of the children was receiving prescribed medication. Though not a test of the Feingold Program, this study is the closest approximation yet of a scientific examination of the method. For the vast majority of children, salicylates were not removed and there was no attempt to control for chemical exposure from nonfoods such as toiletries, toothpaste, and so on.

Unlike food industry–supported studies, the Canadian study was funded by national and provincial agencies. Researchers were Bonnie Kaplan, Ph.D., Department of Pediatrics and Psychology, University of Calgary; Jane McNicol, R.D., Department of Dietetics, Alberta Children's Hospital; Richard Conte, Ph.D., Department of Psychology, University of Calgary; and H. K. Moghadam, M.D., Department of Pediatrics, University of Calgary.

Parents rated their children on a daily basis and observed for such allergy symptoms as skin rashes, red cheeks, dry skin, stomach bloat or cramps, leg cramps, stuffy or runny nose, headaches, earaches, and bad breath, as well as behavior.

> A 10-week study was conducted in which all food was provided for the families of 24 hyperactive preschool-aged boys whose parents reported the existence of sleep problems or physical signs and symptoms. A within-subject crossover design was used, and the study was divided into three periods: a baseline period of 3 weeks, a placebo-control period of 3 weeks, and an experimental diet period of 4 weeks.
>
> The experimental diet was broader than those studied previously in that it eliminated not only artificial colors and flavors but also chocolate, monosodium glutamate, preservatives, caffeine, and any substance that families reported might affect their specific child. The diet was also low in simple sugars, and it was dairy free if the family reported a history of possible problems with cow's milk.
>
> According to the parental report, more than half of the subjects exhibited a reliable improvement in behavior and negligible placebo effects. In addition, several nonbehavioral variables tended to improve while the children received the experimental diet, particularly hal-

itosis, night awakenings and latency to sleep onset. (*Pediatrics* 83(1989):7–17)

Researchers J. Egger, C. Carter, P. Graham, D. Gumley, and J. Scothill treated seventy-six selected overactive children with an oligoantigenic diet; sixty-two improved, and a normal range of behavior was achieved in twenty-one of these. Other symptoms, such as headaches, abdominal pain, and fits, also often improved. Twenty-eight of the children who improved completed a double-blind, crossover, placebo-controlled trial in which foods thought to provoke symptoms were reintroduced. Symptoms returned or were exacerbated much more often when patients were on an active material rather than on a placebo. Forty-eight foods were incriminated. Artificial colorants and preservatives were the most common provoking substances, but no child was sensitive to these alone ("Controlled Trial of Oligoantigenic Treatment in the Hyperkinetic Syndrome," *Lancet* 1 (March 9, 1985):540–45).

Appendix E

Common Offending Chemicals

Exposure to these substances can sometimes worsen ADHD symptoms or trigger an S-R state.

Heating: gas appliances and furnaces; kerosene; oil heat or spills; odorous space heaters; burning of chemically treated wood; smoke from fireplace, wood stove, or coal; propane appliances

Home: moth balls, fresh newsprint, typing correction fluid, holiday decorations of fresh evergreen branches, evergreen trees, formaldehyde from new carpeting, scented candles, menthol cigarette smoke, air fresheners, dog and cat repellent

Kitchen: scouring powders, soaps, waxes, polishes, aerosols, chlorine, disinfectant containing methyl salicylate, pine scent, oven cleaner, rug shampoo, colored dishwasher detergent

HOME WORKSHOP: paint, shellac, varnish, and similar substances; particle board, especially if being sawed; wood coatings; airborne particles from sanding wood; fresh paneling; plaster and dry wall substitutes and fillers; formaldehyde from foam insulation; all-purpose glues; odors from construction of a new mobile home (first seven years after construction); glue used in flooring, wallpaper, and paneling; petroleum products, engine cleaners, and chemicals; damp basements

LAUNDRY: soaps and detergents, especially non-white and heavily scented; scented fabric softeners; fabric softener dryer sheets; freshly dry cleaned clothing; TRIS flame retardant in clothes

PLAYROOM: scented stickers or toys; ballpoint or invisible ink on skin; felt-tip marker on skin; colored chalk or chalk dust; fingerpaint; scratch and sniff stickers; putty- and claylike modeling compounds; caps and fireworks; white powder inside new balloons; Easter egg dyes; art supplies; photographic chemicals; odorous marking devices; glue and paste; modeling clay; paint and other art materials

BATHROOM: deodorant, perfume and cologne, hair spray, alcohol on skin, hand lotion, colored and perfumed soap, facial powder, eye shadow, fingernail polish and polish remover, artificially dyed or flavored toothpaste, lip chapping stick, preshave and after shave lotion, bubble bath, dental cleaning agent, fluoride treatment, adhesive bandages, artificially dyed or flavored medicine

YARD: pesticides, swimming pool chemicals, lawn chemicals, smoke

NEIGHBORHOOD: tar and pitch, smoke from large outdoor fires, exhaust fumes, freshly poured blacktop, roof resurfacing chemicals, tree spraying

SCHOOL: freshly applied waxes and plastic coatings on gymnasium and hall floors, mimeograph paper, duplicating machines, freshly painted walls, formaldehyde from freshly laid carpet, chemically treated paper, school bus exhaust fumes, strong chemical odors from science labs, pets or pet food, moldy odors in lavatories and locker rooms, previously flooded basements or other damp areas of the school, aroma of food to which the child is allergic (such as popcorn), dust, molds, mites

APPENDIX F

SUGGESTED ACTIVITIES

These suggestions were provided by many parents of ADHD children who are successfully using the Fun Idea List to prevent boredom and misbehavior. These activities are effective in helping hyperactive children channel their energy into constructive pursuits and can become the starting point for your own Fun Idea List. You will want to modify it and add to it to fit your family's specific needs.

FUN IDEA LIST

Outdoor or Good Weather Play with Others

Have a popcorn and fruit drink stand; camp in the backyard in sleeping bags or tents; go for a walk or hike;

participate in vigorous activity like swimming, running games, or ball games; do water play with hose and plastic slide cloth; have a water fight with squirt guns and cups, using buckets of water as the source of "ammunition," and trying to douse the other person without getting doused in return.

Indoor or Inclement Weather Play with Others

Play jacks; make a tent with a sheet and a card table; telephone a friend; gather shoes from around the house and play shoe store; using a comb, brush, cup with water, and towel, play barber or hairdresser; put things in a mystery sack and give clues about what is in the sack, allowing the other child to reach into the sack and feel the object as the last clue; play card games; play table games; make up a pretend radio or television interview and talk into the recorder. (Most of these can be moved outdoors in good weather.)

Outdoor or Good Weather Solitary Play

Watch the stars through a telescope; look through binoculars; work on gardening; hug a tree; line up pop cans and throw pebbles at them; feed pets; practice jump-rope stunts; draw pictures of your yard to show the seasons of the year; water some flowers with a sprinkling can; make a collection of leaves from the yard; swat flies; feed spiders; volunteer to sweep a neighbor's sidewalk without pay; draw a portrait of a house, tree, flower, or other outdoor scene on an art pad; play on a climbing structure or swing set; play in a sandbox; roller skate; ride a bike; use a skateboard; go jogging, ice skating, swimming, fishing, horseback riding; build something for backyard (birdhouse, bird feeder); feed bread to birds; train and groom pets; select, clean, and label objects for a garage sale;

earn money by washing cars or mowing lawns; feed ducks, pigeons, songbirds, or squirrels; collect interesting rocks; write or draw on the sidewalk with chalk; play with pets. (Most can be shared with other children, if feasible.)

Indoor or Inclement Weather Solitary Play

Listen to music; try out an electronics kit; punch a punching bag; make muffins; hum; pop popcorn; make an item for a model railroad or toy car set out of frozen fruit sucker sticks, toy logs, or building toys; plan a day trip from the travel drawer for the family to take; write letters to relatives or friends; color in a coloring book; make a crossword puzzle for family members to solve; organize a home slide show; dance; work on a large jigsaw puzzle; play with building toys and construction kits; draw with colored pencils; sing; make a collage out of pictures from old magazines using liquid glue; practice a musical instrument; start or work on a collection (stamps, butterflies, bottle caps, coins, trading cards); play with a flashlight; make shadow pictures on the wall; make new greeting cards using pictures and words from old ones and drawing additional designs; make things with modeling dough; draw a picture of something you would like to do; invent a machine that would help you in some way and draw a picture of it; draw a picture of your house or apartment; draw pictures of inventions we could use in our family, such as something to clean bedrooms or cook or serve meals; put one letter of the alphabet on each card, shuffle, and try to put them back in order faster each time; cut shapes from construction paper and paste them on a large piece of colorful cardboard to make an attractive design; make a standard shape, such as a circle or triangle, then cut into smaller pieces to make a puzzle for family members to put together; paste a pretty picture on cardboard, then cut into pieces for your own homemade jigsaw puzzle; use stencils to write letters, numbers, and designs in pretty or unusual ways; color the ribs around the edge of a paper plate and make an attractive design in the center; stand dominoes on end in a pattern or a long winding line, then knock them down; make a rub drawing by putting something with a distinct texture (such as a leaf or coin) underneath paper and rubbing across the paper with a colored pencil; play Solitaire; juggle three balloons simultaneously; make a tunnel by draping a sheet over the back of a sofa; cook or bake with supervision; write down some good charades titles and topics for the family to use later; use a tape recorder to record sounds around the home; sort family photos and put in album; develop magic tricks; assemble model kits; play with a train or racer set; make drawings with charcoal or colored chalk; make and decorate stationery with stencils for personal use; make personalized gift stationery using stencils; make holiday decorations such as tree or wreath ornaments; measure things with measuring tape, ruler, and yardstick, and write down the measurements; make up a quiz for family members about the measurement results. (Most can be moved outdoors in good weather.)

Whole Family Activities

Have a backward dinner—dessert first; watch home movies; play word games and trivia games; have a story-in-the-round in which each member adds the next passage to the story; tell fill-in-the-blank stories in which each member adds a word when invited to do so by the storyteller; read aloud from a favorite book and act it out; go to a show, sports event, museum, or zoo; do a benevolent project anonymously for a needy person or family; play instruments and sing; go window shopping; drive to a nearby interesting place.

FUN IDEA DRAWER

Arts and Crafts

Crayons, used greeting cards to be cut up and made into new ones, safe paints, pieces of sponge, paint brushes, art and drawing paper, colored construction paper, felt markers, colored pencils, watercolors, play modeling dough, stencils, glitter, white glue, cotton balls, rulers, sequins, buttons, yarn, hole punch, craft sticks, clothespins, oatmeal boxes, cardboard bathroom tissue rolls, stamp pad and stamps (make your own from foot pads), scissors, old magazines with pictures, poster board.

Games

Table game boards, markers, dice, and spinners; children's playing cards; CARROM board (over 100 games and relatively indestructible).

Writing Equipment

Typing paper, notebooks and notebook paper, ballpoint pens, pencils, erasers, stationery for writing to friends.

Glossary

Absorption: Taking a substance (e.g., medicine or food) across tissues, such as through the intestines. Unabsorbed medication is ineffective.

Achievement test: A measure of a person's knowledge level in a particular topic, such as reading or mathematics. Usually expressed as percentile scores or grade equivalents.

ADD-noH: Attention deficit disorder without hyperactivity. Severe attention problems, but without the excitability component of ADHD. See *Hyperactivity.*

ADHD: Attention Deficit Hyperactivity Disorder. A diagnostic term recommended in *The Diagnostic and Statistical Manual of Mental Disorders,* 3rd ed., rev., issued by the American Psychiatric Association in 1987.

ADHD-cd: The conduct disorder subgroup of ADHD.

Reflects the overlapping conditions of ADHD and any conduct disorder.

ADHD imitator disorders: Medical and psychiatric conditions whose symptoms overlap some of the components of the ADHD syndrome. The diagnostic task of the physician or mental health professional includes differentiating between true ADHD and the imitator disorders.

ADHD-ld: The learning disabled subgroup of ADHD. Reflects the overlapping conditions of ADHD and any learning disability.

ADHD-sa: The sensitive-allergic subgroup of ADHD. Reflects the overlapping conditions of ADHD and profound sensitivities or allergies.

Affective education: Formal instruction in how to understand and deal with one's own feelings and be sensitive to those of others.

Alexia: Inability to read written or printed language; sometimes evident in learning disabled ADHD children.

Allergy: An abnormal body response to a substance during which the immune system is mobilized.

American Council on Science and Health: A public information organization promoting the marketing and financial interests of the food industry. It disputes the finding that ADHD symptoms can worsen if food containing artificial chemical additives such as dyes, preservatives, and flavorings is consumed.

Amitriptyline: A tricyclic antidepressant. A trade name is Elavil. Sometimes prescribed to treat ADHD symptoms.

Amphetamines: A group of stimulant medications noted for their enhancement of certain functions of the cortex of the brain. A popular category of medications prescribed for ADHD children; Dexedrine is an example.

Anoxia: Reduced supply of oxygen during the birth process. Can cause damage to the nervous system.

Anticonvulsant: Medication that reduces seizures; also known as antiepileptic medication.

Antidepressant: Medication that reduces depression and uplifts mood and energy in depressed persons. Some antidepressants help control ADHD symptoms though not contributing an uplift of mood. See *Tricyclic antidepressant.*

Anxiety: State of being nervous, worried, tense, and stressed. Should not be confused with eagerness, which is generally a positive condition. Severe anxiety is an ADHD imitator condition.

Aphasia: Impaired ability to understand or express thoughts through ordinary language; also called dysphasia.

Aptitude test: An estimate of ability or capacity for learning.

Assertiveness training: Methods for stating personal needs and wants, setting limits on others' undesirable actions, negotiating, and using refusal skills. See *Refusal skills.*

A through G effects: A summary of the desired effects of biochemical treatment on ADHD children: Activity Control, Brain in Gear, Conscience, Diligence, Emotional Control, Focusing, and Gentleness.

Attention deficit: Impaired ability to maintain alertness, to avoid distractibility, and to select purposeful stimuli to focus on. A key symptom in the ADHD syndrome.

Auditory discrimination: Ability to note differences between similar sounds, such as "bat" and "bet," which is important for learning to read.

Auditory perception: Ability to interpret information coming through the sense of hearing, including discriminating sounds.

Auditory sequential memory: Ability to remember an oral sequence, such as a list of items in alphabetical order or a telephone number.

Autism: A severe form of mental illness in which the individual does not respond to external information or stimulation but centers almost exclusively on internal sensations and thoughts.

Aventyl: See *Nortriptyline.*

Behavior modification: A system of intervention to change a person's behavior by reinforcements of desired behavior (rewards) and extinguishers of undesired behavior (ignoring, punishing).

Biochemical treatment: Treatment of ADHD by attempting to normalize the abnormal brain chemistry causing the disorder, such as with prescribed medications or the Feingold Program.

Breech presentation: An abnormal birth position of buttocks first at the head of the birth canal. Breech presentation is correlated with the occurrence of ADHD.

Caffeine: A xanthene derivative known to speed the metabolism of various substances and drugs, including some prescribed medications. Sometimes used to treat ADHD, though not very effectively.

Carcinogenic: Capable of causing cancer.

Cardiovascular: Pertaining to the blood vessels and heart. A side effect of some of the medications used in treating ADHD is increased cardiovascular rates, reflected in elevated blood pressure and heart rate.

Career education: Educational programs fostering awareness, exploration of alternatives, and vocational and social skills relevant to the world of work.

CBT: See *Cognitive behavioral training.*

Central nervous system (CNS): The brain and spinal cord, which comprise the parts of the nervous system that receive sensory messages and send out muscle-movement messages.

Certified U.S. food colors: Coal tar and petroleum-based dyes added for cosmetic purposes to foods and beverages, and certified to be the exact substances that are registered with the FDA. Certification does not mean safe or unlikely to cause adverse reactions in individuals sensitive to them.

Child abuse: Excessively harsh treatment of children, commonly divided into emotional (rejection), verbal (yelling, name calling, swearing), physical (excessive spanking, slapping, hair pulling, or assaulting), and sexual (force or enticement to witness or participate in sexual activity).

Chlordiazpoxide: A minor tranquilizer sometimes mistakenly prescribed for ADHD individuals in a misguided attempt to slow them down. A trade name is Librium.

Chorea: An infectious disease related to tonsillitis that involves involuntary movements of the limbs and facial muscles accompanied by restlessness, irritability, and insomnia; also known as Sydenham's chorea and acute chorea. An ADHD imitator disorder.

Chorionitis: Inflammation of the outermost of the two membranes completely enveloping the preborn child.

Chronological age: Real age in years and months, as used in psychological testing; often abbreviated CA. A child who is eight years, nine months old would be CA 8–9.

Clinical effect: The desired effect of prescribed medication, as contrasted with side effect. See *Side effect.*

Clonidine hydrochloride: A blood pressure medication useful in reducing the tics of Tourette's syndrome. A trade name is Catapres.

CNS: Central nervous system.

Cognitive behavioral training (CBT): A method of improving performance and self-control with self-reminding statements said silently or out loud throughout the sequence of actions being learned.

Colic: Acute abdominal pains; a term more generally describing digestive upset, crying, and difficult feeding.

Communication disorder: An impairment in the ability to communicate because of a speech problem or the inability to use language effectively; includes difficulty in articulation, voice characteristics (pitch), or fluency (stuttering).

Compulsivity: An irresistible impulse to perform an irrational act; more generally, a tendency to be overly concerned with orderliness to the point of double-checking everything and writing everything down.

Concerns Notebook: A method of anger control, disciplinary supervision, and communication between children and their parents. A special notebook in which the child enters concerns, to be discussed regularly at the PPI. See *Personal private interview.*

Contraindication: A factor impeding the effectiveness of a medication or causing it to create harmful side effects.

Correlated: Occurring together or associated with each other. Many of the predictors and symptoms of ADHD are correlated with each other and with the occurrence of ADHD in any one individual.

Counseling: A type of psychotherapy involving emotional support and reassurance, advice, and education. Intervention includes discussing alternative plans of action, discipline techniques, study skills, and similar topics. See *Psychotherapy.*

Decoding: Converting symbols into understandable concepts, such as reading words or interpreting facial expressions.

Depression: A syndrome marked by sadness, pessimism, low energy for coping with ordinary tasks, lack of zeal or enthusiasm, frequent crying, loosened emotional control, weakened mental alertness, low productivity, and social withdrawal.

Developmental delay: Temporary lag or delay in a child's development of a trait or skill, such as the ability to talk or walk (also known as maturational delay). See *Developmental milestones; Precociousness.*

Developmental milestones: Stages in normal progression of accomplishing increased skills, such as walking or talking. Passing of milestones abnormally late is a developmental delay and abnormally early is precociousness.

Dexedrine: The generic name is dextroamphetamine sulfate. See *Amphetamines.*

Dexedrine Spansule: Trade name for the long-acting form of Dexedrine (also known as Dex-Span). A stimulant medication commonly prescribed for ADHD children.

Dextroamphetamine sulfate: Generic name for an amphetamine stimulant. See *Dexedrine.*

Diagnostic prescriptive teaching: An educational approach that assesses a student's strengths and weaknesses, then designs and implements special instructional procedures to compensate for weaknesses.

Diagnostic test: An in-depth measure of a person's skills, including strengths and weaknesses and style of approach to tasks.

Diazepam: A trade name is Valium. Sometimes mistakenly prescribed for ADHD individuals in a misguided attempt to slow them down. See *Minor tranquilizers.*

Diet Diary: A form for use with the Feingold Program to record chemical exposure through food and beverage intake.

Disinhibition: Difficulty controlling an impulse to act

in a certain way or do a certain thing; roughly equivalent to hyperactivity.

Distractibility: An impaired ability to block out irrelevant stimuli, such as noises while working on a task, and to remain on-task after perceiving the irrelevant stimuli. One of the key traits in the ADHD syndrome.

Dopa: A neurotransmitter derived from tyrosine; transforms into dopamine near the end of the nerve cell (presynaptic cell) prior to the cell's sending dopamine on to the next cell.

Dopamine: A neurotransmitter derived from dopa near the end of the nerve cell (presynaptic cell); migrates to the next nerve (postsynaptic cell), where it transforms into norepinephrine as part of the process of transmitting a nerve impulse.

Dosage: The amount of medication administered at one time; usually expressed in milligrams (mg).

Double blind: A research design in which neither the person giving the treatment nor the person receiving it knows whether the treatment or medication being used is genuine or merely an imitation (placebo). Double-blind experiments eliminate the effects of bias on the research results and are regarded as among the most scientific and reliable forms of research. Can be distorted and abused, as has happened with some of the double-blind research on the effects of chemical exposure on ADHD symptoms.

Drug: Any nonfood substance that affects living tissue and is present in abnormal concentration in the blood. All medications are drugs.

Drug addiction: Persistent drug use and overwhelming

involvement with the drug, securing its supply, and returning to its use after attempts to discontinue using it, despite adverse social and medical consequences.

Drug holiday: A temporary discontinuance of prescribed medication for the purpose of ascertaining whether symptoms reappear and whether continued use of the medication is indicated (also known as a medication holiday or drug-free period).

Due process: A system of legal procedures guaranteeing that persons are treated fairly and can raise issues or objections about the services they are receiving. See *Public Law 94–142.*

Dysarthria: Impaired ability to pronounce words because of difficulty controlling muscle movements in the mouth, resulting in slurred or distorted speech.

Dyscalculia: Impaired ability to perform mathematical computations, either because of perceptual problems (such as aligning decimals) or conceptual problems (such as not understanding a ratio).

Dysgraphia: Impaired ability to handwrite legibly because of difficulty controlling the muscle movements involved.

Dyslexia: Impaired ability to read.

Eclampsia: Convulsions in an expectant mother.

Educational disability: See *Learning impairment.*

Egocentrism: A reaction to every situation from a self-centered or selfish point of view.

Elavil: See *Amitriptyline.*

Emotional lability: Rapidly changing types and severity of emotional display.

Encephalitis: An inflammation of brain tissue, causing a variety of severe symptoms. An ADHD imitator disorder.

Encoding: Transforming ideas into symbols, such as in speaking and writing.

Encopresis: Involuntary defecation while fully clothed, usually without awareness.

Enuresis: Involuntary urination while fully clothed or asleep, usually without awareness.

Epilepsy: Recurring episodes of changing states of consciousness caused by temporary alteration in brain biochemistry, with or without accompanying sensory or muscle involvements. Some epileptic individuals have ADHD, though the relationship between the two disorders is minimal.

Exceptional child: A global term for a child whose needs differ from agemates' and who requires specially designed educational programs.

Expressive language dysfunction: Impaired ability to encode or express thoughts with well-selected words; evidenced by searching for the correct words and stammering (also known as expressive language disability or disorder).

Extreme emotions: See *Emotional lability.*

Failure-to-thrive syndrome: A combination of colic and slow weight gain in an infant.

Family therapy: A form of psychotherapy in which

family members are seen as a group by the therapist; focuses on issues such as sibling rivalry, emotional communication, conflict solving, and power structure within the family.

FDA: Food and Drug Administration. A regulatory agency of the U.S. government responsible for assuring that food is safe and wholesome; drugs, biological products, therapeutic devices, and diagnostic products are safe and effective; cosmetics are safe; and all of these products are honestly advertised and labeled.

Feingold Association of the United States: A nonprofit organization primarily comprising parents of ADHD children. Provides information and resources to assist in using the Feingold Program for biochemical treatment of ADHD.

Feingold, Benjamin, M.D.: Pediatrician and allergist, instructor of pediatrics at Northwestern University, discoverer of the sensitivity reactions underlying some ADHD, and originator of the Feingold Program.

Feingold Diet: Former name of the Feingold Program.

Feingold Program: A method of treating ADHD symptoms by limiting exposure to chemicals to which the children are sensitive.

Fetal alcohol syndrome: A syndrome noted at birth that includes low birth weight, small head size, birth defects, withdrawal symptoms, ADHD, and mental retardation; caused by an expectant mother's excessive consumption of ethyl alcohol.

Figure-ground perception: Ability to differentiate between a prominent item or design and the less prominent background. Auditory figure-ground perception involves hearing the difference between the speaker's voice and other voices or background noise.

Fine-motor coordination: Small-muscle movement ability, such as in handwriting or tying laces.

Formal test: A test that has explicit instructions for administration and scoring, such as an IQ test.

Free agency: An individual's responsibility for and control of his or her own behavior.

Fun Idea List: A list of suggested activities prominently displayed and referred to whenever boredom or misbehavior starts to occur.

Gastrointestinal: Referring to the intestines and stomach.

Generic medication: Medicine manufactured after the developer's seventeen-year period of protected marketing, often by firms who merely copy the formula.

Generic name: The chemical, official, or nonproprietary name for a medication, as contrasted with the trade name.

Grade equivalent: The difficulty level of academic tasks expressed in terms of the average difficulty of similar tasks in U.S. schools (sometimes called grade-level equivalent). A child who scores 5.5 in reading would be able to read as well as the average fifth-grader in the fifth month of instruction (January).

Gross-motor coordination: Large-muscle movement ability, such as in running, balancing, or throwing a ball.

Group counseling: Several counselees and one or two

leaders who facilitate the interaction among group members, with a therapeutic purpose such as social skills training.

Growth rebound: The sudden increase in height, weight, and muscle development that results from cessation of medication treatment for a period of weeks or months; caused by the temporary termination of drug interaction effects with growth hormones.

Guilles de la Tourette's syndrome: A rare disorder characterized by childhood or adolescent onset of jerking muscle movements (tics) and ADHD symptoms.

Haldol: A trade name for haloperidol. See *Haloperidol.*

Haloperidol: A major tranquilizer useful in reducing the tics of Guilles de la Tourette's syndrome. A trade name is Haldol.

Home schooling: An alternative to public education in which the child receives instruction at home usually with the parent as teacher.

Homovanillic acid: One of the main discharge products, along with MHPG, from the neurotransmitter molecules at the junctions of nerve cells. ADHD children have reduced homovanillic acid, which provides evidence for neurotransmitter shortage as the cause of ADHD. Use of stimulants increases homovanillic acid, which provides evidence that medications used to treat ADHD increase neurotransmitter supply.

Hydroxyzine pamoate: Frequently used for quieting colicky babies. A trade name is Vistaril. See *Minor tranquilizers.*

Hyperactivity: In its narrowest sense, excessive movement, excitability, fidgetiness, and restlessness. It represents a key symptom in the ADHD syndrome and often is used as a synonym for that syndrome. Formerly known as hyperkinesis. See *Disinhibition; ADHD.*

Hyperkinesis: See *Hyperactivity.*

Hyperthyroidism: A condition arising from an overly active thyroid; includes high blood pressure and accelerated heart rate. An ADHD imitator disorder.

Hypoglycemia: Abnormally low blood sugar; results in poor emotional control and mental problems. An ADHD imitator disorder. See *Emotional lability.*

I CARE: An acronym for a five-step procedure of disciplinary intervention for use with children: Intervene, Cool off, Affirm, Redirect, and Educate.

Imipramine: Generic name of tricyclic antidepressant imipramine hydrochloride. A trade name is Tofranil. The most popular antidepressant used to treat ADHD symptoms.

Impulsiveness/impulsivity: A tendency to respond too quickly without careful consideration of alternatives and without preplanning. A key symptom in the ADHD syndrome.

Incidence: The number of new cases of a disease or disorder over a certain period of time; often expressed as the number of cases per 1000 live births. For example, the incidence of ADHD during childhood is generally estimated to be 50 to 100 individuals per 1000 live births. See *Prevalence.*

Individualized Education Program (IEP): A written plan for a special education student; includes the student's strengths and weaknesses, goals and objectives, educational services and their starting dates, and procedures for evaluating progress. Devised by a team of school personnel along with the parents and the child.

Individualized instruction: Academic instruction specifically adapted to a given student's learning style and readiness. See *TAPIC; Learning style; Readiness.*

Inflexibility: See *Perseveration.*

Insomnia: Disturbed quantity and quality of sleep. Often included as part of the ADHD syndrome and as a side effect of medication used to treat it, though more appropriately called presleep agitation side effect. See *Presleep agitation.*

Intelligence quotient (IQ): A number expressing the apparent intelligence of a person; determined by mental age, as reported on a standardized test, dividing by chronological age, and multiplying by 100. For example, an 8-year-old with the thinking and learning abilities of a 6-year-old would have a mental age approximately three-fourths the chronological age. Since IQ reflects that ratio as a percentage, the IQ would be 75.

Interaction: In medicine, the modification of the effects of a medication by giving a different medication at the same time, with either desirable (positive interaction) or undesirable (negative interaction) results; the prescribing of medication should always take into account any possible interactions with other substances the patient may be taking.

Kinesthesis: The sense of movement of body parts, such as arms and hands while writing or throwing.

Learning disability: Severe impairment of the ability to learn through ordinary classroom instruction, based largely on difficulties with processing sensory information, memory, understanding and using spoken or written language, listening, thinking, talking, reading, writing, spelling, performing mathematical calculations, refining muscle coordination skills, and developing adequate social skills. Children are classified or approved for learning disability services after a formalized assessment, usually a comprehensive psychoeducational evaluation.

Learning impairment: Mental, physical, or emotional factors impeding the ability to learn and necessitating specially designed instruction. Also called educational disability.

Learning style: The behaviors that characterize a person's approach to learning; includes ability to focus attention, plan ahead, and remain on-task. See *Psychoeducational evaluation.*

Least restrictive environment: A standard established by Public Law 94-142 for placement of students in special education programs. Requires a setting that meets their educational requirements and closely matches the regular education program offered to their schoolmates. The setting must provide maximum participation in a regular classroom and minimum separation from nonhandicapped students.

Levodopa: A precursor of brain neurotransmitters. Some reports indicate that it can have a favorable effect on some ADHD symptoms, though it is not currently considered a viable treatment. See *Precursor; Tryptophane.*

Librium: See *Chlordiazpoxide; Minor tranquilizers.*

Logical consequences: A disciplinary response logically related to a misbehavior, such as paying the offended person back in service for the inconvenience caused by the misbehavior.

Mainstreaming: Placement of an educationally disabled student in a regular classroom.

Mental age: In intelligence testing, a score indicating overall ability to learn, think, and absorb knowledge; expressed as equivalent to the average performance of other children of a given chronological age. See *Intelligence quotient.*

Methylphenidate: A stimulant medication structurally similar to naturally occurring dopamine; seems to work by increasing dopamine and norepinephrine in the brain. It is the most popular medication for treating ADHD. A trade name is Ritalin.

MHPG: One of the main discharge products, along with homovanillic acid, from neurotransmitter molecules at the junctions of brain cells.

Migration: The process of a chemical's movement from one cell to a nearby cell, such as the movement of the neurotransmitter dopamine from one brain cell to the next as part of the process of sending an impulse along a nerve pathway.

Minor tranquilizers: A group of psychotropic medications for reducing anxiety and increasing calmness; includes diazepam (Valium), chlordiazpoxide (Librium), and hydroxyzine pamoate (Vistaril). Often inappropriately prescribed in an attempt to slow down ADHD children.

Motor performance: Ability to perform coordinated movement of large- or small-muscle groups.

Multimodal approach: An instructional technique incorporating several senses simultaneously, as in teaching reading by having the student say the letter, write it in the air with a finger, and read it at the same time.

Natural consequences: A disciplinary approach naturally related to a behavior if no special intervention is provided, such as allowing a carelessly placed bicycle to rust and requiring the child to earn money for a replacement.

Neurologist: A physician specializing in diagnosis and treatment of disorders of the brain, spinal cord, and other parts of the nervous system.

Neurotransmitter: A chemical manufactured in the nerve cells for use in sending impulses along nerve pathways. Deficits in the production of the neurotransmitters tyrosine, dopa, dopamine, and norepinephrine appear to underlie ADHD.

Norepinephrine: One of the four key neurotransmitters undersupplied in the brain of ADHD children. Derived from dopamine that has migrated from a nerve cell (presynaptic cell) to an adjacent cell (postsynaptic cell); its buildup generates the electrochemical energy needed to create a new impulse in the postsynaptic nerve cell.

Norm: The average score obtained by a group on a test, to which any one person's score can be compared.

Nortriptyline: A tricyclic antidepressant. A trade name is Aventyl. Sometimes used to treat ADHD.

Nutrition Foundation: A public information organization promoting the marketing and financial interests of the food industry. Has supported activities to discredit the finding that ADHD symptoms worsen after consumption of food or beverages containing artificial chemical additives such as dyes, preservatives, and flavorings.

Occupational therapist: A specialist in treatment to integrate mental and muscle-movement processes more purposefully and efficiently, especially severe problems of locomotion or coordination.

Off-medication trial: See *Drug holiday.*

Off-task: A descriptive term for someone who is not paying attention to or participating in the correct activity in a classroom setting.

On-task: A descriptive term for someone who is paying attention to or participating in the correct activity in a classroom setting.

Otitis: Abnormal collecting of fluid in the ears. Often occurs as an allergic reaction in infants and young children. See *Allergy.*

Overdosage: An inappropriately high amount of medication taken at one time.

Parent education programs: Training in child rearing methods and philosophy; usually small groups with a leader and resource materials.

Pathway: The series of chemical reactions by which a given chemical affects organs, systems, or other chemicals in the body. Prescribed medication creates pathways or series of chemical reactions to produce its clinical and side effects.

Peer monitoring: Using a classmate or other agemate

to supervise the work and behavior of a certain student at school.

Percentile: A child's test score on a scale of 100; indicates what percent of similar children scored higher and lower. For example, a child in the 90th percentile scored higher than 89% and lower than 10% of comparable children.

Perception: The ability to recognize, process, organize, and interpret stimuli received through the senses.

Perceptual-motor task: An activity requiring coordination of perception (usually vision) and muscle movement (usually hand or foot), such as in batting a baseball, kicking a football, or handwriting.

Perseveration: Continuing to repeat a movement or act when doing so is no longer appropriate; finding it difficult to switch smoothly from one activity to another.

Personal Private Interview (PPI): A technique for monitoring a child's adjustment and maintaining constant parent-child communication; consists of regular brief interviews of the child. See *Concerns Notebook.*

Phenol-based compounds: Substances whose molecular structure is characterized by a benzene or phenol group at the core. Certain phenol-based compounds apparently interfere with neurotransmitter formation within the brains of ADHD sufferers and thereby contribute to ADHD symptoms.

Phenylketonuria (PKU): An inherited disorder in brain biochemistry in which tyrosine is greatly underproduced; results in the severe loss of neurotransmitter functions, including mental retardation and ADHD symptoms.

Phonics: Connecting sounds with the letters and letter combinations that make them.

Physical therapist: A specialist in treatment to improve muscle-movement skills and increase strength and endurance, especially of body parts weakened by injury or disease.

PKU: See *Phenylketonuria.*

Placebo: An inactive medication, inert substance, or therapeutic procedure with no value or potency; false medications often used in double-blind research studies to make the recipient believe treatment is occurring when there is no physical effect.

Placebo effect: An explanation for some improvements that occur with apparent treatment when in fact the treatment had no curative power. The observed changes are assumed to occur because the recipient believed that treatment was occurring (also known as the power of suggestion).

Postmaturity: Being born after ten or more months' gestation.

Postsynaptic nerve cell: A nerve cell that receives dopamine from an adjacent presynaptic cell as part of the process of relaying a nerve impulse from the adjacent cell. Norepinephrine is derived from dopamine in the postsynaptic end of nerve cells. See *Presynaptic nerve cell.*

Precociousness: Acceleration in a child's passing of developmental milestones such as the ability to talk or walk. See *Developmental delay; Developmental milestone.*

Precursor: A intermediary substance along a chemical pathway from which other substances derive.

Prematurity: Low birth weight, generally regarded as less than five pounds.

Pre-post contrast: The observed differences in behavior, thoughts, and feelings between the period prior to receiving biochemical treatment and the period after the treatment is well established.

Presleep agitation: A rebound effect caused by wear-off of medication for hyperactivity near bedtime; often inappropriately called insomnia. The child is agitated and can't get to sleep despite intentions of doing so, for at least an eighty-minute period.

Presynaptic nerve cell: A nerve cell from which the nerve impulse is to be relayed to the next cell. See *Postsynaptic nerve cell.*

Prevalence: The total number of cases of a disease or disorder in a specific geographic area over a certain time period; often expressed as a percentage. For example, the prevalence of ADHD is generally estimated at 5 to 10% of all U.S. children. See *Incidence.*

Proteins: Complex compounds consisting of combinations or chains of amino acids comprising most of the mass in living cells. Neurotransmitters are protein derivatives.

Psychiatrist: A physician who specializes in the diagnosis and treatment of mental and behavioral disturbances and is qualified to prescribe medication for them.

Psychoeducational evaluation: Comprehensive assessment of a child's learning style, academic knowledge, intelligence level, learning disabilities, and related factors; includes formal tests as well as observation.

Psychologist: Holder of an advanced degree, usually a doctorate, in psychology. A clinical or counseling psychologist has specialized training in diagnosis and treatment of mental and behavioral disturbances, normal life-adjustment processes, psychological testing procedures and psychometrics, and research strategies.

Psychometrics: Psychological tests and measurements, such as IQ tests and measures of eye-hand coordination.

Psychotherapy: A general term for intervention into a person's life to improve adjustment; in its narrowest sense, an intense experience involving deep, basic issues such as self-esteem. See *Counseling.*

Public Law 94-142: The Education for All Handicapped Children Act of 1975; the major U.S. federal law providing for free, appropriate public education of handicapped children.

Readiness: The level of skills needed for learning a specific academic subject or task.

Rebound: Temporary magnification of symptoms that occurs when medication wears off. See *Growth rebound.*

Receptive language dysfunction: Impaired ability to understand spoken language (also known as receptive language disability or disorder).

Receptive vocabulary: Understanding of what words mean; expressed as an approximate total number of words understood.

Refusal skills: Methods of resisting invitations and peer pressure to misbehave; one aspect of assertiveness training. See *Assertiveness training.*

Remediation: The processes used to correct or counteract areas of academic weakness; for example, drill, practice, special instructional techniques, and tutoring.

Resource room: A room in which students with academic problems receive remedial instruction from a specially trained teacher.

Ritalin: See *Methylphenidate.*

Ritalin SR (sustained release): Long-acting Ritalin.

Rule of 50–10: A formula for pacing schoolwork; the child studies for fifty minutes, then takes a rest break for ten minutes. Dividing the time periods in half but maintaining the same ratio (25–5) also is part of this rule.

Salicylates: Phenol-based compounds found in various fruits; usually associated with a tangy, bittersweet taste.

School survival skills: Minimal levels of performance required to function in an ordinary classroom with a regular curriculum; includes attendance, class preparedness, remaining on-task, and getting help when needed. See *TAPIC.*

Seizure threshold: The minimal state of disturbance in brain chemistry necessary to create an epileptic seizure; as the threshold lowers, seizures occur more frequently.

Self-centeredness: See *Egocentrism.*

Self-contained classroom: Academic placement of special-needs students of a particular diagnosis or learning style impairment together in one room, often for full-time or nearly full-time instruction. It is an alternative to mainstreaming and is to be minimized under the provisions of Public Law 94-142.

Self-reminders: See *Cognitive behavioral training.*

Semantics: Pairing of words with their meanings.

Sensation: Excitation and activation of nerves designed to help the person be aware of stimuli, such as in the eye, ear, nose, mouth, or skin. Precedes perception during the process of experiencing the environment.

Sensitivity: Abnormal use or processing of a chemical by the body not involving the immune system but creating symptoms of biochemical imbalance or distress.

Sequencing deficit: Impaired ability to perceive stimuli such as letters or numbers in a particular order or stepwise progression.

Side effect: An effect of a drug or medication that occurs in addition to the intended or desired effects; also known as an untoward reaction, a toxic effect, or an undesired effect. See *Clinical effect.*

Six A's of Apology: A method of teaching children how to apologize: Admit, Account, Acknowledge, Affirm, Amends, and Adjust.

Social skills: Ability to choose appropriate actions in social settings, such as being tactful, making friends, and settling conflicts peaceably.

Sociopathy: Lack of normal conscience; results in abusive, manipulative, exploitative, or criminal behavior toward others; also known as character disorders.

Somesthesis: See *Kinesthesis.*

Sound blending: Segmenting or combining components of a word to recognize or pronounce it. See *Phonics.*

Special education: Educational approaches designed to meet the unique needs of a handicapped child; includes comprehensive evaluation, intensive instruction matched to needs and readiness, specialized materials and equipment, specially trained teachers, and ongoing progress monitoring.

Stimulant: A type of medication that increases mental and motor performance and uplifts mood in depressed persons. Generally regarded as the pharmacotherapy treatment of choice for ADHD children.

Support group: A group of interested individuals who meet regularly and provide programs and services to assist each other.

Sydenham's chorea: See *Chorea.*

Symptom-controlled (S-C) state: A temporary symptom-free condition, as when medications are taken at correct dosage level.

Symptom-reactive (S-R) state: A temporary symptomatic condition, as when medication has worn off.

Syndrome: A set or collection of symptoms or traits occurring together and characterizing a particular disorder; several such traits occurring from one person to the next who have the same disorder.

Syntax: Grammatical rules that dictate word order and the function of particular words within sentences.

TAPIC: Taylor Academic Problem Identification Checklist; a simple form to quickly portray a student's school survival skills. See *Individualized instruction.*

Taylor-Latta Diet Diary: See *Diet Diary.*

Taylor S/E/A Checklist: The Taylor Social/Emotional/Academic Adjustment Checklist; a simple form for assessing overall social, emotional, and academic adjustment.

TCDR: Taylor Classroom Daily Report; a method of maintaining daily contact between the teacher and parents of a child whose classroom behavior or academic productivity needs daily monitoring.

THSC: Taylor Hyperactivity Screening Checklist; a simple form for quick, accurate assessment of the severity of hyperactivity in anyone from age two through adulthood.

Tic: Spasm-like movement of a muscle, especially twitching of facial muscles.

Titration: Establishing the correct dosage of a medication by observing the effects created by progressively higher dosages.

TMER: Taylor Medication Effectiveness Report; a method of monitoring the clinical and side effects of medication prescribed for the ADHD individual. Submitted by the parent to the physician. See *TSMER.*

Tofranil: See *Imipramine.*

Tolerance: Decreased response to an identical dosage of a medication after its repeated use. Tolerance toward the clinical effects of a medication is undesirable and usually indicates the need to switch to a different medication. See *Clinical effect.*

Tourette's syndrome: See *Guilles de la Tourette's syndrome.*

Toxemia: Blood poisoning.

Toxic: Causing disturbance in chemistry or function of body tissues or organs.

Trade name: The proprietary or brand name, protected by a patent and trademark laws, under which a medication is sold.

Transition plan: A program for helping a student cope with a change in school environment, as when changing from an elementary school to a junior high school.

Trauma: Extreme stress or shock; results in symptoms such as anxiety or depression. See *Depression; Anxiety.*

Treatment of choice: Preferred method of treating a disease or disorder.

Tricyclic antidepressant: See *Imipramine; Amitriptyline; Nortriptyline.*

Tryptophane: An amino acid precursor of neurotransmitters. Some report favorable effects on ADHD symptoms, when used to blunt the presleep agitation and other rebound effects of prescribed medication. See *Precursor.*

TSMER: Taylor School Medication Effectiveness Report; a method of monitoring the clinical and side effects of medication prescribed for an ADHD child. Submitted by the teacher to the physician. See *TMER.*

Tyrosine: A neurotransmitter chemical that transforms into dopa near the end of the presynaptic nerve cell prior to the cell's sending a nerve impulse on to the postsynaptic cell.

Validity: The extent to which a checklist or test measures what it is intended to measure. The Taylor Hyperactivity Screening Checklist, for example, is valid to the extent that it correctly categorizes children in terms of their level of hyperactivity.

Valium: See *Diazepam.*

Vistaril: See *Hydroxyzine pamoate.*

Visual memory: Ability to retain information obtained through the sense of sight, such as remembering the image of a word when trying to spell it.

Visual-motor integration: A category of perceptual-motor tasks; involves perceiving something visually and reproducing it with the hands, such as copying designs with paper and pencil.

Visual perception: Ability to interpret information coming in through the sense of sight, including discriminating designs or symbols (such as words and letters).

Visual tracking: Following visual stimuli through space, such as reading a line of words from left to right. Difficulty with visual tracking is correlated with ADHD.

Wake effect: The impact of a negative reputation on an individual's social relationships; analogous to the wake that occurs when a boat moves through water.

Wear-off period: The time during which medication

rapidly decreases in its effectiveness and symptoms increase as the medication's molecules are depleted.

Wilson's disease: A rare ADHD imitator disorder first appearing around age ten and involving tremor, loosened emotional control, and mental deterioration; caused by an inherited defect in copper metabolism.

Withdrawal symptoms: Distress occurring after stopping use of a medication or drug, especially after sudden stoppage of medication that was taken for a long time at a high dosage level.

Word finding: Associating an idea with the correct word to express it (also known as verbal encoding). See *Encoding*.

Selected Readings and Resources

Thousands of articles in professional journals have been written on hyperactivity, and hundreds of books have been written on the subtopics covered in this book. The readings listed here supplement the discussion in this book. They were selected because they contain helpful elements, but listing them here does not necessarily imply the author's agreement with or endorsement of all the ideas included in these materials.

Chapter 1

Cohen, Donald, et al. (eds.). *Tourette's Syndrome and Tic Disorders* (New York: Wiley, 1988).

Kavanagh, James, and Tom Truss (eds.). *Learning Disabilities: Proceedings of the National Conference* (Parkton, Md.: York, 1988).

Taylor, Eric (ed.). *The Overactive Child* (London: McKeith, 1986).

Weiss, Gabrielle, and Lily Hechtman. *Hyperactive Children Grown Up* (New York: Guilford, 1986).

Chapter 2

Kerr, Mary, et al. *Helping Adolescents with Learning and Behavior Problems* (Columbus, Ohio: Merrill, 1987).

Taylor, John F. *Diagnostic Interviewing of the Misbehaving Child* (Doylestown, Penn.: MARCO Products, 1989). Available from MARCO Products, Box 1052, Doylestown, PA 18901.

Taylor, John F. *Person to Person: Awareness Techniques for Counselors, Group Leaders, and Parent Educators* (Saratoga, Calif.: R&E, 1984).

Wenc, Charlene. *Cooperation: Learning Through Laughter* (Chicago: Americas Institute of Adlerian Studies, 1986).

Chapter 3

Bosco, James, and Stanley Robin. *The Hyperactive Child and Stimulant Drugs* (Chicago: University of Chicago Press, 1977).

Ferber, Richard. *Solve Your Child's Sleep Problems* (New York: Simon & Schuster, 1985).

SOUNDSCREEN, a white-noise machine developed for blocking noise in offices. Available from T.O.S., 705 College Avenue, Santa Rosa, CA 95404.

Chapter 4

Gadow, Kenneth. *Children on Medication,* vol. 1 (San Diego: College-Hill, 1986).

Chapter 5

Feingold, Ben. *Why Your Child Is Hyperactive* (New York: Random House, 1974).

Feingold, Ben, and Helene Feingold. *The Feingold Cookbook for Hyperactive Children* (New York: Random House, 1979).

Jacobson, Michael. *Eater's Digest: The Consumer Factbook of Additives* (New York: Doubleday, 1972).

Taylor, John F., and R. S. Latta. *Special Diets and Kids: How to Keep Your Child on Any Prescribed Diet* (New York: Dodd, Mead, 1987).

Voodoo Science, Twisted Consumerism (Washington, D.C., Center for Science in the Public Interest, 1982).

Chapter 6

Anderson, Eugene, et al. *Self-Esteem for Tots to Teens* (Deephaven, Minn.: Meadowbrook, 1984).

Arent, Ruth. *Stress and Your Child* (Englewood Cliffs, N.J.: Prentice-Hall, 1984).

Briggs, Dorothy. *Your Child's Self-Esteem* (New York: Doubleday, 1975).

Cautela, Joseph, and June Groden. *Relaxation: A Comprehensive Manual for Adults, Children, and Children with Special Needs* (Champaign, Ill.: Research Press, 1978).

Clarke, Jean. *Self-Esteem: A Family Affair* (New York: Harper & Row, 1978).

Glenn, H. Steven, and Jane Nelsen. *Raising Self-Reliant Children* (Rocklin, Calif.: Prima, 1989).

Hankins, Gary. *Prescription for Anger* (Beaverton, Ore.: Princess Publishing, 1988).

Taylor, John F. *Encouraging the Discouraged Child*

(Doylestown, Penn.: MARCO Products, 1990). Available from MARCO Products, Box 1052, Doylestown, PA 18901.

Chapter 7

Booher, Diana. *Making Friends with Yourself and Other Strangers* (New York: Messner, 1982).

Kirby, Edward, and Liam Grimley. *Understanding and Treating Attention Deficit Disorder* (New York: Pergamon, 1986).

Laster, Thomas. *How to Profit Through Politeness or Good Manners Can't Be All Bad* (Saratoga, Calif.: R&E, 1982).

Newman, Susan. *You Can Say No to a Drink or a Drug* (New York: Putnam, 1986).

Scott, Sharon. *When to Say Yes and Make More Friends* (Amherst, Mass.: Human Resource Development Press, 1988).

Taylor, John F. *No More Sibling Rivalry* (Doylestown, Penn.: MARCO Products, 1989). Available from MARCO Products, Box 1052, Doylestown, PA 18901.

Chapter 8

Simons, Robin. *After the Tears: Parents Talk About Raising a Child with a Disability* (New York: Harcourt Brace Jovanovich, 1987).

Wegscheider-Cruse, Sharon. *Learning to Love Yourself: Finding Your Self-Worth* (Deerfield Beach, Fla.: Health Communications, 1987).

Chapter 9

Diamond, Susan. *Helping Children of Divorce* (New York: Schocken, 1985).

Dreikurs, Rudolph, et al. *Family Council: The Dreikurs Technique* (Chicago: Regnery, 1974).

Eckler, James. *Step-by-Stepparenting* (White Hall, Vir.: Betterway, 1988).

Faber, Adele, and Elaine Mazlish. *How to Talk So Kids Will Listen and Listen So Kids Will Talk* (New York: Avon, 1980).

Wayman, Anne. *Successful Single Parenting* (Deephaven, Minn.: Meadowbrook, 1987).

Chapter 10

Education of the Handicapped Act and Regulations, 1985. Available from CRR Publishing Co., Box 1905, Alexandria, VA 22313.

Gehret, Jeanne. *Learning Disabilities and the Don't-Give-Up Kid* (Fairport, NY: Verbal Images Press, 1990). Available from author, 19 Fox Hill Dr., Fairport, NY 14450.

Greene, Lawrence. *Kids Who Underachieve* (New York: Simon & Schuster, 1986).

Greene, Lawrence. *Learning Disabilities and Your Child* (New York: Fawcett, 1987).

Kavale, Kenneth, et al. *Handbook of Learning Disabilities* (Boston: College-Hill, 1987).

Kinsbourne, Marcel, and Paula Caplan. *Children's Learning and Attention Problems* (Boston: Little, Brown, 1979).

Osman, Betty. *Learning Disabilities: A Family Affair* (New York: Random House, 1979).

Pernecke, Raegene, and Sara Schreiner. *Schooling for the Learning Disabled* (Glenview, Ill.: SMS Publishing, 1983).

Shore, Kenneth. *The Special Education Handbook* (New York: Warner, 1986).

Unlocking Doors: A Guide to Effective Communication (Minneapolis: Parents Advocacy Coalition for Educational Rights, 1982). Available from PACER Center, 4826 Chicago Ave. S., Minneapolis, MN 55417.

Chapter 11

Canfield, Jack, and Harold Wells. *One Hundred Ways to Enhance Self-Concept in the Classroom* (Englewood Cliffs, N.J.: Prentice-Hall, 1976).

Dreikurs, Rudolph, Bronia Grunwald, and Floy Pepper. *Maintaining Sanity in the Classroom* (New York: Harper & Row, 1971).

Hammill, Donald, and Nettie Bartel. *Teaching Students with Learning and Behavior Problems*, 4th ed. (New York: Allyn and Bacon, 1986).

Stewart, William (ed.). *How to Involve the Student in Classroom Decision Making* (Saratoga, Calif.: R&E, 1985).

Taylor, John F. *Motivating the Uncooperative Student* (Doylestown, PA: MARCO Products, 1990). Available from MARCO Products, Box 1052, Doylestown, PA 18901.

Young, Milton. *Teaching Children with Special Learning Needs* (New York: John Day, 1967).

Chapter 12

Ballman, Ray. *The How and Why of Home Schooling* (Westchester, Ill.: Crossway, 1987).

Blumenfeld, Samuel. *How to Tutor* (Milford, Mich.: Mott, 1973).

Fogle, Karen. *Home Schooling* (Woodinville, Wash.: 1989). Available from author. 14241 NE Woodinville-Duvall Road, Suite 243, Woodinville, WA 98072.

Geoffrion, Sondra. *Get Smart Fast* (Saratoga, Calif.: R&E, 1986).

Holt, John. *Teach Your Own* (Boston: Holt Associates, 1981).

Mitchener, Carol, and Carol Newsom. *Have Effective Learning Power: A Self-Directed Study Skills Workbook* (Doylestown, Penn.: MARCO Products, 1987). Available from MARCO Products, Box 1052, Doylestown, PA 18901.

Quackenbush, Ross, and Jerrel Gastineau. *Homework? My Locker Ate It!* (Salem, Ore.: Counseling and Workshop Professionals, 1988). Available from publisher, 965 Ewald Ave. SE, Salem, OR 97302.

Shackelford, Luanne, and Susan White. *A Survivor's Guide to Home Schooling* (Westchester, Ill.: Crossway, 1988).

Chapter 13

Dreikurs, Rudolph, and Loren Grey. *Logical Consequences: A New Approach to Discipline* (New York: Hawthorn, 1968).

Frank, Marjorie. *I Can Make a Rainbow* (Nashville, Tenn.: Incentive, 1976).

Job Sheet (A set of 53 weekly household chore assignment sheets and instructions). Available from Jan Weir Designs, 36834 Happy Hollow Road, Blodgett, OR 97326.

Kelser, Jay (ed.). *Parents and Teenagers* (Wheaton, Ill.: Victor, 1984).

Lees, Dennis. *Successful Parenting for Stressful Times* (Saratoga, Calif.: R&E, 1985).

Nelsen, Jane. *Positive Discipline* (New York: Ballantine, 1987).

Taylor, John F. *Correcting Without Criticizing* (Doylestown, Penn.: MARCO Products, 1989).

Taylor, John F. *Helping Hands and Smiling Faces: Getting Cooperation on Household Chores* (Doylestown, Penn.: MARCO Products, 1983). Both titles available from MARCO Products, Box 1052, Doylestown, PA 18901.

Wilson, Earl. *Try Being a Teenager: A Challenge to Parents to Stay in Touch* (Portland, Ore.: Multnomah, 1982).

Wyckoff, Jerry, and Barbara Unell. *Discipline Without Shouting or Spanking* (Deephaven, Minn.: Meadowbrook, 1984).

Chapter 14

Fletcher, Judy. *Games: Activities for Your Christian Family* (St. Louis: Concordia, 1978).

Guide to Accredited Camps (Martinsville, Ind.: American Camping Association, 1989).

Young, Milton. *Teaching Children with Special Learning Needs* (New York: John Day, 1967).

Chapter 15

Des Jardins, Charlotte. *How to Organize an Effective Parent/Advocacy Group and Move Bureaucracies* (Chicago, Ill.: Coordinating Council for Handicapped Children, 1980). (407 S. Dearborn, Rm. 680, Chicago, IL 60605).

Kuzell, Norma, and Jean Brassington. *Parenting the Learning Disabled Child* (ten-session parent education course with parent's manual and leader's manual). Available from authors, 1355 Bank Street, Suite 301, Ottawa, Ontario, Canada K1H 8K7.

Taylor, John F. *Dynamic Parenting: How to Establish Parent Education Programs* (Doylestown, Penn.: MARCO Products, 1984). (Box 1052, Doylestown, PA 18901).

About the Author

John F. Taylor, Ph.D., is in private practice as a family psychologist, specializing in the diagnosis and treatment of hyperactive and attention disordered children, adolescents, and adults. An authority on diagnosis of children, he is the author of *Diagnostic Interviewing of the Misbehaving Child,* several of the test items on the Wechsler Intelligence Scale for Children-3 (WISC-3), and numerous articles on diagnosis in professional journals.

Author of *Person to Person: Awareness Techniques for Counselors, Group Leaders, and Parent Educators,* he is considered one of the most creative originators of group facilitation and counseling techniques in the United States. He spearheaded a community network of parent education programs that made Salem, Oregon, one of the most active communities in parent education in the United States. He has written the parent educator's guide booklet *Dynamic Parenting: How to Organize Parent Education Programs* and the Family Power series of parent education resources which includes *Helping Hands and Smiling Faces: How to Get Cooperation on Household Chores, No More Sibling Rivalry, Encouraging the Discouraged Child,* and *Correcting Without Criticizing.*

Author of the "Sharpening Your Counseling Skills" column in the journal *Practical Ideas for Counselors,* he has developed many innovative counseling approaches for children, adolescents, and families and is an authority on family relationships and counseling strategies. He has also written the popular counselor's guidebook *Motivating the Uncooperative Student.*

He is co-author of *Special Diets and Kids: How to Keep Your Child on Any Prescribed Diet,* which contains an elaborate discussion of how to manage such programs as the Feingold Program for hyperactive children. His original book on hyperactivity, *The Hyperactive Child and the Family: The Complete What-to-Do Handbook,* was published in the early 1980s.

An entertaining and popular lecturer and frequent guest on broadcast interviews, Dr. Taylor is president of SUN Seminars and frequently gives training workshops to professionals throughout North America. He resides in Salem, Oregon, with his wife Linda and their family of eight children, one of whom has ADHD.

He is willing to come to your conference, convention, public program, or inservice training event. All his presentations contain an experiential in addition to a didactic component.

For information or for making arrangements for training workshops or other programs, write:

SUN Seminars
5406 Battlecreek Road S.E.
Salem, Oregon 97306

INDEX

To Order Books

Please send me the following items:

Quantity	Title	Unit Price	Total
______	______________________________	$ ______	$ ______
______	______________________________	$ ______	$ ______
______	______________________________	$ ______	$ ______
______	______________________________	$ ______	$ ______
______	______________________________	$ ______	$ ______

Shipping and Handling depend on Subtotal.

Subtotal	Shipping/Handling
$0.00–$14.99	$3.00
$15.00–$29.99	$4.00
$30.00–$49.99	$6.00
$50.00–$99.99	$10.00
$100.00–$199.99	$13.50
$200.00+	Call for Quote

Foreign and all Priority Request orders: Call Order Entry department for price quote at 916/632-4400

This chart represents the total retail price of books only (before applicable discounts are taken).

Subtotal $ ______

Deduct 10% when ordering 3-5 books $ ______

7.25% Sales Tax (CA only) $ ______

8.25% Sales Tax (TN only) $ ______

5.0% Sales Tax (MD and IN only) $ ______

Shipping and Handling* $ ______

Total Order $ ______

By Telephone: With MC or Visa, call 800-632-8676 or 916-632-4400. Mon–Fri, 8:30-4:30.

WWW: http://www.primapublishing.com

By Internet E-mail: sales@primapub.com

By Mail: Just fill out the information below and send with your remittance to:

Prima Publishing
P.O. Box 1260BK
Rocklin, CA 95677

My name is ______________________________

I live at ______________________________

City ____________________ State ______ ZIP __________

MC/Visa# ______________________________ Exp. __________

Check/money order enclosed for $ __________ Payable to Prima Publishing

Daytime telephone ______________________________

Signature ______________________________